The Homeopathic Treatment of Children

The Homeopathic Treatment of Children

Pediatric Constitutional Types

Paul Herscu, N.D.

North Atlantic Books
Berkeley, California

Homeopathic Educational Services
Berkeley, California

The Homeopathic Treatment of Children: Pediatric Constitutional Types

Copyright © 1991 by Paul Herscu, N.D.
ISBN 1–55643–090–6

Published by
North Atlantic Books
2800 Woolsey Street
Berkeley, California 94705
and
Homeopathic Educational Services
2124 Kittredge Street
Berkeley, California 94704

Cover photograph of Andrew and Sarah Ullman by Gayla
Hachenberger of Honeybee Photo, Woodland Hills, California
Cover and book design by Paula Morrison
Typeset by Campaigne & Associates Typography
Indexed by S. Rosko Rossoff

Printed in the United States of America

The Homeopathic Treatment of Children: Pediatric Constitutional Types
is sponsored by the Society for the Study of Native Arts and Sciences,
a nonprofit educational corporation whose goals are to develop an educational and crosscultural perspective linking various scientific, social, and
artistic fields; to nurture a holistic view of arts, sciences, humanities,
and healing; and to publish and distribute literature on the relationship
of mind, body, and nature.

Library of Congress Cataloging in Publication Data
Herscu, Paul, 1959-
    The homeopathic treatment of children : pediatric constitutional
types / Paul Herscu.
        p.   cm.
    Includes index.
    ISBN 1-55643-090-6
    1. Children—Diseases—Homeopathic treatment.   I. Title.
    [DNLM: 1. Drug Therapy—in infancy & childhood. 2. Homeopathy—
in infancy & childhood.   WS 366 H571h]
RX501.H58 1991
615.5'32'083—dc20
DNLM/DLC   91-2390
for Library of Congress   CIP

To Durr Elmore and Kai Palmqvist—it is for your spirit in homeopathy that I write this book—as well as to Sophia Doris Herscu, my beautiful daughter, and to Misha Harrison Herscu, my newborn son.

Contents

Foreword ix

Note to Parents xi

Introduction xiii

Acknowledgments xx

Calcarea carbonica 3
    Notes on Infants 35
    Outline 38
    Confirmatory Picture 47

Lycopodium 49
    Notes on Infants 80
    Outline 83
    Confirmatory Picture 90

Medorrhinum 91
    Notes on Infants 129
    Outline 131
    Confirmatory Picture 138

Natrum muriaticum 139
    Notes on Infants 165
    Outline 167
    Confirmatory Picture 174

Phosphorus 175
    Notes on Infants 205
    Outline 206
    Confirmatory Picture 213

Pulsatilla 215
    Notes on Infants 246
    Outline 248
    Confirmatory Picture 254

Sulphur 255
    Notes on Infants 292
    Outline 294
    Confirmatory Picture 302

Tuberculinum 303
    Notes on Infants 341
    Outline 343
    Confirmatory Picture 351

    Index 353

Foreword

There is at present a great necessity for information on the homeopathic treatment of children. We do not actually have enough literature on the subject apart from Borland's booklet which is quite good but not sufficient for the needs of our time. I feel that Paul Herscu's book goes further than any other homeopathic book in giving detailed information which will be very useful to any practitioner who treats children.

Homeopathic care is a great benefit for the healthy development of children. In my thirty years of practice I have seen children who were treated homeopathically for a long period of time and who have developed and become healthier than their siblings who did not receive homeopathic treatment. I continually observe that children who have been treated well with homeopathic medicines usually exceed in height their parents and siblings who have not been similarly treated. This simple observation shows how deeply homeopathy can affect the body, most probably reaching to the very genetic level of the body.

I would also like to say that I consider Paul Herscu to be a person who is not only deeply devoted to homeopathy but also is an excellent practitioner.

George Vithoulkas

A Note to Parents

Homeopathy is a system of medicine that treats the entire pattern of physical, emotional, and mental characteristics of children and adults who are ill. This book describes eight of the most common patterns of illness that children experience and the corresponding homeopathic medicine for them. It is the intent of this book to demonstrate the extent to which homeopathy can significantly help in the prevention and treatment of illness in children.

I find several reasons why parents should know about homeopathic constitutional types described in this book. The primary reason is to find out what your child's constitution is at present. This information is most important, as it will tell you what your child's susceptibilities are. It can show you what stresses are most likely to bring about illness. Avoiding these stresses comprises what we term "primary prevention" in health care, and these avoidances will help keep your child healthy.

Learning the child's constitution will also help you to know the parts of the body that are weakest. These areas can be protected, again helping the child to stave off illnesses.

Understanding the child's constitution aids in identifying the ailment from which the child is complaining, thereby helping you and your physician understand the disease more quickly than before. For instance, if you know that your child has a *Phosphorus* constitution, you know that the pancreas is commonly a weak organ for that constitutional type. Then when the child complains of pain in the head, trembling, weakness, and hunger, you may be able to help the doctor diagnose hypoglycemia.

There is yet another reason to know these types. Different remedy types respond differently to various methods of parenting, disciplining, and communication in general. Better understanding of your child through homeopathy should enhance your relationship with him or her and create the most fertile environment in which the child, as well as you the parent, can blossom. As an example, some children need "time outs" while others need only a parental glance to understand that they are misbehaving—and in this second type, time outs can cause emotional scarring. Likewise, some children have strong fears of animals, others of abandonment, while others have unmentioned fears for the parents' welfare. Knowing your child's constitutional type can help you build up the child's self-confidence and dispel the child's fears.

It has become increasingly popular for parents to treat their children at home for a wide range of common acute problems. This is to be encouraged. However, if your child is suffering from a chronic ailment—a frequently recurrent problem or a deeper emotional or mental imbalance—then homeopathic care is best left to someone who is trained in classical homeopathy, as well as someone who has more objectivity in perceiving your child's condition.

This is not a self-help book; rather, it is a reference guide for parent and doctor alike. It is hoped that by reading this book you will better be able to report recognizable symptoms and personality traits to your homeopath, so that he or she in conjunction with you will be better able to find the remedy that will help your child.

Paul Herscu, N.D.

Introduction

During my first years of studying homeopathic materia medicas, I often found myself going over the same pages again and again, unable to grasp and retain enough of the information to apply it easily. Bits of information often seemed unrelated to each other and therefore hard to remember.

Later, after poring over these texts so many times that the material seemed second nature to me, I was able to look at them from a different perspective and notice patterns not easily discerned up close. For instance, if one were to organize the most valuable materia medicas chronologically, one would find that they parallel the evolution of homeopathy itself.

The first materia medicas written contained mostly provings organized according to the various sections of the body. What they amounted to, in fact, was a "laundry list" of symptoms. Lacking the wisdom that comes from the oft-repeated experience of many, these books nevertheless provided something priceless to the practice of homeopathic medicine: the raw materials with which future homeopaths could build. Doctors read these materia medicas, began to apply the remedies successfully, and recorded their findings.

The next generation of materia medicas consisted of these ever-growing records of clinical experience grafted onto the older laundry lists.

Finally, by the late nineteenth century, some materia medicas contained primarily clinical experience and little else. For example, Hering's *Guiding Symptoms* and Kent's *Materia Medica* are both rich treasuries of clinical experience and are very valuable as such. More complete knowledge on how the remedies should be applied in actual practice, rather than theory, was made available in books like these.

This transformation of elemental data into practical wisdom through the process of analyzing and compiling one's own and others' clinical experiences continues to this day with the writing of modern materia medicas, which usually contain scant theory but ample experiential knowledge. Yet there is still something important missing from this continuum: materia medicas that vividly describe whole syndromes, whole symptom complexes, just as they appear in real patients and as they are commonly treated in practice today. I have approached the material with this in mind and have attempted to present it in a manner that makes it easily accessible to the reader. It is my belief that this book, and books following this concept, represent a necessary next step in the further evolution of materia medicas.

This book is also intended to help solve another problem with existing materia medicas: the dearth of theoretical, experiential, or any other type of homeopathic information available regarding children. Remedies are usually described primarily in the context of adults, leaving a large and treacherous gap in the literature. Attempting to apply that knowledge to an infant or a child has frustrated many homeopaths, myself included. We have often found ourselves prescribing solely on the basis of keynotes, which we were loath to do because keynotes do not adequately reflect the totality of the youngster's presenting symptoms and underlying weaknesses.

Because we could not fully recognize the remedy picture of a child from the available inadequate descriptions, we floundered and were sometimes left unsure of the correctness of our prescription. This situation is particularly unfortunate because such a large number of homeopathic patients are children—and tragic as well, because the early and proper homeopathic treatment of children can contribute greatly to sound development and lead to a healthier adulthood.

Borland advanced the cause of pediatric materia medica with a short discourse, *Children's Types*, published as a monograph on materia medica for the treatment of children. It consisted of brief compilations of clues upon which he would prescribe a polychrest remedy. Since his first step early in this century, no great strides have been made in the field of pediatric materia medica.

To my great fortune (though I thought it misfortune at the time), early in my career as a homeopath I was thrown into a busy practice that served hundreds of children. Overwhelmed by an unceasing flood of pediatric cases, I struggled to find the simillimum with tools and training that were inadequate to the task. The struggle lessened as I began to find the correct remedies by careful observation, long hours of study, and the grace of God.

In retrospect, I saw that the correct remedy was eventually found in countless cases without recourse to information contained in any materia medica. Talking with colleagues, I found that many of them wrestled as I had with this pediatric dilemma and craved help that might make this part of homeopathic practice easier. I proceeded to gather information from a great many successfully cured cases in my wife's and my practice, which has evolved into this book. It is my fondest hope that others will add to this body of knowledge with their own experience, and in so doing continue to build a strong and eminently useful pediatric materia medica.

With this book, then, I wish to accomplish two things: first, to help fill the gap in pediatric materia medica; and second, to write a materia medica that I myself would like to read. Such a book, I thought, would describe syndromes just as they are seen in real patients. Psychologically, it would offer behavioral profiles of patients not in theory, but exactly as seen in office visits, complete with all their attendant expressions and actions. Physically, it would describe how individual diseases present in actuality. A student or practitioner would not need to memorize a list of disparate symptoms or compile symptoms to fit the patient sitting in front of him or her; the complete state of the patient could be read about here in its entirety, just as it presents itself in nature.

I decided to focus on eight remedies—*Calcarea carbonica*, *Lycopodium*, *Medorrhinum*, *Natrum muriaticum*, *Phosphorus*, *Pulsatilla*, *Sulphur*, and *Tuberculinum*—rather than a more extensive or exhaustive selection on the basis of a simple discovery: these eight remedies make up the constitutional simillimum for nearly eighty percent of an average general pediatric practice. I decided that writing a book that would help other homeopaths get to know these remedies very well and enable them to cure at least eighty out of one hundred cases easily, efficiently, and with confidence was more important than presenting a longer, more comprehensive book that would dilute the information I have found to be essential in my practice. There are at least another thirty remedies that are also deep-acting constitutional remedies in pediatric populations, but all are much less commonly employed than the ones listed here.

There are three major sources of symptoms in our homeopathic literature: provings, poisonings, and clinically verified symptoms. To my knowledge, this is the first book that is exclusively devoted to the third source—the clinic. I wrote each chapter with as full and clear a clinical image as I could so that one would not discount a possible remedy merely because a symptom in question had not been attributed to the remedy before. I have excluded material that was not personally observed in countless cases, even if that material was something I was taught to be theoretically important to these remedies. Nor have I added symptoms extraneous to my experience, as they are written about extensively in other books.

Because I am most interested in clinical experiences—in the patients themselves—I have begun to alter my personal copy of Kent's *Repertory* by changing the grading of symptoms and adding rubrics that reflect what I see in my office. I understand that this may become a hotly debated topic in the future, but it is a process that began long ago and must continue into the future. If materia medicas become more refined, it must follow that repertories will mirror these new developments.

Ultimately, there are two purposes to a repertory: first, to record symptoms indicative of the remedies; and second, to aid the homeopath in finding the correct remedy for a given patient. While these two points may sound as though they are the same, they are not. If one is most interested in the patient, then all the books must become tools, personalized with wear and tear and showing the path trodden by the practitioner through the pages. Toward this end, one must make one's copy of the *Repertory* one's own to reflect what is actually experienced in the clinic.

As I have mentioned, there are at least thirty other remedies about which I wish to write. Because these types are much rarer than the remedies in this book, neither I nor my colleagues have seen hundreds of each kind, and consequently it is not yet possible to write a clinical materia medica of those remedies. I am currently in the process of collating the clinical findings of many homeopaths into a complete living picture of each of these remedies for future publication.

Looking back on the process of writing this book, two thoughts about the nature of homeopathy continue to amaze me. First, how fantastic it really is that a homeopathic remedy can effect a cure on so many levels. Second, how wonderful it is that a mere handful of such remedies can do so much of the work. Armed with only these few remedies, a homeopath can fulfill the deepest mission of the work: to aid in healing and preventing illness in the shortest, surest, least harmful, and most permanent fashion possible.

Some notes on the format of the book:

I have reorganized the sections in the materia medica in a way that is easier to use and follow while reading the book. The sections are as follows: Mental/Emotional Characteristics, Sleep, Vertigo, Physical Symptomatology, Fevers, Physical Generals, Notes on Infants, Outline, and Confirmatory Checklist.

I placed Sleep immediately following the Mental/Emotional Characteristics section because much of what I had to write about sleep involved the child's emotional state, and so it seemed fitting to place these sections near each other.

Physical Symptomatology is divided into four main sections: the Head, the Torso, the Musculoskeletal System, and the Skin. The Head area contains the Head, Eyes, Ears, Nose, Face, Mouth, Throat and Neck subsections. The Torso contains the Lower Respiratory System, the Alimentary System, and the Urogenital System. The Musculoskeletal System includes the Back and Extremities. The Skin is usually the shortest of the sections, concentrating as it does on just the skin itself.

I began the Torso subsection of the Physical Symptomatology section with the Lower Respiratory System, breaking with tradition for a reason. It is traditional to present the material with the symptoms in descending anatomical order, beginning in the head and working down the torso. But when I got to the throat, I had a choice to make: should I stress the pharynx and esophagus and then go down the torso and describe the digestion, or should I stress the pharynx and larynx and go down the torso and describe the lower respiratory tract? I naturally assumed at the beginning that I would follow my predecessors and begin with digestion. On reviewing the pediatric ailments that I have written about in these pages, I found I had a great deal to say about the pharynx and larynx but very little to say about the esophagus. Since I began by describing the upper respiratory system, it was only fitting to keep the subsections together, and so I followed the Throat and Neck subsection with the Lower Respiratory System. Upon reading it over, I found that this arrangement works well for the material presented here.

After the Physical General symptoms for each remedy, I have included some notes in a special section on infants for easy reference. This is for study purposes only. If one is treating an infant, one should refer primarily to the material in the main body of the text, as it is richer in information.

At the end of each remedy description I have included a brief summary outline. Sometimes, while reading many pages of material, one can get lost in all the details, especially if one is new to homeopathy and does not yet grasp the larger picture inherent in diagnosing and prescribing. An adequate philosophical understanding is essential to make sense of it all and to structure and prioritize the information, such as which symptoms are most essential and must be prescribed upon.

These condensed summaries are meant as an aid to beginners and should serve as a skeleton of knowledge to be fleshed out with the information in the main body of the chapter. Conversely, the reader may wish to refer to this final section in order to cross-check symptoms that are indicated in the chapter as mainstays of the diagnosis. After the book has been read, the practitioner may refer to this section for easy reference while interviewing a patient and return to the main body of the text for more complete information on specific syndromes.

I have also added a confirmatory checklist following the outline at the end of each chapter. These are points to look for in the case and questions to ask each patient once a remedy is selected. The more points that are strongly confirmed by the patient, the more likely it is that the remedy will be efficacious.

Throughout, I have endeavored to present as many objective symptoms as possible. Symptoms that we can easily observe often lead to the correct remedy quickly. These telling vignettes make up a major portion of the book, but they also represent a major aspect of case-taking in general, illustrating once again the aptness of the old adage, "A case well taken is half cured" when applied to the art of homeopathic medicine.

The reader should also bear in mind that throughout the book, unless gender is specified for a particular case or characteristic, statements apply equally to both girls and boys.

The information that is contained in these pages was gathered at our offices. Amy Rothenberg, N.D., my wife, is half of our joint medical practice and has contributed a great number of the cases and observations. It became cumbersome to distinguish who had observed a particular trait first, so the book is written in the standard first person form. Although the text refers only to me, "we" is implied throughout. But to say more here would give away the acknowledgments that follow.

The complete title of Kent's *Repertory* is *Repertory of the Homeopathic Materia Medica*.

The complete title of Kent's *Materia Medica* is *Lectures on Homeopathic Materia Medica*.

The complete title of Boericke's *Materia Medica* is *Pocket Manual of Homeopathic Materia Medica Comprising the Characteristic and Guiding Symptoms of All Remedies*, Ninth Edition. (This book is often titled or referred to as the *Materia Medica with Repertory*.)

The complete title of Hering's *Materia Medica* is *The Guiding Symptoms of Our Materia Medica*.

This book is the first volume of a series on the homeopathic treatment of children.

Paul Herscu, N.D.

Acknowledgments

I want to express great gratitude and thanks to Amy Rothenberg, N.D., my wife and partner, whose many observations, ideas, and long hours of work are represented in these pages. Her initial editing made my ideas decipherable to a professional editor. Her encouragement, support, and unending love wove the fabric that held me together. Without Amy, this book would still be just another idea in the mind of a dreamer.

Abraham and Clara Herscu, my parents, taught me to care for others and supported me in the writing of this book. Thank you.

Marta Herscu, my sister, introduced me to homeopathy in the first place and encouraged me on my life path. Thank you.

My friends Durr Elmore and George Guess helped to edit the chapters on *Calcarea carbonica* and *Lycopodium*. Thank you both.

Dana Ullman oversaw this project and brought the book to fruition. I relied on Dana to see it through from manuscript to the finished text. Thank you.

Robin Bishop provided considerable editorial assistance. A gifted editor, she found English somewhere in my writing. Thank you.

Thank you also to S. Rosco Rossoff for his comprehensive index.

A special thank you to George Vithoulkas, who has taught a generation of homeopaths how to see what they are looking at.

For a referral to a classical homeopath nearest you, please contact:

New England School of Homeopathy
356 Middle Street
Amherst, Massachusetts 01002

Homeopathic Academy of Naturopathic Physicians
11231 SE Market Street
Portland, Oregon 97216

National Center for Homeopathy
801 N. Fairfax #306
Alexandria, Virginia 22314

International Foundation for Homeopathy
2366 Eastlake Drive East #306
Seattle, Washington 98102

Homeopathic Educational Services
2124 Kittredge Street
Berkeley, California 94704

The
Homeopathic
Treatment of
Children

Calcarea carbonica

Mental/Emotional Characteristics

Every homeopathic practitioner who treats children will thank heaven for the remedy *Calcarea carbonica*; thus, it is fitting to begin the book by describing this remedy. Children expend a great deal of energy on growth and therefore often need remedies that correspond in symptomatology to growth difficulties. During these times the thyroid gland and calcium metabolism are inextricably tied together. It is then no wonder that *Calcarea carbonica*, a remedy that **cures problems of the thyroid and calcium metabolism**, is so frequently needed. Illness for these children may begin when either system is stressed, as may be the case during dentition, growth spurts, learning to walk, and bone injuries.

Slowness

One may observe difficulties related to growth by taking note of the state of mental development. One finds in *Calcarea carbonica* cases a child who is **delayed in developing mental as well as physical skills.** With babies, this manifests as a delay in walking or talking. There is a slowness of comprehension and a delay in acquiring new skills much like that seen in *Baryta carbonica*. The subtle difference between the two remedies is that in *Calcarea carbonica* there is a **deliberate, even willful, slowing of development** on the part of the child in order to understand and assimilate new information more carefully, whereas in *Baryta carbonica* apparent retardation is just that and is not under the control of the child. It may require so much from the *Calcarea carbonica* child to study that he or she may refuse to do it altogether. This is not the procrastination of a *Sulphur* or a *Lycopodium*, but rather the

3

inability and frustration involved with trying to focus the mind on learning.

Adding to the similarity of *Calcarea carbonica* and *Baryta carbonica* is the fact that there is often a **problem with memory**. Brad, a teenager who responded well to the remedy *Calcarea carbonica*, came to see me because of a chronic sinus infection. Along with the infection, he complained that his memory was severely impaired. If told to do three things, Brad could recall the first two but not the third. He kept a written list of all the chores he needed to do. So affected was his mind that it was very hard for me to differentiate between *Baryta carbonica* and *Calcarea carbonica*. Had not the rest of the case fit the *Calcarea carbonica* picture so fully with symptoms such as a fear of heights and spiders, and perspiration of the scalp, he might have fared well enough with the other remedy. (If forgetfulness is the *major* problem associated with mental slowness, forcing the child to repeat lessons over and over, and is accompanied by a fear of strangers, *Baryta carbonica* is usually more indicated.)

With respect to mental aptitude, two types of children need the remedy *Calcarea carbonica*. **Due to mental strain**, the first type does not try hard enough in school. Even if pushed by their parents, they still do not really apply themselves and usually receive poor grades. At school the child cannot keep up with the rest of the class. This slowness may be classified inaccurately as a mental handicap or as a learning disability. *Calcarea carbonica* children make mistakes in all language skills: reading, writing, and speaking. They may work hard when they go home, spending hours on their homework often developing headaches and eyestrain in the process, but still manage to only barely keep up with their classmates.

The second type of *Calcarea carbonica* child is **brilliant**. These children work hard, plod along, and often receive the best of grades, maintaining a B average or higher. However, the great amount of time they must commit to study far exceeds that needed by other remedy types to earn comparable grades. Such children need structure, need to incorporate and classify each piece of information, and as a result may **appear slow**. Their learning ability is such that they need to **learn step by step**, word by word, paragraph by paragraph. Material is therefore learned solidly and will not be soon forgotten. They build up their knowledge slowly but surely on a strong foundation, unlike other remedies such as *Lycopodium* or *Sulphur* that procrastinate and then only learn enough to pass the next test. *Calcarea carbonica* could never do this; the ideas would be too many and the time too short.

Slowness of comprehension is easily **observed in the office.** When explaining to the child how to take the remedy, the doctor may have to repeat the instructions two or three times, slower each time, even to a teenager, until the youngster finally understands the process. It is amazing how often this happens with *Calcarea carbonica*, especially as the teen becomes an adult. The parents of such a child may notice the puzzled expression on the doctor's face and may add when their offspring is out of earshot that the child is very bright but has his or her own speed of assimilating new information. This last statement is exact. The child may be the most intelligent in the class, but information must come in slowly and systematically.

Introversion

Calcarea carbonica children discover early in life that they are slower than others their age. During play, they find themselves slow at games and sports—perhaps to the extent that other children taunt and laugh at them. **To avoid** this **ridicule,** they may become quiet, withdrawn loners who play by themselves and do not seek out friendships with others.

At this early stage of the interview they can seem shy, chuckling self-consciously after answering each question. While this may appear to be similar to *Natrum muriaticum*, it is not due to grief and one will not be able to elicit the *Natrum muriaticum* cause for this fear of others approaching too closely to their sensitive emotions. In *Calcarea carbonica*, the turning inward accompanied by a sense of self-assurance allows them to become self-reliant. This **self-reliance** is illustrated by the child who can be left for an hour to play alone while his mother cleans the house.

During illnesses, *Calcarea carbonica* children become quiet and withdrawn. This introversion is especially observed in obese teenagers who become chronically lethargic and mope about feeling sorry for themselves.

Cautiousness

The child is cautious and **refuses anything new for a length of time** until he can assimilate the new information and then structure and categorize it in his mind. Toby, a boy of two with a streptococcal infection of the throat, personified this trait. He would not pick up a toy given to him. After staring at it for a long time, he picked it up, played with it for a minute, and then put it down again. Even though the desire to pick up the toy was plainly evident, he had to stare at it first; then at me, the provider of the toy; then at the toy again—back and forth until his curiosity won out over caution.

Likewise, a *Calcarea carbonica* child may refuse to take the remedy. As with *Tuberculinum*, it may become a battle of wills and physical prowess to get him to open his mouth and take the remedy. The child screams, "No! I don't want it!" The parent counters with, "Take it, it's sweet, it's good for you." The child repeats, "No!" and kicks and tries to pull away.

Four-year-old Melissa, brought in for enuresis, showed this trait in a subtle way. When asked to do anything, she would say no, wait ten seconds, and then do it. She clearly exemplified the need for more time in order to integrate new demands and fit them into a larger frame of reference.

Closure/Inflexibility

Extra time is also **needed to finish tasks** the child has begun. When parents, looking in on the child, think she seems to be pleased, enjoying herself with her projects, the child is actually hard at work trying to finish what she started. Anything left undone nags at her consciousness; she feels compelled to finish it. As a result, it may seem to the parent at times that the child is deliberately disobeying or being obstinate.

Whenever the mother of four-year-old Alan came along and asked the child to do something, he would say yes, but continued to plod along, working on his current project. Alan's mother was angered, thinking that the child was deliberately disobeying her. In actuality, the child simply needed to finish his task before moving on to another. **Structure and scheduling** are very important for these children. They must have each activity or encounter finished and categorized in their minds or it haunts them constantly.

An **inability to change their minds quickly** is characteristic of *Calcarea carbonica* toddlers. They are **self-willed** and desire to do things at their own pace and at a time of their own choosing. When the parent or sibling interferes with the choice made, the child is unable to change his frame of reference, unable to give up what he is doing. As a result, he begins to yell, cry, or throw a tantrum, not budging until the other gives in or until he becomes interested in something else.

The following scene is common in the *Calcarea carbonica* home. When refused something, eighteen-month-old Carla would point to the desired object and scream. When the parents continued to say no, she too remained steadfast and stood there crying, pointing at what she wanted. The parents of such children must forget insisting upon having their own will obeyed. Instead of having a continual no-win situation, the substitution/distraction method is the best way to stop these behavioral nightmares. If the parent offers something else to change or distract the child's focus from the current object of fascination, the child usually becomes engrossed in examining the new object or exploring the game and is satisfied.

Obstinacy

Obstinacy is a major clue to the remedy. Martin, a one-year-old boy who was usually fussy if a parent interrupted his play, began to demonstrate an intense temper. Any time he was teething or having problems with earaches, this behavior manifested as an escalation of his usual **intolerance to contradiction**. This aspect of his emotional makeup—so strong for one so young—led me to choose the remedy *Calcarea carbonica*. When a part of the body becomes ill, it is as if the whole person becomes ill. Individual responses to physical ailments offer clues to the correct remedy; in this case, the extreme obstinacy pointed to *Calcarea carbonica*.

7

Samuel, another one-year-old brought in during dentition, was forbidden to continue an activity. In response, he became angry, cried, threw himself on the floor, fussed for a minute, and then got up and tried to do what he was not supposed to do— again. For this child, as for many of those needing *Calcarea carbonica*, it was easier to use all his energy to obstinately get what he wanted and be done with it than to have "unfinished business" weighing on his mind. Another child may try to finish a project without permission, as did fifteen-month-old Linda, a patient who waited until her mother turned her back before restarting the waiting room game from which she had been forbidden.

Obstinacy, then, is one of the main personality characteristics of the child. It is extremely unfortunate that most parents are unaware of this kind of innate mental structuring and persist forcefully with their own agendas and schedules for the child. As a result, instances of irritability, crying fits, and tantrums that crop up whenever the child is interrupted, opposed, or contradicted come as a complete surprise to the parents. Responses seem disproportionate to the magnitude of the request asked of the child. This is sometimes compounded by the fact that the child may not be talkative because of an introverted nature, so the parents cannot tell what is happening inside the child's mind and are therefore required to ineffectively muddle through endless tantrums and fights.

The nature of the **tantrum** is also telling. While some *Calcarea carbonica* children throw a short tantrum to show displeasure only to give in at the end, more characteristic are children who are unable or refuse to stop their tantrums. These children cry and stomp longer than those needing other remedies. Long after other remedy types realize that they will not get what they want and surrender, the *Calcarea carbonica* child is still kicking and pounding the floor with his fists. Ironically, the tantrum often continues so long that the parent gives in at the end, therefore reinforcing the behavior and ensuring that the child will continue to hold out with tantrums in the future.

At times the obstinacy may be observed in other ways. One boy who was extremely delayed developmentally began to talk in short sentences only when his younger sister was old enough to speak. Apparently he had some speech skills, but only pushed himself to use them when sibling rivalry demanded. Fifteen-month-old Barry seemed unable to walk, not from physical inability but simply because he did not wish to. Four days after the remedy was given, Barry was no longer stubborn and coincidentally began to walk with ease. This **delay in walking** is classic behavior for the *Calcarea carbonica* child. Obstinacy may also show itself whenever *Calcarea carbonica* youngsters are pushed to perform extemporaneously. There is a primal response consisting of obstinacy, refusal, and delay until they can process the new material at their own pace. What parents say about these children is that they do not try new things easily, but when they do make such an attempt they often show perfect mastery.

Another common scenario may be enacted when the child is tired. Instead of lying down or falling asleep, the child whines and cries and cannot be calmed down. It is as if the child is stuck in the obstinacy of **staying awake**, even if the urge to go to sleep is overpowering.

Strong Character and Independence

Obstinacy is a sign of the basically strong character of the child. One can also observe this in the interview. The children look directly at the doctor with a **strong, serious stare** rather than relating with the shyness of a *Lycopodium* or the timidity of a *Pulsatilla*. They just sit quietly, looking directly at the doctor. This little clue can prove to be very important to accurate case analysis. A typical example of its usefulness may be demonstrated during a fevered state, when the *Calcarea carbonica* resembles *Pulsatilla* greatly. The first and major differentiating clue will be the intensity and duration of the stare.

As mentioned before, the child is **independent by nature.** One mother was pleased to say that wherever she put her toddler down, he stayed where he was placed and played with his toys. As his mother told me this, little Vincent sat on the floor happily rummaging through his mother's purse, emptying it bit by bit. Henry, another toddler, loved to play with his father's wallet, playing, stacking, and rearranging his credit cards. This is the same toddler who toilet trained himself at twenty months of age. No longer tolerating soiled pants, he took matters into his own hands and trained himself—to his parents' great surprise.

In the office, emotionally healthy *Calcarea carbonica* children with only a few or no fears may give in to their **natural curiosity** and begin to investigate and **categorize things**. They go about the office touching everything, pulling books off the shelves, and trying to open doors. If the mother tries to halt this independent exploration without channeling the curiosity into a more appropriate game or toy, the child may whine, fuss, or scream. At the same time, the child continues to try to look at books or open drawers until there is a concession by the mother. She has to take his hand, talk to him about what a drawer is, have him touch it, and then have him go on to something else.

It is a good practice to step back during the interview and simply observe how the parent and child are interacting and what they are doing in the office. These observations may often be enough to reveal what the prescription should be. The *Calcarea carbonica* children who later need *Tuberculinum* do one peculiar thing: if there is a large plant in the office, *Calcarea carbonica* children who have an **underlying tubercular miasm** invariably **reach for the plant** and proceed to tear at it, pulling off leaves and sometimes pulling the whole plant down. A defenseless potted palm in our office has helped to confirm many diagnoses of *Calcarea carbonica*.

The parent may become exasperated by the child's behavior, having to repeatedly restrain the child from straying in the plant's direction. This behavior stops with the taking of the remedy, although it may return later when the child requires the remedy *Tuberculinum*.

Seven-year-old Charlotte's mother had her daughter's ears checked several times to make sure that she could hear. The mother said, "The child is so independent she only does what she wants. It got to the point where I seriously wondered if she ever heard me say no!"

Another illustration of this independence, **evident even in the very young**, was recently provided me by a seven-month-old boy who stubbornly wanted things his own way. He wanted to eat with a spoon unaided. He grabbed the spoon with both hands and tried to feed himself. After a while, he gave up on the spoon and started to shovel the food into his mouth with his free hand. He nevertheless held onto the spoon with a strong grip and would not let go, fearing interference by the parent.

This fierce independence can be distracting to the parent. Two-year-old Patricia decided when it was time to end the interview. She stood up, took her mother's wrist, and said over and over again in an increasingly louder voice, "Let's go, let's go!" while attempting to drag her mother toward the door. With a *Lycopodium* child, this sort of scene would have the overtone of bossing the mother around. In contrast, the child needing *Calcarea carbonica* is not bossy, but rather shows the need to express the fact to the parent, often strongly, that he or she is done and ready to go.

The child has a **mind of her own** and **"sticks up" for herself**. The parents say the child's own ideas and opinions are not easily encroached upon. Fourteen-month-old Jennifer screamed at the top of her lungs at her older brothers when they tried to take away her toys. Although she could not yet speak, she still made her views known loud and clear on the unjust acts.

Concentration

This individuality combined with slowness can benefit the *Calcarea Carbonica* child as it often leads to very **deep and lengthy concentration**, even in the very young. Babies only several months old can play by themselves for long periods of time. My wife and I saw an eighteen-month-old boy during a social engagement a week after *Calcarea carbonica* was prescribed for him. In a room full of active children and loud adults, the child managed to remain intensely focused on his play, apparently unaware of anything around him.

Fears

The fears are many in this child, possibly more than in any other polychrest remedy type. Several fears are common. Most have fears of **the dark** and of **shadows**, as does *Phosphorus*. These children often want to sleep with a light on because they are susceptible to **nightmares** in the dark. They fear **spiders and insects**.

Toddlers may point at insects and scream hysterically, "Bug! Bug! Bug!" They often fear **heights, dogs,** and **thunderstorms** as well.

Infants have a fear of **loud-voiced people** because they are startled by them. The *Calcarea carbonica* infant is also frightened by people approaching too quickly, as are *Baryta carbonica* and *Lycopodium* infants. Older children and teens may develop a fear of mice and of narrow, enclosed spaces.

Fear that something unpleasant will happen leads *Calcarea carbonica* children to be apprehensive when they do not know the plans, or if plans are changed unexpectedly or at the last minute. Because of their **apprehension about the future** and the need to finish tasks, they do not like breaks or changes in routines. They also **want to know everything** that might happen in a new situation. Like good journalists, they want to keep abreast of who, what, when, where, why, and how—particularly in unfamiliar territory. They virtually interrogate the parents with questions, trying to flesh out their understanding of unfamiliar places, activities, or guests. In a new classroom or in any **new group**, the child appears **nervous,** often to a degree inappropriate to his tender years.

If the parents are not home on time, they **fear a calamity.** If they learn of an accident through the television or newspaper, they immediately project the event onto their own family members. This anxiety about others is most often seen in *Calcarea carbonica* children who have had a recent emotional loss.

They also have a fear of being **alone in the dark.** They may not wish to go to bed alone, as their fear of **ghosts** and **monsters** mandate that a parent tuck them in. Others merely need a parent to be somewhere in the house, even if they do not interact directly. This may mislead some homeopaths to prescribe the remedy *Lycopodium*. If the rest of the case lends itself to a *Calcarea carbonica* diagnosis, prescribe it and you will find that these and other fears will disappear. Later on, in children who have had these *Lycopodium*-type fears, the fear of being alone in the dark may return with a constellation of new symptoms. This will most likely point to a new remedy picture; namely, *Lycopodium*, which often follows *Calcarea carbonica*.

Bad news, ghost stories, masks, and **fright for any reason** upset these children very much. They are overly sensitive and vulnerable to these experiences, and become very frightened. Nightmares are likely to follow watching scary movies or television programs, or hearing ghost stories. When they watch something frightening on television, they usually try to change the channel or leave the room.

One girl would close her eyes and begin to sing and shout at the top of her lungs to drown out the sound of the television. This annoyed the family to no end. In fact, it was her brother who volunteered the details of all her fearful behavior. If the children are unfortunate enough to have watched frightening programs, the fright is compounded every time they close their eyes at night, as the image returns to frighten them anew.

Many *Calcarea carbonica* children become **clingy during illnesses**. This is especially true of those who are very fearful or who have experienced a deep grief. During fevered states the children want to be very close to the mother or father for security. These toddlers may cry and scream, follow the mother around the house, and demand constant attention. The child's screaming, though intense, stops immediately upon being picked up. One sick thirteen-month-old cried whenever the mother left the room, wanting to be held on her lap the entire time. After the remedy helped this child, she stopped acting so dependent and began to show curiosity, exploring and getting into everything. While the initial behavior is similar to that of *Pulsatilla*, including crying, wanting to nurse, and wanting to sleep with the parents, the child appears basically strong. Once the parents are established as an anchor, the little one is able to confront the rest of the world easily. This can be observed in the strength of character and the gaze.

Many **chronic fearful behaviors** may have their etiology traced to specific frights. Either seeing a stimulus or hearing of it draws the child back into a remembered state of fear. Continued worry can also produce this state. For example, the slow child who needs to take a school entrance exam in order to get into a good school may develop this syndrome. He or she will have studied and studied and worried continuously up until the time of the test. While other students may be able to handle the stress, the *Calcarea carbonica* may collapse with it.

Sadness

Sadness and seriousness may also be major factors of the *Calcarea carbonica* personality. In the office, sad *Calcarea carbonica* teenagers may be incommunicado and taciturn. They may answer questions with a lackluster, monotone yes . . . no. . . . They turn to their parents and say, "Let's go home. I want to go home now." This may seem similar to *Natrum muriaticum*, bu. the immense feeling of sadness or grief behind the presentation is lacking. There is only the feeling that they obstinately refuse to answer, that the doctor cannot move them to reply completely to queries. Again, the sadness is intertwined with their obstinate behavior.

In the slow child, sadness may also stem from **self-doubt** and low self-esteem. Because the child is slow, he may be ridiculed early on by schoolmates and siblings, or even parents and teachers. He cannot stand this criticism and becomes sad, quiet, and withdrawn; he stops many public activities that might give others a chance to make fun of him.

Insulation from others and **not wanting to be laughed at** in the adult leads to the familiar keynote of *Calcarea carbonica* in Kent's *Repertory*: Mind; Fear; confusion, that people would observe her. They fear that others think them incompetent or inadequate, even if it is not the least bit true. Mandy, a girl of nine, developed this complex when her mother was ill for several months. She not only worried constantly about her mother, but also about what other people thought of her. When others looked at her, she assumed that she was doing something wrong and consequently tried to escape the situation.

Fascination with the Supernatural

Calcarea carbonica children may become extremely curious about supernatural phenomena. Kent writes in his *Materia Medica* under *Calcarea carbonica*: "'Whimpering. Low-spirited and melancholy.' It is a strange thing to see a bright little girl of 8 or 9 years old taking on sadness, melancholy, and commencing to talk about the future world, and the angels, and that she wants to die and go there, and she is sad, and wants to read the Bible all day. That is a strange thing; and yet Calcarea [carbonica] has cured that. . . . They are a little inclined to be precocious, and they have attended the Sunday-school, and they have taken too seriously the things they have learned."

The hereafter is a major topic of interest to these children. They ask many questions about God, about heaven and hell, about death and ghosts: about **all things that are unknowable.** One child asked a series of questions when his aunt died that are typical of the *Calcarea carbonica* mind. He wanted to know where his aunt had gone after she died. What did it mean to die? Why did she die? How did it happen? Why were all the people crying over her? And why was Uncle not crying?

Calcarea carbonica children are not able to put this subject down. They think about it, talk about it, and have nightmares about it. One boy was treated for depression. Along with the rest of the case, he had developed a fear of dying after a family member had passed away. From the time of this death onward, he had had many nightmares and a continuous fear that one of his parents would also die. This fear occupied his mind to a great extent until the remedy *Calcarea carbonica* brought him back to his old cheerful self. The reason these children seem to get stuck on such weighty questions is that they **must categorize this information** mentally—as they must categorize everything—yet these issues are not readily sorted out or labeled, so they struggle with them.

Capriciousness

Capriciousness, though not a major factor in most cases, does affect a portion of *Calcarea carbonica* children. Children may moan, not knowing what they want and not wanting to be touched, resembling *Tuberculinum* or *Chamomilla*. This is especially to be **found in a few circumstances:** during colic, fever, after vaccinations, and after an epileptic attack, the child becomes very **irritable and difficult to please.**

When asked where it hurt, a little girl with stomach pains answered, "I won't tell you. It doesn't hurt. Give me water. No, I don't want it. I will get it myself." The conversation went back and forth like this, just as might be found in *Tuberculinum.*

One toddler who suffered from epilepsy became not only

capricious but irritable as well, and cried for a few hours after every seizure. She also became obstinate and mean, hitting her mother and disobeying every request, yelling back any orders given her.

Influence of the Underlying Remedy

Calcarea carbonica seems to **frequently intertwine its symptomatology with the remedy underneath**: the constitutional picture yet to emerge. For instance, tantrums, obstinacy, and destructive tendencies may fit the underlying *Tuberculinum* layer. In another example, a reading of the physical symptoms of *Calcarea carbonica* will reveal that these children produce many symptoms that are similar to those of *Pulsatilla*, a remedy which may follow *Calcarea carbonica*. Yet another example, as previously described, points to the fears that fit both *Calcarea carbonica* and *Lycopodium*, the latter being a remedy that may indeed follow as an appropriate remedy prescription in a particular *Calcarea carbonica* case.

In all of these cases, there are strong symptoms indicating the two remedies that help to form a **bridge** between them and later lead to the prescription of the complementary remedy. Key symptoms shared by two remedies often disappear with a *Calcarea carbonica* prescription only to reappear later when *Tuberculinum*, *Pulsatilla*, or *Lycopodium* is needed. Symptoms that are covered well by two remedies should be carefully recorded, as they offer an easy clue to the possible underlying remedy.

Sleep

The characteristics of sleep give us many symptoms to examine. *Calcarea carbonica* **babies like to be rocked** as much as those needing *Pulsatilla*. To contrast the two, the *Calcarea carbonica* infant likes to be rocked very hard with the parent bobbing up and down quickly and with a degree of force. *Pulsatilla* requires the quite different gentle, swaying type of motion.

By far the most common remedy for **night terrors** is *Calcarea carbonica*. Children may fear to close their eyes and go to sleep because they imagine monsters, ghosts, and all sorts of creatures attacking them. Others experience these dreams in the middle of the night, causing them to wake up screaming. They awake terrified and screaming and are hard to quiet down. This behavior resembles *Stramonium*, though usually the child does not become violent, as would *Stramonium*. They often have nightmares after frightening stories have been read to them or after watching a scary show on television. A good example of this is the nightmares that occur after watching the flying monkeys scene from *The Wizard of Oz*, which usually leaves a lasting impression on these children.

The children occasionally become **overheated in bed**. They **perspire quite profusely**, especially the infants, during the first few minutes to hours of sleep. Perspiration is greatest during dentition and other acute conditions and may tend to be sour. Some children stick their feet out of the covers, while others completely throw off all their covers in the middle of the night.

The children occasionally grind their teeth or gums, moving their mouths as if they were breast-feeding—especially tubercular children during dentition. Some of the children may sleepwalk, though not as commonly as is found with *Natrum muriaticum* or *Phosphorus*.

A good differentiating point for *Calcarea carbonica* is that the child **wakes up refreshed** and in a good mood and is usually the first one up, which is unlike *Lycopodium*, *Tuberculinum*, or *Nux vomica*.

Physical Symptomatology

Head

The head offers a number of valuable symptoms for the *Calcarea carbonica* prescription. First, the shape of the head is quite distinctive: in the infant, we find a **large**, **round head** due to the late closure of the fontanelles. Kent's *Repertory* lists *Calcarea carbonica*, *Calcarea phosphorica*, and *Silicea* in bold type in the rubric: Head; Open, fontanelles. In practice I have found that around two-thirds of these infants need *Calcarea carbonica* while the other third need *Silicea* or *Sulphur*. The other possible remedies listed are needed quite infrequently. *Lycopodium* infants may seem to have large heads as well. However, this appears to be so only in relation to the smallness of the body, not because of the absolute size of the head.

It is common to find a *Calcarea carbonica* baby with a huge, perfectly round head that is either completely bald or covered with a very thin, sparse carpet of hair. The look can be somewhat amusing: a toddler with such a large head being held by the mother while struggling with its little legs to wobble away and staring at you with wide open, good-natured eyes.

The next point is the ease with which the child develops **eruptions of the scalp**. The infant may be born with cradle cap that is unresponsive to orthodox treatment. The rash tends to be very wet, exuding a thick yellow or white discharge that crusts over to form thick scabs, making way for new ones each time they fall away or are removed. The eruption can be offensive with a sour odor in some children, while in others it is odorless. The eruption may also go through phases of being dry and crusty and then wet and weeping, only to crust over again.

The cradle cap may be an early precursor to eczema of the scalp, face, or ears. The remedy *Lycopodium* (and less so *Natrum muriaticum* and *Sulphur*) should also be considered, especially if the eruption is behind the ears.

The parent may state that the eczema appeared as soon as the cradle cap disappeared.

Eczema that covers the whole head and face may occasionally become life threatening to the child. The eruption is present from birth and exudes much pus and liquid. The child loses flesh due to the leakage of serum protein and enters a state of marasmus. It is also worth noting that the eruption often occurs or appears worse in the areas where the child perspires the most, which is often the occiput. Even in healthy *Calcarea carbonica* children, one often observes a reddish discoloration in this area. The destructive nature of the eruption may cause the child to lose all the hair at the site of the problem.

A history commonly told by a parent is that the child now being treated for asthma or chronic sinusitis had this type of eruption as an infant and that the respiratory symptoms came only after the rash was treated and had disappeared. It is also common to give the remedy and then to find that the child develops skin disorders as the respiratory symptoms disappear. This response to the remedy should be viewed as positive and should not be interfered with.

The *Repertory* lists over fifty subrubrics under Head; Eruptions. *Calcarea carbonica* is found listed in italics or bold type in almost half of these subrubrics, showing the frequency with which this disorder appears in practice. In the primary rubrics, *Calcarea carbonica* ties with *Sulphur* as the most common remedy for this complaint. *Calcarea carbonica* should be upgraded in the subrubric Head; Eruption, crusts, as well as in the subrubrics Head; Eruptions, crusts, bloody, moist, white, yellow; lifting the remedy to bold type in all cases. Likewise, *Calcarea carbonica* should be upgraded in the rubric: Head; Eruption, moist; to bold type and should be added in italics to Head; Eruptions, moist, yellow.

The ease with which the head **perspires** is one of the most famous symptoms indicating this remedy. The head perspires in most of these infants and children, especially upon the slightest exertion. In the infant the act of nursing is usually enough to start the perspiration flowing. The child also perspires during sleep, especially while falling asleep or during the first period of sleep.

Another time a parent is prone to notice the perspiration is when the child is put in a car seat and a small puddle forms beneath the sweaty baby. The infant also perspires quite easily if too warm, as when wrapped too well. The mother may be terrified, however, not to wrap up the child, because she hates the thought of cold air against the wet head and knows how often and easily the child develops colds. Even with the child who does not perspire in droplets, clumpiness or a wet appearance of the hair on certain parts of the head may be noticed.

It is important to realize that when one asks the parent if the child perspires, the parent may mistakenly claim that the child does not, and yet the matted hair and the damp scalp will be observed. I always try to feel the scalp, as that may give me the clue I seek.

These children also perspire profusely with every acute illness, especially during dentition. They perspire most commonly on the occiput, but perspiration may be seen dripping from any-where on the head or face. The perspiration may have a sour odor and should be added to the rubric: Head; Perspiration, sour, in italics. It should be noted that of the thirty-four subrubrics under the rubric: Head; Perspiration, *Calcarea carbonica* is found in ful-ly a third, and most often in bold type or italics.

Headaches

Headaches are common complaints and fall into three major group-ings. One common cause of headaches is from **intense study** during school, as is found in *Natrum muriaticum, Phosphorus, Pulsatilla, Sulphur,* and *Tuberculinum.* These headaches may be caused by eyestrain, like *Natrum muriaticum, Pulsatilla,* and *Tuberculinum* all experience. These remedies should all be added in italics to the subrubric: Head; Pain, school headaches. While *Calcarea phos-phorica* is in bold type in this rubric, these other remedies are much more commonly employed in practice.

Congestive headaches are next. These headaches occur most frequently before the menstrual flow and involve the right eye or the right forehead area. A differentiating point is that, unlike many of the remedy types that commonly have congestive headaches of the right side, *Calcarea carbonica* headaches may be ameliorated by the application of hot packs to the head.

Headaches that develop from **sinus colds** leading to sinusi-tis form the third group. A common etiology is that sinusitis occurs after a chill to the head. The parents notice that if the child overexerts himself, the head becomes quite hot and flushed and begins to sweat. Clothing is loosened in order to cool down, but instead the child chills too quickly and develops a respiratory tract infec-tion accompanied by a headache.

Because of this sensitivity, a leading indication for *Calcarea carbonica* is that the children **love hats,** as do *Silicea* children, and keep them on unless they overexert themselves. This makes the differentiation from *Pulsatilla* easier, because *Pulsatilla* children hate to wear hats. The rubric: Head; Uncovering head, aggravates, lists *Calcarea carbonica* in italics and *Silicea* in bold type. The opposite rubric below it, Head; Warm covering on head, aggra-vates, also lists *Calcarea carbonica* in italics but also *Pulsatilla* in bold type. While *Calcarea carbonica* is included in both rubrics, it is listed in the latter rubric because of all the symptoms the remedy type develops upon exertion. With any stress, exercise, play, or illness, the head becomes congested with blood, making it hot. Therefore, anything that increases this vasomotor instability, creating more heat to the head, will be aggravating.

Eyes

The **gaze** of the child shows the underlying natural **strength** and, at times, the characteristic obstinacy. The toddler playfully struggling to escape the arms of a protective mother will look directly at the doctor; the child who traipses through the office looking for mischief continues to look directly at the doctor in a way that a *Lycopodium* or *Pulsatilla* could never manage. The eyes show fierce determination as the mother struggles with the child to retrieve the book or piece of equipment that was on the doctor's desk.

The eyes of *Calcarea carbonica* are frequently affected in the adult but less so in the child, although there are a few affections that may be observed in the child. As in *Pulsatilla*, they often develop **colds** that extend to the eyes, accompanied by bland, yellow-green, thick mucus.

Occasionally a parent seeks care for an infant with a closed lacrimal duct, the eye producing the same kind of bland, thick pus. These symptoms are curable with *Calcarea carbonica* and are shared with *Pulsatilla* and *Silicea*.

Also in common with *Silicea*, *Calcarea carbonica* will be one of the remedies for **fistulous lacrimal duct**. The rubric: Eye; Fistula, lacrimalis, lists *Calcarea carbonica* and *Silicea* in bold type while the rubric: Eye; Stricture of lacrimal duct, lists *Calcarea carbonica* in plain type and *Silicea* in bold. In this last rubric, *Calcarea carbonica* should be elevated from plain type to italics.

The other major affection of the eye is the **weakness of the eye muscles** and the ease with which the child develops eyestrain. Overuse leads to headaches that are especially aggravated by reading, watching television, and writing. All of the eyestrain symptoms will resemble those of *Natrum muriaticum*, and like that remedy, *Calcarea carbonica* may develop photophobia with eye complaints. To differentiate between these two remedies, it will be noted that photophobic *Calcarea carbonica* children and adults still love the sunshine and enjoy being out in it, quite unlike *Natrum muriaticum*.

Some of these infants may be born with **congenital cataracts**. In others, a pediatric ophthalmologist may have a difficult time controlling **juvenile glaucoma**. The ophthalmologist may finally pronounce that the child has been born with a "bad eye." Older materia medicas discuss the ulcers commonly found on the cornea, but these are seldom seen in pediatric practice today.

Ears

The ears are a **constant source of illness** for the *Calcarea carbonica* child. The child's history often contains many episodes of otitis media. The mother commonly reports how an earache began following a bout of bronchitis, tonsillitis, or even a cold, and how quickly the infection found its way to the ears. The earaches described are very similar to *Belladonna* earaches. In fact, *Calcarea carbonica* children develop many acute illnesses that the remedy *Belladonna* will cure.

The complementary nature of *Belladonna* and *Calcarea carbonica*, as well as the possible confusion between two such similar remedies, is well illustrated in the case of **earaches**. In *Calcarea carbonica*, the child develops a very high fever, especially with a hot head and cold extremities. The ears become quite painful, throbbing and perhaps turning red in color; these symptoms are shared with *Belladonna*. A mistake may be made here if the child is treated with the incorrect remedy. For instance, if the *Calcarea carbonica* otitis is treated with *Belladonna*, thinking that the earache needs an acute remedy and in the hope of either ending the illness or stopping the inflammatory process, one finds that the fever drops, yet the illness is not ended. The ear may still throb, but now there is also pus and discharge that would typically not be found if the *Belladonna* prescription was correct and ended the inflammation.

A good differentiating point that may indicate the child still needs *Calcarea carbonica* and not *Belladonna* is the amount of moisture found. The head perspires greatly with the fever and the nose and chest are full of mucus: symptoms that are not found strongly in *Belladonna*. In fact, it is the intense heat and dryness of the scalp that should lead one to grasp the fact that the child no longer needs *Calcarea carbonica* but rather its complement, *Belladonna*. Using these symptoms, it is easy to differentiate between the two remedies and thus give the correct one. *Belladonna* is often called for in the treatment of true acute otitis in constitutional *Calcarea carbonica* children, but will later need to be followed up with the constitutional remedy.

In *Calcarea carbonica* the **discharge** tends to be thick, yellow, and very smelly. At times this discharge may last for weeks or months after the acute episode has ended. It seems as if the body cannot combat the infection successfully, and so the discharge continues on with the eardrum never quite healing.

The otitis and the discharge are **aggravated by cold wind**, even if only the ears are exposed. These children, unlike *Pulsatilla* or *Natrum muriaticum*, like to keep their hats on lest their ears begin to hurt. On palpation the doctor may find many large, tender cervical nodes. Scarring and sclerosing of the tympanic membrane may develop, causing mild to severe deafness. With this history, many of the children also develop fluid in the ears that may lead to a **chronic hearing loss**.

Calcarea carbonica is one of only a few remedies in the *Repertory* listed in bold type under Ear; Catarrh, eustachian tube, and Ear; Hearing impaired, catarrh in eustachian tube. This **fluid buildup** is often noted in allergic children who have a nasal obstruction, breathe through their mouths, and develop one respiratory infection after another.

The other common finding in the ears of the infant is **cracking of the skin** behind them, much like that of *Lycopodium* and *Sulphur*. There is a predilection for moist eruptions or eczemas that cause fissures in this area. These cracks may disappear without any sort of treatment as the child grows. Therefore, direct questioning is the best way to learn of this problem if it is past history.

Nose

The nose is **very often affected** in these children. Even in good health they often have **runny noses**. Whenever the children go outside to play, clear, watery mucus spills out their noses as soon as they exert themselves in the cold air. This discharge seems to aid them in establishing and maintaining an internal balance that promotes health.

Many worried parents give a child unwarranted antibiotics that do not work for this watery discharge, and then antihistamines that succeed in stopping the discharge, but to the detriment of the real health of the child. With the suppression of the discharge, respiratory infections become commonplace; the child must weather one bout after another. It is not uncommon for a *Calcarea carbonica* child to be ill every two or three weeks, first with tonsillitis, then otitis, and finally bronchitis. One would typically discover in such cases that, as a toddler, the child had a runny nose that was suppressed with medication, after which these infections all began.

The best-case scenario for some of these children is one in which the prescription is given and all the infections end, only to be replaced by the constant but "normal" runny nose once more. The beauty of homeopathy is that one can either prevent such interference in the health of a child or, if it has already happened, bring the child back to the level of well-being he or she had before the suppression of natural mechanisms by pharmaceuticals.

As mentioned, the child tends to **contract frequent coryzas** that greatly resemble those of *Pulsatilla*. The nose becomes obstructed with thick, yellow puslike mucus that may smell sour. If the child is old enough to say so, he may complain of a bad odor in his nose. The mucus obstructs the nasal passages, especially at night, preventing normal breathing. The thick mucus crusts over and eventually creates sores in the nose. This last point, along with the offensive odor, aids in differentiating *Calcarea carbonica* from *Pulsatilla*.

These colds occur when it is cold outside or when, as with *Dulcamara*, the weather changes from warm to cold, damp days. These children, like *Lycopodium* youngsters, are chronic snufflers who are aggravated by drinking milk.

Boericke states at the end of the nose section for *Calcarea carbonica* in his *Materia Medica*, **"Coryzas alternate with colic."** This has been confirmed often in practice and should be considered a good indication for *Calcarea carbonica*.

The other major affection of the nose is epistaxis: frequent **nosebleeds**. Plethoric, obese *Calcarea carbonica* individuals are the ones who often complain of nosebleeds in the morning.

Face

Typically, the *Calcarea carbonica* **baby has a round face** with fat rolls around the neck and jowls. The skin has a thick quality to it, having the appearance of a great deal of **underlying fat**. They seem pasty and pale, and many are born with red "**stork bites**" on the face, especially between the eyes and in the middle of the forehead. These fade as the child grows and are often only visible when the child is straining, such as during a bowel movement or while crying.

The problem of **cradle cap** described under **Head** may extend to the face. Another keynote observed, especially in undersized babies, is a **swollen upper lip** that protrudes.

Infants suffering from failure to thrive and who lose weight often develop the **wrinkles** for which the *Calcarea carbonica* adult is so well known. The infants begin to look like the little old men or women that the early books describe. Many of the more obese toddlers scratch their faces, leaving behind nail marks. They usually do this when they are tired, have just awakened, or have eaten a food to which they are sensitive. Active obese teens blush easily and turn red with the slightest exertion.

Mouth

The oral mucosa is very sensitive to damage in *Calcarea carbonica*. The child develops **canker sores** and **aphthous ulcers** readily with any small puncture of the inner lip or mild trauma to the area. Many of these same children also develop **thrush**. The mother may state that the child first developed the problem, passed it to the mother's breast, and then became reinfected again. The two end up bandying the thrush back and forth for a length of time.

The other main complaint of the mouth revolves around **dentition**. The developmental time line of tooth eruption in children is somewhat dependent on the status of the thyroid gland. Since

25

many *Calcarea carbonica* children are functionally **hypothyroid**, dentition **tends to be late**. The typical delay in dentition ranges from three months to one year late. Teething is often accompanied by many difficulties such as colds and croup, colic and diarrhea, irritability, and, much more rarely, epilepsy.

Tooth eruption is often **painful**. The child may wake up at night screaming and tossing about in bed. The keynote of perspiration of the head at night may begin during this time. The pain is ameliorated if the child is given cool water to drink; this is a point that may confuse one into giving *Chamomilla*.

At the other end of the range of possibilities, a minority of *Calcarea carbonica* children are functionally **hyperthyroid**. What one finds in these cases is that some of the skull sutures close early and, more commonly, dentition is very early. The child belonging to this subgroup is often tubercular and may need the remedy *Tuberculinum* at some point of the treatment.

The **teeth** may be **soft**, lacking enamel and decaying quickly.

Throat and Neck

Calcarea carbonica children **develop sore throats easily**. It is common to elicit a history of repeated streptococcal infections of the throat. They develop sore throats when exposed to cold winds or if they are caught even briefly in the rain. The etiology is similar to that described under earaches. The child goes out to play, becomes overheated, begins to perspire, and perhaps takes off some clothes. Later that night the child awakes in the middle of an acute infection. The tonsils grow to an enormous size, becoming red and swollen and throbbing with pain. The uvula is also often inflamed. The child may respond to the remedy *Belladonna* every time this acute situation develops. As a general statement, if the sore throat is severe in a *Calcarea carbonica* child and is accompanied by dry, painful swallowing, one should give the remedy *Belladonna* if one cannot decide on which acute remedy to use, as this will almost always stop the acute symptoms and clear the way for the constitutional remedy to do its work.

With these sore throats one is always able to palpate many **swollen glands**, be they the submaxillary, posterior, or anterior cervical chains. The glands may be hard, swollen, and tender to the touch for the first few days of the illness. While rarely found in general practice today, the remedy *Calcarea carbonica* may be considered for any disease involving the thyroid gland itself, its functioning, or any fistulas or ducts that are connected to it.

Lower Respiratory System

The **chest** takes the brunt of the allergies and respiratory infections by producing **coughs**. A keynote of *Calcarea carbonica* shared by *Pulsatilla* is found in the cough, which is dry at night but loose with easy expectoration in the morning. The cough is triggered by a variety of food allergies, cold weather, and pollens in the air. Oftentimes, colds progress easily into **lung congestions** as the ability to isolate infections to the throat fails and the infection drops into the lungs. In toddlers, the congestions may be accompanied by high fevers, a desire to be held by the parents, lethargy, crankiness, a hot head and cold extremities, perspiration on the scalp, and weight loss due to disinterest in food. These last symptoms are similar to *Belladonna* and *Pulsatilla*, so be careful. The expectoration tends to be thick, yellow, and, occasionally, foul smelling.

Chest infections may ascend and bring about painless **hoarseness**, especially in the morning. The children may also develop asthma that is aggravated by cold and exertion (especially climbing stairs). Although these symptoms seem common to many, *Calcarea carbonica* is one of the most frequently used remedies for childhood asthma and bronchitis.

Alimentary System

Food Cravings and Aversions

Calcarea carbonica youngsters **love all the carbohydrates:** sweets, ice cream, pasta, bread, and potatoes (even if raw). They also crave **salt** and **fish**. The children also crave **cheesy foods** such as pizza, macaroni and cheese, and lasagna.

Eggs are the big favorite and serve as a very strong keynote for this remedy, confirming most prescriptions. They particularly crave soft-boiled eggs, but eggs in almost any form are considered desirable. Some *Calcarea carbonica* infants, when just beginning to eat solids, only want eggs. Even more peculiar is that in acute febrile conditions the *Calcarea carbonica* child may suddenly begin to crave eggs even more than usual, even if eggs were formerly disliked.

They **dislike meat** in general and **fat** in particular. They dislike **slimy foods**. If an egg is too soft and slimy on top they may refuse to eat it, even though they love eggs. They also may dislike **mixed foods**, liking each food to remain separate and not in contact with other foods on the plate.

Some toddlers develop **pica**: they begin to nibble on sand, chalk, lime, dog bones, glue, and other found substances. Most of these materials contain calcium, for which the child must instinctively feel a need.

They tend to **crave cool or cold water and foods.**

A few may desire milk, though most develop upset stomachs from it. **Many do not like or tolerate milk** at all. Vomiting, diarrhea, respiratory infections, or respiratory allergies may occur after drinking milk, occasionally even mother's milk. The child reacts the same way if breast-fed and the mother drinks milk. Digestive upsets of this nature are prevalent at the time of dentition. With each new tooth eruption the child may have a period of vomiting and diarrhea.

Stomach

The stomach offers **many keynotes** for the prescription. As a general rule, the vast majority of these children tend to have **slow digestion**, with the exception of the children with failure to thrive. **Babies** tend toward **chronic vomiting**, with or without pain. It is as if the cardiac sphincter at the bottom of the esophagus and top of the stomach does not function properly for these infants. Clinically, *Calcarea carbonica* is to be thought of for babies who nurse and then, within five minutes of unsuccessful burping, regurgitate the undigested milk. They may open their mouths and, without any effort or commotion, find that the milk spills out, much to their mothers' amazement and frustration. Such infants again act as if they are hungry, and the mother must repeat the feeding. The vomitus may have a sour odor or be preceded by sour, empty eructations. If not vomited right away, the milk will be curdled. The vomiting may be associated with hiccoughs in infants. *Calcarea* *carbonica* should be added in italics to the new rubric I created: Stomach; Hiccoughs; eating, after, in infants; with *Pulsatilla* in bold type, *Lycopodium* in italics, and *Nux vomica* in plain type. In older children motion sickness and car sickness are the main causes leading to vomiting, much like *Natrum muriaticum*.

While some of the children may be picky eaters, most **wake up hungry** and demand to be nursed or to have breakfast. This is particularly common in children with failure to thrive. The appetite of many of the older children wakes up with them in the morning, unlike *Sulphur* who usually does not need to eat for a number of hours after rising.

Abdomen

These children often have large abdomens that pouch out as if there were no musculature to hold back the intestines. It is quite distinctive to see such a **big belly**, especially in children who have failure to thrive, as they begin to resemble truly starving children.

The abdomen is soft and has poor tone, which allows the separation of the rectus abdominis muscles, thereby leading to the easy development of **umbilical hernias**. While doctors may wish to operate on these hernias, they are easily treated by mechanical means along with the remedies. A skein of yarn with a knot in it does well as a truss. Place the knot over the hernia and tie the ends of the skein behind the child's back. Then tape over the knot. Tape vertically and then from side to side. Keep the tape in place as much as possible. The forced proximity of the two long muscles held in position this way allows cross-fibers to form. The hernia will begin to heal in two or three weeks.

While *Calcarea carbonica* is listed only in italics in the rubric: Abdomen; Hernia, umbilical, with *Nux vomica* in bold type, one finds clinically that *Calcarea carbonica* is the main remedy and should be elevated to bold type. *Nux vomica* is called for and used mainly if and when the hernia strangulates and the child begins vomiting, straining, or developing other *Nux vomica* symptoms. One should keep in mind that a strangulated hernia is a medical emergency, and although the remedy may help or even reduce the strangulation, the child should be taken to an emergency room as quickly as possible.

Rectum

Constipation is the chief complaint for many of these children. The stools are large and hard, and may fill the whole toilet bowl. Parents are amazed at how much stool a little child can pass at any one time. The constipation may be so severe that these children only have a stool every week to ten days. Many materia medicas describe the stools as whitish and bileless. Although this would certainly confirm a diagnosis of *Calcarea carbonica*, it is not frequently seen in practice today.

The most unusual characteristic described in old materia medicas is that the child does not seem to mind being constipated—in fact, seems **cheerful when constipated**. In many cases, the parents will be the ones who complain about the child's constipation, the child seeming placid and only complaining when the parents give a laxative or cathartic. For some of these children, however, there are great pains along with the constipation. The large girth of the stool may bring on hemorrhoids and, on occasion, fissures that are exquisitely painful during a bowel movement. The pain in turn causes the child to try and hold back the stool against the natural urge to eliminate, which only exacerbates the problem.

The other main bowel complaint is **diarrhea**. Those children suffering from **celiac disease or lactose intolerance** illustrate the tendency best, though other children in subclinical states may also share this symptomatology. Abdominal colic followed by explosive diarrhea is the usual pattern. These loose stools are often triggered by drinking milk or eating bread products. In the lactose-intolerant infant, the milk becomes sour and curdles in the stomach. A short time after drinking milk, gurgling can be felt and the child develops colic that ends with explosive diarrhea. If the process continues for a short time, the child develops a voracious appetite but loses everything eaten to the diarrhea. Should this continue for too long, the child's mental and physical growth can be greatly stunted.

Occasionally a child with celiac disease may experience constipation for a few weeks, followed by severe diarrhea with mucus; the diarrhea always alternates with constipation as the child wastes away. *Calcarea carbonica* has cured many such children.

Diarrhea also **accompanies many acute diseases** such as otitis media, bronchitis, and difficult dentition. Such diarrhea may have a sour odor and may have green mucus as a constituent. It tends to be worse in the evening, a good point for differentiating such cases from those requiring *Sulphur* and *Podophyllum*, who are worse in the mornings.

A last point that may lead to confusion is that the diarrhea often causes a **diaper rash due to yeast overgrowth**, making the anus red. A careful observer finds the redness and may assume that the stool is very acrid and excoriating, and may incorrectly prescribe a remedy such as *Sulphur*. Aiding in this incorrect prescription is the fact that *Calcarea carbonica* is not listed in the rubric: Rectum; Redness of anus. Clinically, one finds that redness accompanies many *Calcarea carbonica* diarrheas and should be added in italics to the above rubric. More specifically, one may find the remedy listed in italics under the rubric: Rectum; Eruption about anus, and Rectum; Excoriation. Since there are no subrubrics that give the color red to the eruption, the only place to list the yeast infection is under Rectum; Redness.

Urogenital System

Boys

The boys tend to develop **hydroceles** almost as often as *Pulsatilla* does. **Rashes and eruptions** around the genitals caused by the action of strong urine may also occur. The rashes are often yeast infections that turn the scrotum and surrounding parts bright red, similar in this way to *Medorrhinum*. Some of the more obese boys also experience nocturnal enuresis, though more commonly this will be cured by *Tuberculinum, Pulsatilla, Natrum muriaticum,* or *Medorrhinum*.

Girls

Recurrent vaginitis caused by yeast occurs mostly in obese infant girls. The vaginal discharge is thick and milky yellow, resembling thick breast milk. It tends to be acrid, itchy, and odorous, smelling like mold.

The first **menstrual cycle** may begin early or late, starting as early as the tenth year or as late as the seventeenth. The flow, occurring every twenty to twenty-eight days, may be quite profuse and last a long time. The first and succeeding menses may be preceded by strong symptoms. Most girls develop breast swelling and tenderness as well as fluid retention all over the body. Coryza, vaginitis, and headaches may also be part of the premenstrual package. Occasionally a patient who complains of seizures that occur before the flow will be cured by the remedy *Calcarea carbonica*.

Musculoskeletal System

Back

The older materia medicas list *Calcarea carbonica* as one of the main remedies used in the treatment of bone problems such as rickets, as is *Silicea*. Although rickets is no longer frequently seen in the Western world, when found it will often respond to the remedy *Calcarea carbonica*. More prevalent now is a calcium imbalance that shows up as a **weakness of the back and/or scoliosis**, especially of the thoracic vertebrae. A more serious condition is **spina bifida**. Children with these spinal anomalies seem to respond well to *Calcarea carbonica*.

As also noted under **Throat and Neck**, the **cervical region** shows swollen glands that are indurated, forming a necklace about the neck, found in *Silicea* and *Tuberculinum* as well. This region also perspires a great deal, especially during sleep. As the toddler passes through growth spurts, the neck thins down as if it had elongated.

Extremities

Materia medicas commonly describe *Calcarea carbonica* as though all the babies are tardy in **walking**. In fact, less than half have this complaint; most children learn to walk at the normal time. Some simply do not try to walk until they are fourteen or fifteen months old, at which time they get up and easily walk over to get something, shocking a parent who had no idea the child was even trying to walk. Others seem to be born with **weak ankles**; one or both feet may turn in. In most cases the foot condition will correct itself without intervention. In others, the parents may take on a vigorous massaging and stretching program for the baby that helps too little and is followed by braces or corrective shoes. The remedy, however, will strengthen the ankles very quickly.

Weakness of the ankles is also observed in plethoric, obese teenage girls. In these girls the combination of weak, easily turned ankles and the swelling of the ankles before each menstrual flow helps point to the correct prescription.

The weakness also affects the **long bones**; children tend toward rickets, osteogenesis imperfecta, or more commonly, bowleggedness. The growth plate of the tibia weakens in the adolescent, leading to Osgood-Schlatter disease and its resulting pains near the head of the tibia. The child with this disease wakes up at night with pains in the shins or knees and possibly cramps in the calves.

Weakness of the extremities is observed in the **nails** as well. The growing child develops many problems with brittle, cracking, or ingrown nails.

Even the infant is plagued with nails that grow slowly or break easily.

The **fingers** can **hyperextend** as much as the **ankles** do. In infants and toddlers you can demonstrate the weakness of tendons by bending the fingers backward to a wide angle.

Another common keynote is the ease with which the **hands and feet perspire**. The child perspires even when cold or at rest. While this is less commonly found in children than in adults, the toddlers may have wet socks that require constant changing. The perspiration may or may not smell sour. The same uneven temperature and blood regulation observed in the head is also found in the extremities. The feet, though wet with perspiration, may feel as cold as ice during the day. Although the child does not complain of **cold feet**, the doctor may touch the feet and not believe how cold they are. As soon as the feet are wrapped up in blankets at night they begin to heat up and eventually become too hot to remain covered.

The last complaint of the extremities is **juvenile rheumatoid arthritis**, which is aggravated by first motion and by cold and wet conditions and is ameliorated by continued motion and heat. As a point of differentiation, one should recall that the arthritis of a

Calcarea carbonica adult is aggravated by continued motion, unlike the more flexible child.

Skin

This remedy type has a propensity for **eczema**; many infants are born with it. The scalp is most often involved, but it may extend to the face and extremities. They may also be born with heavy **cradle cap** consisting of thick, white crusts that resemble chalk. Older children may develop chronic recurring hives, as do those needing *Natrum muriaticum*.

They often develop **Candida rashes** that are bright red and have a sharp line of demarcation. These rashes most often occur around the diaper area, front and back. As mentioned in the respiratory section, Candida rashes may return to the allergic or asthmatic child a few months after the remedy is initially prescribed. The respiratory symptoms disappear but the parents may insist on treatment for the nasty diaper rash the child now has. Do not be coerced! The rash is the body's way of overcoming an imbalance. The eruptive state should absolutely not be interfered with homeopathically or with strong antifungal medications, as the rash will disappear but the respiratory symptoms will surely return. Simple applications of Calendula ointment, perhaps with acidophilus supplementation, is all that should be recommended. Many a successful case has been destroyed by trying to get rid of a rash. Be patient and explain the healing response carefully to the parents. Parents should likewise explain it to their anxious doctors.

The other main skin symptom found in some *Calcarea carbonica* children is **warts**. These occur usually on the palms and fingers. The warts are round and skin colored and tend to erupt in crops rather than singly.

Something unique to be observed in infants and toddlers is that they often **scratch their faces**. When they eat something to which they are allergic or when they are tired, they begin to scratch in a mechanical, clawlike fashion. They may also do this upon rising from sleep.

Physical Generals

Calcarea carbonica is by far the most common remedy for **epilepsy**, especially if it occurs during dentition. Birth trauma that causes calcification in the brain may also be an etiologic factor in these early seizures. The child becomes a little more reclusive before an attack, and afterward may moan and whine and not want to be touched. During these episodes the child seems like a *Tuberculinum* type, but *Calcarea carbonica* will cure the case. In older girls the seizures may be most common premenstrually.

To restate the generalities, *Calcarea carbonica* children show a **poor assimilation of calcium** as well as malfunctions of the thyroid gland, which lead to slow mental and physical development. These children tire easily and seem malnourished, sometimes to the point of rickets or marasmus.

Many symptoms may develop when metabolism changes, such as during dentition or learning to walk. The hair, nails, and bones often grow poorly and the glands enlarge and indurate easily. Children may become anemic and chilly as they age, and characteristically perspire even though they are cool.

They become allergic and tend to get sick, at which point they develop discharges that are offensive and sour smelling.

In general, they are **aggravated by dentition**, exertion (especially climbing stairs), **cold and wet weather, a change of weather** from warm to cold, and the beverage **milk**. They are helped by warm, dry air, and love the summertime.

Notes on *Calcarea carbonica* Infants

Calcarea carbonica infants are obstinate, especially when tired. Instead of falling asleep, they whine and cry and cannot be calmed down. It is as if they become mired in obstinacy, forcing themselves to stay awake even if the urge to sleep is overpowering.

They are independent. They stay wherever they are placed and play contentedly with their toys. They like to do things their own way and in their own time. An example of this independence in the very young is the seven-month-old who wanted to eat with a spoon by himself and would not give up, even though he finally had to cling to the spoon with one hand while shoveling food into his mouth with the other.

Even the very young are capable of long, deep concentration. Babies only a few months old can play contentedly by themselves for long periods of time, apparently unaware of anything around them.

Infants are easily startled by loud people. They are also frightened by people approaching them too quickly, as are *Baryta carbonica* children.

They cling to parents for security during illnesses and fevered states, especially when already fearful. They near the parents during fevered states as if they offered a base of stability. These infants may demand attention by crying and screaming. The screaming, though intense, stops immediately upon being picked up.

Infants and young toddlers wake up screaming with fear as if from nightmares.

Irritability is common, and even more likely to occur during illnesses such as colic and fevered conditions, after vaccinations, and after an epileptic attack. This irritability can be accompanied by moaning, indecisiveness, and an aversion to consolation; all this mimics *Tuberculinum* and *Chamomilla*.

Infants are born with large, round heads (due to the late closure of the fontanelles), and are either completely bald or have very thin, sparse hair. Infants may be born with cradle cap that is resistant to treatment. The rash tends to be very wet with a thick, yellow or white discharge that crusts over. The scalp perspires easily, especially from the slightest exertion. Nursing is characteristically enough to bring on copious perspiration. Infants also perspire during sleep (especially upon falling asleep), acute illnesses, and dentition.

Colds often extend to the eyes and produce thick, greenish mucus there. Babies may be born with closed or fistular lacrimal ducts and sometimes congenital cataracts.

Frequent earaches throb with pain and cause the head to become hot. They are similar to *Belladonna* earaches but with more mucus or discharge and with enlarged cervical glands. The skin may crack around the ears.

The children have frequent runny noses even in health, and

colds accompanied by thick, yellow-green mucus occur whenever they become chilled. Chronic snuffles are also common and may be due to a milk allergy.

A fat, round face with "stork bites" is characteristic. Wrinkles appear on the faces of babies suffering from failure to thrive. Babies scratch their faces when tired or awakening or after drinking milk.

Thrush and recurrent canker sores are common mouth problems. Slow dentition is accompanied by a myriad of infections and diarrhea.

Many swollen cervical glands may be palpated in the neck. The thyroid gland may be subject to congenital disorders.

Babies chronically vomit milk they have just swallowed and become hungry again afterwards. They hiccough after nursing. Babies have strong, healthy appetites. Often they cannot tolerate milk and develop colic, diarrhea, flatus, or vomiting in response. Children crave eggs and cheese and sometimes exhibit pica. They often have distended abdomens with weak muscles.

Infants are subject to umbilical hernias. Constipation with large stools; diarrhea with colic, especially in the lactose intolerant; and diaper rashes of yeast overgrowths with very red discoloration of the skin are all common.

Boys are sometimes born with hydroceles. Yeast infections can be found on and around the penis.

Recurrent vaginitis occurs in obese infant girls.

These children are susceptible to epilepsy, especially after head trauma causing calcification within the brain. Epilepsy can also manifest during dentition.

Babies may learn to walk late and may be born with spina bifida or develop various bone deformities. The joints hyperextend with ease. The extremities tend to perspire.

Babies develop eczema, especially on the scalp. They also develop cradle cap and yeast infections of the skin.

Babies can be obese.

Calcarea carbonica is the remedy most often called for to aid in curing growth difficulties of infancy and early childhood, especially those due to malfunctions of the thyroid and the calcium metabolic process.

Calcarea carbonica Outline

I. Mental/Emotional Characteristics
  A. Delayed or faulty development
    1. Delayed skills
      a) Walking and talking
      b) Comprehension of new skills
      c) Willful delay of acquisition in order to categorize new information
    2. Slow comprehension in school
    3. Poor recall
    4. Mistakes in reading and writing
  B. Plodding
    1. Slowly plod from one project to another
    2. Study methodically and receive top grades
    3. Cautious
      a) About anything new
      b) Until subject is understood
    4. Able to play patiently with one object for a long time
  C. Inflexible and obstinate
    1. Due to a plodding nature
    2. Because of a need to finish what is started
    3. Will have tantrums in order to be allowed to finish tasks
    4. Obstinate
      a) If interrupted
      b) If plans are suddenly changed
      c) If forced to change
    5. Desire structure
      a) To categorize things
      b) To complete things
    6. May sustain a tantrum for a long time
    7. Refuse to do anything extemporaneously
  D. Strong character
    1. Willfulness
    2. Easily seen in the strength of the stare at observers
  E. Independent and curious
    1. Curiosity evident in the doctor's office

      a) Characteristically tear at plants in the doctor's office
      b) Touch and play with all things in order to categorize them
  2. Independently play with anything fancied
  3. May wish to feed themselves at a very young age
  4. Have minds of their own

F. May become a loner
  1. Due to a slow, plodding nature
  2. May become sad and withdrawn
  3. Seen the initial interview
      a) Serious
      b) Quiet

G. Fascination with the unknown
  1. Death, especially brought on by the death of a family member
  2. The supernatural
      a) Attempt to categorize the unknowable
      b) Many questions about God

H. Fears
  1. Many
  2. The dark
  3. Insects
  4. Animals
  5. Ghosts and monsters
  6. Startle easily
  7. Fright from scary stories
  8. Worse from frights
      a) Nightmares
      b) More fears
  9. Generalized foreboding that something "bad" will happen
  10. Clingy during illness

I. Sleep
  1. Babies like to be rocked
  2. Night terrors and nightmares from the day's scary events
  3. Become too warm in bed

a) Perspire and uncover until eight or ten years of age.

b) After eight or ten years old they may stay chilly and covered at night.

4. May grind the teeth at night during dentition

5. Sleepwalking common

6. Wake up refreshed

II. Physical Symptomatology

    A. Head Area

        1. Head

            a) Large, round shape due to late closure of the fontanelles

            b) Eruptions such as cradle cap are common

                (1) On the occiput

                    (a) Often located or worse there

                    (b) Where perspiration is greatest

                (2) Exudate

                    (a) Thick

                    (b) Yellow

                    (c) Sour smelling

             c) Copious perspiration

                (1) Especially on the occiput

                (2) During sleep

                (3) While nursing

            d) Headaches

                (1) Due to mental strain from study

                (2) Eyestrain

                (3) Congestive

                    (a) Premenstrual headache

                    (b) During upper respiratory tract infections

                (4) Due to a head chill after becoming too warm

                (5) Localized congestion with exertion

                    (a) Causes the head to throb

                    (b) Hot head

        2. Eyes

            a) Expression

    (1) Shows strength of character
    (2) Patients look directly at the physician, even
       if very ill
  b) Colds often extend to the eyes, giving rise to
    mucus
    (1) Bland
    (2) Thick
    (3) Yellow
  c) Lacrimal canal problems
    (1) Closed
    (2) Fistulous
  d) Weak eye muscles lead to eyestrain
  e) Congenital cataracts
  f) Glaucoma

3. Ears
  a) Otitis
    (1) Frequent
    (2) Accompanies respiratory tract infections
    (3) Discharge
      (a) Thick
      (b) Yellow
      (c) Offensive
      (d) With a ruptured ear drum
    (4) Aggravated by cold wind
    (5) Scarring of the tympanic membrane
    (6) Pus and fluid in the ear cause impaired
      hearing
  b) Cracking of the skin behind the ears

4. Nose
  a) Runny nose
    (1) Even when healthy
    (2) Especially when playing outside
  b) Many colds
    (1) With otitis
    (2) With tonsillitis
    (3) Nose is obstructed with mucus
      (a) Thick
      (b) Yellow

(c) Offensive odor
(4) During the change of seasons to cold and
wet weather
(5) Alternate with colic
c) Frequent nosebleeds
5. Face
a) Characteristic appearance
(1) Round
(2) Fat rolls on the neck and jowls
(3) "Stork bites"
(a) Anywhere on the face
(b) Especially on the eyelids and forehead
b) Cradle cap spreads to the face
c) Swollen upper lip in infants
d) Failure to thrive in babies causes many facial
wrinkles
e) Infants and toddlers scratch the face
(1) When tired
(2) Upon awakening
6. Mouth
a) Frequent sores
(1) Canker sores
(2) Aphthous ulcers
b) Thrush develops easily
c) Difficult dentition
(1) Delayed
(2) Accompanied by respiratory infections
7. Throat and Neck
a) Frequent sore throats
b) Enlarged cervical glands
(1) Many
(2) Hardened
c) Enlarged tonsils
d) Frequent illnesses due to exposure to cold when
overheated
B. Torso
1. Lower Respiratory System
a) Many coughing fits and infections

(1) With dry coughs at night

(2) Loose, productive coughs in the morning

b) Asthma aggravations

(1) From exertion

(2) During cold and wet weather

(3) From climbing stairs

2. Alimentary System

a) Food cravings and aversions

(1) Cravings

(a) All carbohydrates

i) Bread

ii) Pasta

iii) Potatoes

iv) Sweets

(b) Eggs, especially soft-boiled

(c) Ice cream

(d) Salt

(e) Fish

(f) May develop pica: craving of odd substances

i) Sand

ii) Glue

iii) Found substances such as chalk

(2) Aversions

(a) Slimy foods

(b) Mixed foods such as casseroles

(c) May dislike milk

i) Even if other dairy foods are craved

ii) Babies may chronically regurgitate after nursing

b) Stomach: problems after nursing in infants

(1) Hiccough easily

(2) Vomit sour curds

c) Abdomen: Poor musculature

(1) Large and distended

(2) Umbilical hernia

d) Rectum

(1) Constipation that may or may not be

painful
(2) Very large, bulky stools
(3) Diarrhea accompanies many conditions
    (a) Malabsorption syndromes
    (b) Celiac disease
    (c) Milk allergies
    (d) Acute respiratory tract infections
    (e) Dentition
3. Urogenital System
    a) Diaper rashes in infants
        (1) Due to yeast overgrowth
        (2) From acidic urine
    b) Boys
        (1) Tend to develop hydroceles
        (2) Rash around the penis from acidic urine
    c) Girls
        (1) Recurrent vaginitis
            (a) Even in very young girls
            (b) Discharge
                i) Thick
                ii) Milky
                iii) Smells like mold
        (2) Premenstrual syndrome
            (a) Fluid retention
            (b) Breast swelling
            (c) Colds
            (d) Vaginitis
            (e) Headaches
            (f) Seizures
C. Musculoskeletal System
    1. Many spinal disorders
        a) Scoliosis
        b) Spina bifida
    2. Cervical region problems
        a) May become very thin
        b) Swollen cervical glands
            (1) Many
            (2) Hard

(3) Sore

(4) From repeated infections

3. Extremities

a) Slow learning to walk

b) Bowlegged

c) Weak ankles that turn easily

d) Hands and feet perspire

(1) Profusely and easily

(2) Even if they are cold

e) Arthritis aggravations

(1) From first motion

(2) During cold, wet weather

f) Problems with nails

(1) Grow slowly

(2) Brittle: they crack and break easily

D. Skin

1. Eczema

a) Babies tend to be born with eczema or cradle cap

b) Develops easily on the head

2. Candida skin infections develop readily

3. Warts

a) On the palms and fingers

b) On the soles

4. Face-scratching

a) After eating allergenic food

b) When tired

c) Upon awakening

III. Physical Generals

A. Epilepsy

1. During dentition

2. From birth trauma

3. Premenstrually

B. Problems with metabolism

1. Poor assimilation and utilization of calcium

2. Thyroid malfunction

3. Failure to thrive in small babies

4. Obese babies and children

C. Slow development

      1. Mental

      2. Physical: hair, nails, and bones grow poorly

D. Many swollen glands

E. Profuse perspiration

F. Offensive discharges

G. Chilly as they grow older

H. Easily tired

I. Aggravation

      1. From exertion

      2. During dentition

      3. During cold and wet weather

      4. From change of weather

      5. From drinking milk

J. Amelioration

      1. From rest

      2. During dry, warm weather

Calcarea carbonica Confirmatory Picture

These are healthy children with strong personalities that lead to strong wills, obstinacy, and independence. They tend to be plodders and have delayed mental development. They fear insects, scary stories, and ghosts; they are fascinated with the supernatural.

Confirmatory Checklist

- Night terrors, sweat during sleep
- Perspiration on the head
- Headaches
- Frequent upper respiratory tract infections with copious mucus
- Canker sores
- Problems with dentition, which is often delayed
- Many swollen glands
- Crave eggs, carbohydrates, salt, and sweets
- Avoid slimy or mixed foods
- Babies spit up food just eaten
- Failure to thrive in small babies
- Tend toward constipation with large stools
- Epilepsy
- Calcium metabolism and thyroid problems causing bone disorders; hair, nails, and bones grow poorly
- Slow physical and mental development
- Tire easily
- Obese
- Profuse perspiration, offensive discharges
- Many yeasty infections anywhere on the body
- Chilly
- Aggravation from exertion, dentition, cold and wet weather, change of weather, and drinking milk
- Amelioration from rest and dry, warm weather

Lycopodium

Mental/Emotional Characteristics

The descriptions of the remedy *Lycopodium* as presented in the old materia medicas may mislead the prescriber because they tend to fit only the adult. The *Lycopodium* youngster may be an entirely different experience.

Two distinct types of behavior can be observed in *Lycopodium* children. In one type, **fear and apprehension** affect every aspect of the child's life. In the other, the child is **bossy** to the point of being dictatorial and strives to control those close by, be they parents, siblings, or friends.

In the waiting room, the first child sits very near his mother and watches everything from that secure vantage point since the office visit is a strange, new situation. The second child, in contrast, can be heard loudly voicing variations on a theme: "Bring me that toy!" "I don't want to be here!" "Take me home!"

What this demanding child *says* is only part of it. It is the tone in which these commands are spoken and the attitude that it reveals that prompts one to first think of *Lycopodium*. The child speaks irritably to the parent and the parent answers weakly, almost apologetically; one quickly grasps that the normal parent-child dynamic has been reversed. The child, not the adult, controls the relationship. Furthermore, it is as if all the members of the family have become the *Lycopodium* youngster's inferiors, there only to meet the little tyrant's needs and gratify his whims.

From these brief initial observations, the doctor can deduce the major thematic elements that will shape the behavior of *Lycopodium* people throughout their lives.

In the first example, we see a lack of self-confidence and the presence of many overriding fears. In the second, we find an irritable nature and a great desire for power. While these two types may be found in different individuals as described in this chapter, they also represent a continuum that may be expressed in one person.

First I will discuss the aspects of fear, then the lack of self-confidence, and finally the emergence of the desire for power.

Insecurity/Fear

Fear is an essential factor in the development of the *Lycopodium* psyche. In Kent's *Repertory*, one finds only *Baryta carbonica* and *Lycopodium* under the rubric: Fear; People, in children. Even the **babies are apprehensive.** Infants need to be near the mother or on a parent's lap, as they become especially afraid when alone and when around other people, especially loud strangers. Fear is immediately observable in the facial expression, set off by the distrustful look in the eyes and a stare. While most three-month-old babies smile back at a doting parent, the most pleasant expression a *Lycopodium* child of that age can muster is often a mild **frown.** There may be clearly visible wrinkling of the forehead proportionate to the degree of apprehension the child is feeling. For example, in the office, the closer the doctor gets to the baby to pick her up, the more numerous and deeper the creases become. The eyes, too, stare out at the world with an expression of fear unusual for such a young person, making the observer wonder what the child is so worried about.

This illustrates the fact that one of the main ways in which fear is elicited, even in very young *Lycopodium* children, is as anxiety caused by the presence of strangers. Whereas most children go through a "**stranger anxiety**" phase at some time within the first couple of years, *Lycopodium* babies develop this from birth and experience it throughout most of their childhood. It seems as if these infants and children only like what is already known; in this case, only those people with whom they are intimately familiar.

Such a strong fear of strangers may often be conjoined with a **fear of being alone** that becomes evident in many circumstances.

50

The parents may describe it in the interview if the child does not. The child keeps track of the parents' whereabouts throughout the day, following them around the house and constantly querying the parents: "Where are you going? When will you be back? Are you upstairs or downstairs?"

While in *Natrum muriaticum* this same behavior exists, it stems from a concern and fear for the parents' safety. In *Lycopodium*, the fear is that if the parent is not nearby, they themselves will not be safe. They may need to be in the same room or at least next door to a parent, as with *Pulsatilla*. In *Pulsatilla* the fear is of abandonment, whereas in *Lycopodium* the fear is that something "bad" will actually happen to them.

Happier *Lycopodium* children wish to stay in the room with a parent and will be quite content with that setup. Conversely, the irritable child wants to be alone, yet is afraid. When expressed fully in the irritable child, this fear leads to the famous symptom and keynote in the *Repertory*: Mind; Company; aversion to, yet dreads being alone.

Fear of being alone is greatly **accentuated in the dark.** They often do not like to go to bed alone, wanting a parent to go along to check the area and turn on the lights. A *Lycopodium* baby will begin to cry as soon as the parents turn off the lights and leave the room, just like those needing *Pulsatilla*. Some fear may be allayed by keeping a light on, but many of these children continue to scream until they are allowed to sleep with their parents or siblings.

This is especially true after they have watched a scary movie, listened to a ghost story, or even just viewed the six o'clock news on television. *Phosphorus, Pulsatilla,* and *Calcarea carbonica* are also unusually sensitive to horrible stories and have fears in the dark. *Lycopodium* children may wake up with a fright and go to the parents' bed, as do *Phosphorus, Pulsatilla,* and *Stramonium.* Some children go to sleep more easily than described, but if they wake up at night for any reason, such as to urinate, they may check all the beds to make sure that the family members are each where he or she should be and that they have not been left alone.

Fear of being alone in the dark may arise at other times as well. For instance, the child will refuse to bring something up from the basement. The thought of going into the dark underground, unprotected and alone, is unendurable. The fear of being alone, aggravated by being in the dark, is a good clue to other remedies as well, such as *Causticum*, *Phosphorus*, *Pulsatilla*, and *Stramonium*. In *Phosphorus*, one encounters many other fears the likes of which only an intensely active imagination can create; in *Stramonium*, this fear will be seen in a violent child.

Fear of New Things

The child may also develop a fear or aversion to new things, not due to stubbornness, as is found in *Calcarea carbonica*, but because he fears the new thing itself. The parent states that in new places and situations (as in the interview) and in crowds, the child will be fearful and timid at first. Once the situation is better understood by the child, he becomes more comfortable and is able to interact with others more normally. In brief, anything new will be regarded with suspicion until it can be understood.

In contrast, a *Calcarea carbonica* child 's dislike of new things is due to slow assimilation and comprehension. Mothers say that the *Calcarea carbonica* children cannot be budged to start activities in a new situation because their stubbornness prevents it. However, when they finally understand what is going on, they join in and often cannot be stopped! The *Calcarea carbonica* child is obstinate and unyielding, while the *Lycopodium* child is fearful and anxious. Even though similar behavior is noted in their dislike of new things, the root causes are radically different for each of these remedy types.

Fear of new situations may be **observed in the clinic**. If there are several chairs from which to pick, the first-time *Lycopodium* patient will often pick the chair farthest from the doctor and will have to be coaxed to sit any closer. The child, squirming in her seat, will neither talk to nor establish any eye contact with the doctor. Others whisper, mumble, or look at the parent for cues or for whole answers. Some giggle nervously before or after every answer. Some will be very adultlike and answer properly (if stiffly, due to nervousness), looking at the mother only when they do not know the answer. Toddlers may sit on their mothers' laps frowning at the doctor and screaming whenever the doctor or the mother asks a question.

During the follow-up interview some weeks later, the child knows the doctor and what to expect and so is much friendlier and acts more comfortable all around. At this point the practitioner may be misled to think that the remedy given has acted, based on the changes observed in the office, but these changes will occur even if the wrong remedy was prescribed simply because the situation is no longer new and therefore not threatening. A good way to determine accurately whether or not it was the remedy that caused a change in the child is to ask the parent how the child behaved in other new situations during the interim or in situations that previously made the child anxious.

Often the fear of new things leads to a predictable **lack of initiative**. The parents state that the *Lycopodium* child is "not a spur-of-the-moment type of person." For example, every time the family goes out for supper the child may order the same meal. Parental attempts to convince the child to choose something else are usually in vain. If forced to pick a new food, and if the food is liked (as it often turns out to be), the new item will be added to the menu of acceptable choices.

I am reminded of eight-year-old Roger, who was brought for treatment of his frequent colds. Along with the rest of the symptoms was a strong fear of new things. He would invariably cry and hide when presented with new tasks or new choices in clothes, foods, or activities. If he had not shown all the other fears and physical general characteristics of *Lycopodium* such as a fear of the dark and of being alone, right-sided sore throats, and stomachaches, I would have given the remedy *Baryta carbonica*, so marked was this behavior of hiding from new situations.

Fear of Public Failure

If one perceives why and how the child exhibits these fears, the case becomes greatly simplified. The fear of new situations in *Lycopodium* is intimately bound to a prominent fear of failure. This pattern grows more and more pronounced as such children mature into adulthood. The exact description of what I have observed is that they **fear the decision-making process and the repercussions of any decisions made.**

For the most part, the fear of failure is felt only before an upcoming event, not during it. They **anticipate** that something will go wrong, something bad will happen, or that they will be ridiculed in some way. However, once they begin the activity, the fear diminishes and they accomplish the task with ease. The type and degree of apprehension is second only to that found in those responding to the remedy *Silicea*. These children also experience fear before an activity or event that disappears as soon as the event begins and they find that they perform well. *Argentum nitricum*, *Gelsemium sempervirens*, and *Phosphorus* may likewise greatly fear upcoming events.

It should be noted that this fear is not merely a fear of failure; rather, it is a fear of failing in public. What the child may tell the doctor is that she does not mind trying new things if she is alone, but does not wish to do them in front of others, especially her peers.

This **sensitivity to ridicule** should be explored carefully, as it leads the prescriber to understand the *Lycopodium* child's personality more fully. Each constitutional remedy type is affected by the same stresses in different ways. Compare the *Lycopodium* child to *Natrum muriaticum* and *Pulsatilla*. The *Natrum muriaticum* child can be destroyed emotionally by ridicule. *Natrum muriaticum* children have such strong emotions, which they try to control, that the thought of being made fun of is itself overwhelming. They become severely traumatized, something that will not be easily resolved once they are made fun of. The *Pulsatilla* child also has an emotional base of existence, being also easily hurt; especially if the ridicule threatens to take love away from him. If he does not feel that this will happen, however, the *Pulsatilla* child will usually resolve the situation easily. The *Lycopodium* child is concerned about something quite different. He does not have the strong, deep emotions of the *Natrum muriaticum* and so will not be so easily crushed emotionally. However, he is **sensitive to social ranking** and will not wish to lose status. For this reason, the *Lycopodium* fears new situations, people, and activities that can potentially reveal his inadequacies. He resists new projects, new ideas, and even new games. He fears that he will get up in front of the class, make an error, and look foolish.

Herein lies the *Lycopodium* fear of ridicule. Later in life these individuals learn to bluff their way through situations such as this, but as youngsters, they resist putting their rank on the line.

We can conclude that in *Natrum muriaticum* the criticism and condemnation comes from within. In *Pulsatilla* the fear of losing love is the major threat felt in being made fun of. In *Lycopodium* the child is most concerned with how he or she is perceived within the group.

As a corollary to this concern about what others think, one finds that the *Lycopodium* child may **compromise easily**, dress neatly, and maintain a tidy appearance in general. Such behavior shows that her energy is spent on climbing the social ladder, doing everything right so as to secure a desirable position within the social strata.

Lycopodium children are **preoccupied with their looks**. The children may be sloppy in their rooms and messy in the bathroom but they groom themselves well, always concerned about their "show." *Lycopodium* will often prove to be the remedy needed for seven- to ten-year-old girls who are preoccupied with clothes, hair style, jewelry, and makeup, even though her family does not encourage this behavior.

A memorable case illustrating this aspect involves sixteen-year-old Jody. She complained of allergies, a postnasal drip, and sore throats that had become more or less constant during the past two years. The case fit *Lycopodium* in the time and temperature modalities, becoming aggravated in the morning and late afternoon and in the cold. When asked what had happened in the two previous years, the answer confirmed a *Lycopodium* diagnosis. When she was fourteen years old, she became pregnant. This shock seemed to place her not in grief or in sadness, but rather in a deep *Lycopodium* state. She became so concerned about what others might think that she starved herself. For eight months no one suspected that she was pregnant. Finally, when she could hide the truth no longer, she was found out and married the father of the child. As usual in *Lycopodium* pregnancies, she developed constant stomachaches. And what is also usual for *Lycopodium* pregnancies, though unusual for one her age, she developed extensive varicose veins and hemorrhoids. She became severely constipated as well and needed strong laxatives to have a bowel movement during the two months following the birth.

It was impressive to hear how the emotional shock of this unwanted pregnancy, which put an unbearable strain on maintaining social status and appearances, expressed itself physically. Even two years later, when she was first seen in our clinic, all the symptoms of her physical pathologies still fit the *Lycopodium* picture.

Fear Somaticized

Apprehension and anxiety are often felt by *Lycopodium* children in the **stomach and abdomen.** They develop frequent stomachaches, nausea, vomiting, and loose stools or diarrhea. I remember a teenager who complained of frequent sore throats. Along with all the *Lycopodium* modalities of the sore throats, food desires, and skin problems, she also described herself as having had a "weak stomach" her entire life. She was a very good student who maintained a high grade average. Her scholastic abilities, however, did not lessen the anxiety she experienced before every test. Whenever she studied for any test she would develop stomachaches so intense she would eventually vomit.

Physical problems may also lead to emotional changes. Charles, a boy of seven, became very crabby and challenged all of his mother's requests and argued with the neighborhood children with no apparent provocation. This behavior began immediately after a hernia operation and persisted until given the remedy *Lycopodium* years later. It seemed that the physical *Lycopodium* symptomatology transferred to the emotional state after the operation. Another *Lycopodium* patient of mine developed similar irritability, along with fears of the dark and of being alone, after receiving allergy shots to cure a chronically stuffy nose.

In **arthritis** cases, as the inflammation increases, so too do the fears and irritability. Parents of arthritic children bemoan the transformation, saying that the child used to be more "happy-go-lucky" until the physical changes occurred. Changes in emotions can be an especially important clue in diseases that have exacerbations and remissions. These slight changes on the emotional level can indicate to the parent that a flare-up is eminent even before the physical symptoms are fully expressed. One little girl who responded well to the remedy *Lycopodium* in the treatment of juvenile rheumatoid arthritis became increasingly insecure in the weeks before a relapse, needing to be near her parents all the time and being unbearably sensitive and crabby with her siblings. Whenever her moods would change to fit this remedy, we would repeat the remedy, thus preventing any relapse of her arthritis.

Flat Affect

Parents often talk about their *Lycopodium* children using descriptions that are flat; that is, lacking any enthusiasm. They describe the child as a "considerate little girl," or say that she is "nice." Others volunteer that the child does all the right things, and yet it is as if the child has little "soul" or charisma; as if she lacked a personality. In trying to maintain her social rank, **she has abdicated anything that sets her apart from others.** While this *Lycopodium* offspring may be a relief for the parents of, say, a *Tuberculinum* child (because the *Lycopodium* is at least not out of control), most parents are apt to favor children of other remedy types and feel neutral or negative about the *Lycopodium* child.

Indecisiveness

A hallmark of the combined lack of self-confidence and insecurity is seen in the child's indecisiveness. In the office, the child presents a very **weak handshake** at best, and that only after the doctor has offered a hand first. The child often answers in a **timid voice** that lacks any expression of self-assurance. She anxiously looks at the mother for every answer, as does *Pulsatilla*. The indecisiveness may even make a *Lycopodium* child run away and hide her head or cry if forced to make a decision. The child may need to have the parent decide what should be worn to school the next day. While speaking with such children, it may be noticed that they giggle before every answer and never look up at the doctor. The doctor may do a double take on the age that is written down on the information intake form because the child seems so much younger than the age reported.

Timid, fearful boys may often be mistaken for *Pulsatilla* youngsters. One differentiating point will be that a *Lycopodium* boy will have nasty, irritable moments with the family whereas *Pulsatilla* will rarely show this negative trait. Likewise, *Lycopodium* teenaged girls will at times be closed and shy, resembling *Natrum muriaticum*, but will not have the callous or oversensitive emotions and special sensitivity to grief found in the latter.

Love of Power

To restate the characteristics of the *Lycopodium* psychology mentioned thus far, we may safely say that the children fear being alone and being around new people and situations. They rarely develop a strong sense of self and remain plagued by a feeling of powerlessness. Since they feel that the parents will take care of them in difficult situations, *Lycopodium* children try to stay very near them.

The natural outcome of this is that the child is surrounded by adults who do not make fun of or criticize her. An interesting phenomenon occurs as she realizes that there are times when she can be in absolute control of situations. The child needs something; namely, protection, which the parents offer. In her mind, the *Lycopodium* child translates this into the belief that the parents are under her control. When this occurs, the child now realizes that, for the first time, she can exert some power.

Kent describes this situation in his *Materia Medica* thus: "It is a dread of people, and when that is fully carried out in the Lyc. patient you see that she dreads the presence of new persons, or the coming in of friends and visitors; she wants to be only with those that are constantly surrounding her."

Occasionally this dread may be taken to some strange extremes. The child may appear rude whenever he is around strangers. The parents say that the child will totally avoid a stranger, as though pretending that the unknown person did not exist. He will not look at the person or respond to any attempts at communication. Looking at the quote from Kent, one can deduce the source of this desire for company and yet not for strangers. Since one never knows how a stranger will react, they are to be avoided. He wants to only be around family members, the ones who can be controlled and will not put up a fuss. This is what "unconditional love" means to many *Lycopodium* children. A more conscious decision is then made to **have only people around who they can control**, since this is the first real feeling of power that they have felt. It is only external power, though; internally, they still feel weak.

I once treated a toddler, Lisa, just over one year old, for respiratory tract infections. When asked about the girl's temperament, the mother bemoaned the fact that the child would respond to any attempted request by her mother by screaming at the top of her lungs. The noise would automatically stop the mother's request and she would capitulate. This description of domination by one so young combined with the fears mentioned above and the modalities of the respiratory tract infections confirmed the prescription for the remedy *Lycopodium*.

Because the feeling of power allays insecurities, it becomes **addictive** to *Lycopodium* children, and they develop what can be found in Kent's *Repertory* as a rubric: Mind; Power, love of. This desire for power is strong and takes many forms. One may hear parents complain of the the headstrong, cranky *Lycopodium* who controls the household. The bossy child orders around parents and siblings alike. During this phase of the interview, a description of the child's behavior may become confused with that of *Nux vomica*, as this particular trait can become quite pronounced in both remedy types.

In one case, the child whined constantly and ordered his mother around. "Get me this book." "Turn on the television." "Give me that toy." The homeopathic prescription was confirmed by the fact that the same child was also fearful and would not play by himself, always following the mother about the house instead. It is a peculiar combination: a **domineering yet needy**, fearful person. When these characteristics are found together, it will most often point to *Lycopodium*.

Lycopodium children grow **irritable if not obeyed** or if not obeyed quickly enough. As alluded to above, this behavior can be already manifest in the infant who early on grasps the fact that if he yells, screams, or acts badly, he can manipulate this loving adult to do anything he wishes. The child becomes **critical and faultfinding**, chastising siblings for doing this and that wrong or even accusing the mother in a similar fashion. In the interview it is this sort of *Lycopodium* child who constantly corrects and insults the mother in a way that implies the parent is but a peon. This is an important point to remember as it keeps one from confusing *Lycopodium* with *Pulsatilla*, as exemplified in the following story.

While eliciting a case history from seven-year-old Janice, I found that all the symptoms fit both *Lycopodium* and *Pulsatilla*. Each remedy was considered and questions were asked and answered. As I pressed on, the manner in which the questions were being answered was noted and recognized. Though the answers came forth easily and with the eagerness one would expect to find in a *Pulsatilla* child, the ease with which the girl also corrected her mother's responses (in a tone of voice somewhere between good-natured and condescending) helped to confirm the *Lycopodium* diagnosis.

The "love of power" syndrome will also manifest in the manner in which the child plays. A *Lycopodium* child with this trait often **prefers to play with younger children** so that he will be "king." He can then decide what and how they will play, give directions, and set the tone for all events.

The power dynamics may also be seen in the interaction between siblings in relation to toys. The child becomes manipulatively **possessive**, requiring brothers or sisters to *ask* permission or pledge obedience before using his toys. *Lycopodium* at this stage of development is frequently confused with *Tuberculinum*, as they both may hit other children. The *Lycopodium*, however, only hits younger or weaker playmates. When the child is forced to play with older children, the weakness of character shows itself readily. In these circumstances the *Lycopodium* child tends to be a follower, quieter and more compliant to what others wish. This again shows a painful awareness of social standing and the fear of making mistakes.

In later stages of *Lycopodium* psychopathology, this love of power leads to a strong **intolerance of contradiction**. The child is not able to handle the slightest degree of criticism or correction from others, yet with ease he picks on and finds fault with other children or family members, especially those deemed weaker.

Many **teenaged *Lycopodium* girls become hypercritical** and faultfinding. After being with one of them for half an hour or so, one begins to feel that they can find something bad to say about everyone. One such teenager, a sixteen-year-old suffering from chronic sore throats and hay fever, was sure to tell me about her brother. "My brother is a bum. All he ever does is watch television and play sports. He's so lazy." The degree of unelicited criticism and nastiness led me away from a *Natrum muriaticum* prescription, although it initially seemed from the girl's ailment to be equally called for.

In both the fearful and the domineering types of *Lycopodium*, as the interview proceeds there is a growing feeling that these young women take themselves entirely too seriously. These girls are usually very neat and proper in their attire, hair, manners, and speech, but the judgements and disgusted feelings they express toward others will confirm *Lycopodium* over other possible remedies, resembling the remedy *Nitricum acidum* most closely.

Irritability

One definite *Lycopodium* characteristic is intense irritability. *Lycopodium* children who tend to be domineering also tend to be irritable. They become **impatient, cranky, and demanding.** If they are not obeyed they fly into a rage, as one would expect to see in a *Nux vomica*. They become annoyed easily with what the parents claim are insignificant things. One eventually realizes that this irritability is yet another tool that the children use to manipulate situations for their own ends.

The little *Lycopodium* tyrant must have his way without any contradiction or he throws a fit. He does not wish to speak to the offending parent, and in this mood exaggerates every little thing. For instance, he may act as if he is very sensitive to physical contact. At a busy shopping center the parent may request something of the child; for example, to put down a toy; asking over and over again while the child ignores both the parent and the request each time. As the parent pulls at the child's arm to lead him away, he will scream something like, "Ow! You're hurting me! Let me go! Ouch!" The child complains as if the parent had committed an atrocity against his body. Bystanders turn to see what is happening while the parent sinks in disgrace, lest others suspect child abuse. As the parent releases the arm, the child feels victorious once more and occasionally smirks in defiance. I should add, however, that these children may also truly be very sensitive to pain and can become as irritable as *Hepar sulphuris* does when they are in true physical pain.

They may become more **irritable when constipated**. They are easily frustrated, hitting younger children or perhaps telling the mother that she is stupid. After a bowel movement they may become reasonable for another few days until the constipation returns. The parents, not the children, are the ones who must be convinced to stop giving cathartics so that their systems might have a chance to come back into balance. One can commiserate with the poor parents' predicament as their child's irritability holds hostage everyone in the household.

The child often **wakes up in an irritable mood** and does not wish to talk or get out of bed. The parents state that the child's worst time is in the morning when she first gets up, especially if she did not get enough sleep or is hungry. These cranky youngsters become much more civil after they have eaten and have been awake for a while. They are also quite grumpy around **four in the afternoon**, a classic *Lycopodium* aggravation time, when they return from school. When the parent asks the child how school was, the child, in a hypoglycemic state, growls and goes to the kitchen for some sweets and then lies down in front of the television for a couple of hours.

Babies are also typically irritable, and frown and scream at the slightest provocation. The crankiness has a demanding tone to it. They are, of course, especially cranky when they are hungry upon awakening or if they are tired, ill, or colicky.

Dyslexia

In *Lycopodium* there can be an inability to integrate the left and right sides of the brain. It is as if the corpus callosum has been severed and does not transfer information from one hemisphere to the other as it should.

Lycopodium **infants** commonly have difficulty mastering the sucking reflex. They likewise have difficulty **developing a coordinated pattern of crawling** ("cross-crawling") and learn to walk later than their siblings. They are found to be, along with *Medor-*

rhinum, the most prone to dyslexia, both as children and as adults. Indeed, dyslexia often first indicates a need for this medicine. They make **mistakes in reading and writing**, inverting or leaving letters out or using the wrong words; and in arithmetic, adding up columns of numbers incorrectly.

Frustration with these disabilities naturally causes **apprehension** any time they need to demonstrate their mental skills either in front of classmates or in homework. In order to avoid being laughed at by their peers or receiving a poor grade from the teacher, the child needing *Lycopodium* procrastinates instead of doing assignments. They put off doing their schoolwork as frequently as does the *Sulphur* child. While *Sulphur* resists doing homework out of laziness, for *Lycopodium* it is due to fear of failure and lack of self-confidence.

A peculiar behavior pattern may develop in these children: they hurriedly write their work but **cannot bear to read what they have just written**. This is seen particularly in those who have a history of making many mistakes. Reviewing the work means having to come to terms with the mistakes made, a task that is anathema to the *Lycopodium* psyche as it deflates the ego as well as makes the child fear a loss of status. Also, refusing to review the mistaken work is a type of procrastination. They feel that since they must write it down, they wish only to be finished with the torture as quickly as possible.

The more immature *Lycopodium* children also exhibit this symptom when they do not care at all about the work but are forced to do it by a parent or teacher. The attitude that the child portrays in this case is, "Fine. I did it. Now leave me alone, I want to play." Younger children will not care about schoolwork at all and will prefer to play most of the time. In *Lycopodium* the extent to which children are "lazy" reflects the degree to which they fear failure, while in *Sulphur* it reflects a breakdown in the ability to concentrate.

Sensitivity

Some *Lycopodium* children cry easily. They can be **moody and tearful** when offended. They cry involuntarily and say they "can't help it" when a parent demands that they stop. This is especially true after admonition. If the child did something objectionable and the parent raises his or her voice to tell him why it was wrong, the child begins to weep, forcing the parent to cut short any planned discourse. In addition, a low pain threshold will cause some to cry from the slightest injury.

Hyperactivity

There are some hyperactive children who respond beautifully to the remedy *Lycopodium* and who exhibit many of the traits discussed here. They are hurried and unrelenting in everything they do. They rush through their homework, make many mistakes, have a poor attention span, and are often dyslexic. They scribble down anything as long as they can say they are finished. As mentioned before, these children hate to read what they have written.

They are very **restless** and unable to sit still, and nervously touch whatever they can in the room. They must eat every two or three hours and especially crave sweets, sometimes screaming at a parent, "Give me, give me," as if their lives depended on it. Their hands are often in their mouths and they lick their lips until dry, red, and irritated.

When reprimanded, they weep. If a parent grabs them, they feign pain, screaming as if they had been struck with force. The hyperactive *Lycopodium* child is also very messy in his environment.

Fears in General

The main fears of the *Lycopodium* child discussed so far are **of being alone (especially in the dark), failure, making mistakes, new situations, and strangers.** Other strong fears include those of **ghosts, skeletons, monsters, large animals, and robbers.** The way the child often describes it is that he hates to be alone "because of the monsters out there," or that "the bears will kill me." While there are many examples of how a child might express this, the common element of all these fears is that the child feels too weak to overcome these external forces. This is confirmed by the fact that most of these fears disappear or do not arise if the parent is nearby.

They may also fear snakes, insects, and especially spiders, though not as intensely as do the remedy types *Calcarea carbonica*, *Natrum muriaticum*, or *Phosphorus*.

Correcting the Past

There are two other symptoms that the old materia medicas describe in great detail that I have not found to be as important as was previously thought.

Early books describe the behavior of crying all day and sleeping all night as a major keynote of *Lycopodium* in infants and toddlers. This symptom is rarely found among *Lycopodium* babies in practice, and in actuality, many *Lycopodium* infants with colic have exactly the opposite modality, waking up and crying the whole night through and sleeping soundly during the day.

The other symptom often described in the past is an overall weakness of the body combined with a keen mental aptitude that encourages the child to sit and read all day. This, too, is rarely observed now. In the past, because the aggravation time of *Lycopodium* is from four o'clock in the afternoon to eight o'clock in the evening, they were too tired to play after school like other children. Afternoon reading was thus not so much because of a brilliance of the mind as much as from a dullness of the body. Now what is reported is that the child comes home from school and sits down to watch television or plays with a coloring book until dinnertime, activities that show that the child is in a passive mode both physically and mentally.

Sleep

Some children develop insomnia during anxious times such as before a test, play, or singing performance. One common time is due to apprehension before school begins. Many have trouble sleeping after summer vacation ends, just as school is about to start again. During these anxious times the child may again need to sleep with a parent or sleep with the lights on. Some girls who have a fear of monsters and of the dark will not be able to fall asleep unless a parent sleeps with them. I remember charming little Caroline, who would sneak into her parents' bed during the middle of the night, but defended it, stating that "I surely must be asleep when I do that because I cannot remember any of it at all." I remember trying to maintain composure as she spoke, having doubts about this last comment.

Occasionally one finds a child who **wakes up at night frightened and not knowing where he is**, which causes him to scream and yell for his parents. The parents come in, calm the child, and stay with him until he falls asleep again. This is noted to be without the violent characteristics of *Stramonium*, the clinginess of *Pulsatilla*, or the night terrors of *Calcarea carbonica*.

They frequently **need the lights on and may need to sleep with others** in the room. The children sleep on their **right side**, as do *Phosphorus* children, or on their **abdomens**. In their sleep they frequently **talk or laugh**. Even the infants will babble or coo. They **remain covered**, well cocooned under their blankets, even in the summertime.

They **suck their thumbs** until they are quite old, sometimes into their teens.

They **awake unrefreshed** in a terribly irritable mood and do not bounce out of bed like *Pulsatilla*, *Calcarea carbonica*, or *Natrum muriaticum* children. As well as being ill-tempered, the characteristic strong hunger directly after rising makes *Lycopodium* the first child to arrive in the kitchen. This is in sharp contrast to those children needing the remedy *Sulphur* or *Natrum muriaticum*, who may skip breakfast completely.

Physical Symptomatology

Head

The head of the *Lycopodium* child may appear similar to the *Silicea* head by **seeming too large for the size of the body**. This apparent disproportion is only in relation to the smallness of the rest of the body, not because of the absolute largeness of head that is often evident in *Silicea* or *Calcarea carbonica* children. Curiously, many *Lycopodium* girls often draw people with gigantic heads, tiny or insignificant bodies, and spindly limbs; similar in appearance (at least as a caricature) to some needing the remedy *Lycopodium*.

The scalp develops **eczema** quite easily, *Lycopodium* being the main remedy for eruptions appearing on or behind the ears. The eruption oozes a clear to yellow watery discharge that forms sheets of itchy, cellophanelike material that can be pulled off in strips.

Occasionally, teenaged girls may complain of slow hair growth or of gradually thinning hair. This is not usually a major complaint, rather being mentioned only during a follow-up interview as an observation that, since the remedy was taken, the hair has been filling in and growing much faster than before.

Headaches

Lycopodium children occasionally complain of one of **two types** of headaches. The first is **common to adolescents who crave sugar.** If they miss a meal or are late for one, they develop a headache that subsides as soon as they eat. While the same will also be found with *Phosphorus* and *Sulphur*, the differentiating point is the sensitivity to noise and the irritability that accompanies a *Lycopodium* headache. During headaches they become extremely **sensitive to noises**, shouting at offenders in a bossy tone to "cut it out!" or to "shut up!"

This sensitivity to noise may not be seen in younger children with such headaches. What may be described in these cases is their irritable mood upon awakening, accompanied by a voracious appetite and a demand for food. *Tuberculinum* also becomes very irritable with a headache, but the greater intensity of the irritability prompts one to consider the nosode instead of *Lycopodium*.

The second type of headache about which a *Lycopodium* teenager is likely to complain is nondescript in comparison. It tends to be located in the right temple area, aggravated by heat and worse at night when the sufferer lies down or in the morning if he or she sleeps too long. It is ameliorated by taking a walk in the cool air. These headaches may resemble those of *Natrum muriaticum* and *Pulsatilla*, but the rest of the symptoms should be used to dictate the remedy.

Lycopodium should be added to the subrubric: Head; Perspiration, night. While this symptom is not as commonly found in *Lycopodium* as it is in *Calcarea carbonica*, it can help point to this remedy.

Eyes and Ears

The **eyes are relatively free of problems** except for an occasional **stye**. In contrast, the **ears are frequently affected**. The child often develops painful **cracks behind the ears,** as if the ears were trying to detach themselves from the scalp. *Lycopodium* is the main constitutional type with this symptom, although *Calcarea carbonica* and *Sulphur* share this complaint. The cracks are so prevalent in *Lycopodium* children that they can be used as a confirmatory symptom in prescribing. I am commonly told by parents that the child had these ear cracks as an infant and toddler. The lesion may only be a crack or there may be a full-blown case of **eczema** behind the ears. Such eczema exudes a clear, yellow, watery discharge that coagulates into thin, transparent sheets that can be peeled away to expose raw skin, which may bleed.

The *Lycopodium* child may also develop middle ear infections that resemble those of *Calcarea carbonica*. The **otitis media** tends to be on the right side and often causes the tympanic membrane to rupture and the ear to discharge thick, yellow pus that has a strong odor. Infants become very irritable with this condition. After the membrane heals, some fluid or mucus may remain in the middle ear that thickens and causes gradual deafness in that ear. The common combination of right-sided otitis media with cracks behind the ears will almost always be cured by the remedy *Lycopodium*. Kent's *Repertory* gives the rubric: Ear; Discharge, purulent, with eczema, and lists five remedies, one of which is *Lycopodium*.

Nose

The nose is **affected in almost all *Lycopodium* children**. Infants, toddlers, and young adults almost all have **obstructed nasal passages**. The babies will not be able to nurse properly because they cannot breathe through the nose. Infants must pull off the breast, breathe through the mouth, cry, and then try to nurse again. The mother of such an infant may show the doctor the bulb syringe that she carries around in the diaper bag with which she suctions out the baby's nostrils. The obstruction may also consist of swollen nasal turbinates that accompany dry snuffles.

The mucus resembles the discharge from the ears: thick and yellow to green in color, similar to that found in *Kali bichromicum*. The mucus may form hard crusts, also found in *Kali bichromicum*, that the child picks at all day. The difference with *Kali bichromicum* crusts is that once they are pulled away they leave the nose very raw and sore. In *Lycopodium* the nose does not become so sore. The other differentiating key is that this thick type of discharge is seen more in acute *Kali bichromicum* sinusitis cases, whereas in *Lycopodium* it is found in chronic ailments.

A case of **snuffles** in infants or children is cured most frequently by the remedy *Lycopodium*, which should therefore be raised in grade in the *Repertory* to bold type in all the appropriate rubrics. The nasal obstruction is much worse at night when the child lies down, as is found with *Pulsatilla*. It is aggravated in the morning due to mucus accumulating overnight. It is commonly made worse by taking dairy products, summertime heat, and pollen. Those prone to nasal obstructions develop frequent head colds with these symptoms.

The nose may be completely dry and the snuffles described only as "sniffing," but which drives the parents to distraction. They ask the child to blow the nose but no mucus comes out. This **chronic, dry snuffling** is even more infuriating for parents who compare this child to another of theirs who needs the remedy *Calcarea carbonica*. This other child "sniffs and blows and mucus pours effortlessly out the nose," so they cannot understand why the *Lycopodium* child sniffs and sniffs and rubs the nose, but reports that "there is nothing there."

This incessant need to sniff is commonly observed in practice and can confuse the prescriber who may mistakenly try to repertorize each of the little rubrics in the nose section, leading to many obscure remedies that do not work or work only partially for a short time. The symptom of dry snuffling is observed frequently in *Lycopodium* children and should alert the prescriber to look for other confirmatory symptoms during the interview and exam.

The other keynote of the *Lycopodium* nose is the **flaring of the nostrils**. Though all the materia medicas describe this symptom as a common finding, in practice it is rarely observed in children; it is more commonly found in adults. Flaring nostrils will be observed in pediatric practice in nervous teenagers and in infants and children with severe respiratory tract infections who require *Lycopodium* as a remedy to regain their health. In both cases, **wrinkling of the forehead** will also be observed.

Finally, the remedy *Lycopodium* should be considered for **nosebleeds** and should be listed in italics under a new rubric I have created: Nose; Epistaxis, summer.

Face

The face may be quite **distinctive**, especially in children with malabsorptive syndromes. Those with such conditions tend to lose weight from the head area and upper torso, so that the skin hangs a little more loosely there and begins to **wrinkle**. The materia medicas describe infants showing such a failure to thrive as having the countenances of very old people. What they were referring to was the degree of **wrinkling combined with the wasting of flesh** that one would expect to find in someone over sixty years old.

In practice, this extreme example is not frequently seen. More commonly found is the infant who sits on the mother's lap looking right at the prescriber with an **anxious look on the face**, eyes full of apprehension and forehead lined with wrinkles proportionate to the anxiety felt. As the doctor approaches to reach for the child, the anxiety increases, the eyes widen, the wrinkles deepen, and the grip on the mother's arm tightens.

This type of fear may confuse one, thinking that it is a *Pulsatilla*-type fear of abandonment, but the extensive wrinkling and yellowness of the skin common in *Lycopodium* will aid in differentiating the two.

Babies may be **jaundiced at birth** and may never lose a yellowish tinge around the nose and cheeks, similar to the *Sepia* skin color, even as adults.

Lycopodium children with allergies, eczemas, and respiratory problems develop dark blue circles under their eyes and "adenoidal" faces. This expression, characterized by slight to moderate buck-toothedness and a mouth that is always slightly open, reflects the need to breathe through the mouth instead of the obstructed nose.

The **boys** often **lick the lips** causing a chapped appearance with a red discoloration or eruption around the mouth.

Lycopodium children also often have freckles.

Mouth

One of the few oral conditions found here is the speedy **yellowing of teeth.** This may be seen not only in children who do not like to brush their teeth but also in the ones who brush their teeth religiously.

Even the older children often put their fingers in their mouths, showing an **oral fixation.**

Throat and Neck

Recurrent sore throats and tonsillitis plague this group. Perhaps eighty percent of those who complain of sore throats that begin on the right side and extend to the left, or that affect the right side only, and that are ameliorated by warm drinks, benefit from a dose of *Lycopodium*. This is especially true if one confirms the time modality that the child worsens upon awakening and during the late afternoon, beginning at about four o'clock in the afternoon.

The tonsils enlarge and repeatedly exude smelly white pockets of hardened pus from deep crypts within the tonsillar surface. These are offensive and strong enough to smell up an entire room, resembling *Hepar sulphuris*. After the patient leaves, the doctor often wants to air out the examination room.

Swollen, tender cervical glands develop with pharyngitis that coincide with the above modalities of right-sidedness and aggravation in the morning and at four o'clock.

It is very unusual for a child to **desire warm drinks** in general, but *Lycopodium* leads the list in that respect, as it ameliorates the pain in the throat. The child will likewise desire and will be momentarily soothed by a warm compress to the neck. It is common for a postnasal catarrh associated with subacute sinusitis to either bring on the sore throat or be concomitant to it. The mucus not only obstructs the nasal passages but also irritates the mucous membrane of the pharynx.

Torticollis is a neck complaint that the remedy *Lycopodium* frequently cures in the adult. While the disease is less common in children, *Lycopodium* is frequently called upon to cure it when it does occur. Though a full-blown case of torticollis is rare, the prescriber may more frequently see the child who does not hold his head straight. In the office the child's head moves from being vertical to leaning toward one side. It is as if there is a weakness of one of the sternocleidomastoid muscles so that good posture of the head cannot be maintained.

Mononucleosis

Lycopodium should be one of the first remedies considered for the treatment of mononucleosis. The right side of the throat will be most affected, and the glands will be more swollen on the right. Offensive-smelling pus produced from the throat and obstructed nasal passages is also present. The child becomes very chilly, weak, and tired. Pains develop in the abdomen and nausea and vomiting follow.

The abdominal pain is ameliorated by bending over and by eating. As the acute infection progresses, the child begins to lose weight, especially in the upper torso. The skin begins to look translucent with a greenish hue and the face becomes ashen with dark circles under the eyes. One should also think of *Lycopodium* if the child has a history of frequent upper respiratory tract infections, an obstructed nose, and stomachaches ever since an episode of mononucleosis.

Lower Respiratory System

The *Lycopodium* child is susceptible to colds and flu that descend easily into the bronchi, leading to **bronchitis, bronchiolitis, or pneumonia.** Recurrent bronchitis produces scant expectoration or, in serious cases, thick yellow mucus. After the acute infection is over, a lingering dry cough often remains, which keeps not only the child but the parents up at night. It is aggravated at night when lying down, resembling the cough found with *Pulsatilla* children.

Infants develop chest colds that are accompanied by much mucus, causing rattling in the chest with breathing. The cough rattles so much it may be mistaken for a *Kali sulphuricum* or

Antimonium tartaricum infection. With the congestion the pre-scriber has an opportunity to observe two keynotes of *Lycopodium*: the wrinkling of the forehead and the flaring of the nostrils. The right lower or middle lobe of the lung is most often involved.

This acute infection becomes a problem later in life if the bronchitis or pneumonia is not addressed quickly and properly. From that time onward, whenever the child develops a cold it descends and becomes bronchitis easily. This is one of the rea-sons *Lycopodium* can be found listed in bold type in the rubric: Chest; Inflammation; lungs, neglected.

Other *Lycopodium* children develop **asthma** after such an acute respiratory infection. This asthma presents as shortness of breath that begins when a cold drops into the lungs and sets off the attack. Exertion, such as climbing steps or running, may also set off an attack, as it does in *Calcarea carbonica*. The asthma attacks are aggravated at night.

Alimentary System
Food Cravings and Aversions

By far the most **enjoyable** foods for *Lycopodium* children to eat are **sweets**. This overwhelming desire in a child is a forecast of blood sugar problems in the future. Tendencies toward hypo-glycemia or diabetes are also heralded by intense hunger and irritability upon awakening and by headaches that come on after missing a meal and are dissipated by eating. The importance of sweets and treats in these children's lives becomes obvious when the doctor suggests to the parents to stop giving sweets in order to improve the child's overall well-being and the child bursts into tears.

They **crave ice cream, soda pop, and warm food and drink.**

Some of the following foods they simply **dislike**; others wreak havoc on their digestive systems, causing gas and colic: **beans, bread, fat, cheese, onions, oysters, and any vegetable of the cab-bage (Brassica) family.** If a nursing infant or mother needs the remedy *Lycopodium*, the child reacts to these foods in the mother's diet as well.

Oysters may act as a poison to them, causing diarrhea, vom-iting, or hives.

They **might not show much evidence of thirst**, especially being averse cold drinks, except for a desire for sweet drinks like soda pop.

Stomach

The **stomach and abdomen are the most symptomatically rich areas** of the *Lycopodium* body. The children are often described by the parents as having a **sensitive stomach**. The *Lycopodium* child develops stomachaches during all illnesses, from colds to flu to asthma. Children needing *Lycopodium* feel anxiety in the stomach *more than any other remedy type discussed in this book*. The stomach becomes affected by frequent stomachaches, nausea, and vomiting with the slightest degree of stress. These children say that they develop such symptoms before any test or performance. The discomfort is ameliorated by eructation or by passing flatus.

This line of questioning should always be pursued, as the responses may confirm a number of remedies. It must be explored especially if the remedy *Lycopodium* is being considered. It may be that the child does not have these symptoms now but indeed did have them in the past. This history of symptoms can also be used for the confirmation. The child may also complain of stomachaches if she **eats too much**; something *Lycopodium* children are often guilty of doing.

Appetite

The adult has either a voracious appetite in which "the more I eat, the hungrier I become and the more I want to eat," or a very small appetite: "I can come to the table hungry, eat only a mouthful or two, and suddenly feel full." In the child, we find mostly the former.

The infant has a huge appetite and screams when it is hungry. Unwilling to wait patiently for the mother to unfasten a nursing bra or heat up a bottle of milk, the baby fusses and screams until fed. The baby may wake up during the night to nurse with a **big appetite** every hour or two and not voluntarily stop until the morning. Mothers have to call it quits each nursing session.

The baby may be described by the mother as a "wild nurser." As the infant breast-feeds, it sucks forcefully, almost greedily, naturally taking in a lot of air along with the milk. The air becomes one of the ingredients adding to digestive problems.

In the child or teenager, the appetite verges on the voracious. This is especially marked upon awakening, in the afternoon when the child returns from school, and in the evenings. During these times the child must be fed or there will be no peace in the house.

Occasionally the parents may only complain that the child eats too quickly, not chewing food properly. In these situations the prescriber must ask directly about the level of hunger, as the parents may not be able to gauge it accurately. Ask how this child compares in food consumption with others his age or with adults in the household.

Lycopodium babies often **hiccough after nursing**. Some women say that they have felt their *Lycopodium* babies hiccough in utero. *Lycopodium* should be added in italics to a new rubric I have created: Stomach; Hiccough; after eating, in newborns. *Pulsatilla* should be listed in bold type, *Calcarea carbonica* in italics, and *Nux vomica* in plain type.

Colic

Babies are often good sized at birth but become underweight quickly. Problems begin with infantile colic. Trapped gas in the stomach causes pain and fussiness all day and/or all night. The parents may report that the trouble begins in the late afternoon or evening. They may say that there are times in the evening when the child begins to scream and roll back and forth, trying to find a comfortable position. This may continue for as long as two hours, with the parents unable to console their suffering infant. Finally the baby passes flatus or stool, and then is hungry again and wishes to nurse. During this time the baby looks very unhappy, with a wrinkled forehead and a scowl.

The infant may also wake up in the middle of the night with a howl and continue screaming until the gas passes. The parents may report that hot compresses applied to the abdomen or warm baths enable the baby to eructate more easily, alleviating the pains. The child can be rocked in any direction to try to help with the passage of flatus. The colicky *Lycopodium* infant may only appear contented during feedings and while being held. At all other times the baby becomes irritable and fidgety, and experiences episodes of screaming. The parents state that they cannot put the infant down for five minutes without the child crying.

Abdomen

After infancy the abdomen continues to fill with gas frequently, becoming a constant source of discomfort. The gas passes up or down or becomes trapped within the digestive tract. The pain is ameliorated when hot compresses are applied to the abdomen or with abdominal massage, both of which encourage the gas to pass. With malabsorption syndromes the flatus actually distends the abdomen, making it tympanic. Even young babies pull the clothes away from the abdomen and stretch this way and that, screaming, until the gas passes. After these children eat or directly before passing stool, loud intestinal rumbling may be heard that ends with the passage of flatus. In the evening this often precedes a bowel movement.

Although this book, as well as other materia medicas, describe digestive symptoms in great detail, these discomforts are not necessary for the prescription of the remedy. Many children who need the remedy *Lycopodium* will not have any digestive complaints. One should not hesitate to give the remedy if this is so, as it covers such a multitude of symptoms. Many children who develop pathology in other physical systems still benefit greatly from the administration of *Lycopodium*.

Rectum

The child tends to be **constipated**, having a bowel movement every two, three, or even five days. The constipation can be traced to anxiety or the lack of effective bowel urges. The difficulty in passing stool may occur in situations that cause anxiety for the child, such as may occur in public rest rooms. The child finds it difficult to relax the anal sphincter muscles when anxious, and may have to read for an hour or more while sitting on the toilet to have a bowel movement.

Lycopodium children may not feel any urge to stool or have urges that are unproductive. Passing stool may be painful, though; the infant or child may fuss and cry and be averse to anything and everything until relieved by a bowel movement. One differentiating point between *Lycopodium* and *Calcarea carbonica* is that some children needing the remedy *Calcarea carbonica* may feel fine when they are constipated, while *Lycopodium* children are disturbed during constipation. The child may exhibit the keynote commonly found in adults that the first part of the stool is hard and the last part is soft.

Lycopodium children, even infants, may develop hemorrhoids that remain the same, rarely becoming symptomatic, enlarged, or bleeding; unlike those of *Nux vomica* or *Muriaticum acidum*, which do become very painful.

Urogenital System

Older materia medicas describe many symptoms in the kidneys and urinary tract. In practice, the kidneys are adversely affected in only a small minority of *Lycopodium* youngsters. The oft-quoted symptoms of "red sand" in the urine and screaming with pain before urinating are very rare indeed. The former symptom was easier to find in the early part of the century when there was no indoor plumbing. This meant that the child urinated into a receptacle that allowed the urine to settle overnight, and so one could easily spot the red sediment. The latter symptom is found in the atypical child who has a **uric acid** diathesis and passes gravel, screaming before urinating, and eventually develops either gout or (right-sided) kidney stones.

A confirmatory symptom that may be elicited is the curious fact that the **boys have to urinate more frequently in the evening** than during the day.

There is a great propensity toward **birth anomalies** involving the urogenital tract. These anomalies include structural problems of the kidneys or ureter, such as a ureter attaching at an improper location, hypospadias or epispadias (where the urethral meatus is not in the proper location), and urethral stricture.

Many of these problems are surgically corrected and the patients granted normal function, so the information is only elicited in the history taking. Others, however, may have some lingering symptoms after the repairs, such as frequency and urgency to urinate as well as dribbling profusely after urethral repair.

Perhaps it is this urogenital weakness that causes these boys to commonly be **bed-wetters.**

Boys

I have found that *Lycopodium* is the most frequently prescribed remedy for infant boys born with **undescended testicles,** and should be added to the appropriate rubrics. Boys also develop **right-sided inguinal hernias.** Many adults who need *Lycopodium* mention this symptom in their health history. It is interesting and curious to note how many of these children develop a new condition, such as hay fever or chronic sinusitis, after the hernia repair.

Girls

The girls may not develop secondary sexual characteristics until fifteen or sixteen years old. The menarche may arrive quite late. **Premeñstrually,** the adolescent experiences an increase in her appetite, especially for sweets, as well as an increase in constipation and irritability. A smaller percentage develop a slight case of acne just before the flow, and may weep easily. The menstrual flow is accompanied by pains that begin in the right lower abdomen and extend to the inner thigh. Right-sided ovarian pain at the time of ovulation may also be elicited.

A thin neck and upper body atop wide hips for some teen girls resembles the characteristic shape so commonly seen in *Lycopodium* adults. At first these girls appear very thin while sitting in the waiting room, until they stand up and the heavy buttock and thigh area can be seen.

Musculoskeletal System

Extremities

A *Lycopodium* prescription should be considered for **rheumatic pains and arthritis** in the childhood years when it is worse on the **right side.** The modalities are identical to those of *Rhus toxicodendron*: the pains are ameliorated by motion and heat and are aggravated by rest. Nodular swellings will be observed in the affected limbs, especially the joints of the hands and feet. A characteristic feature of *Lycopodium* rheumatoid arthritis is painless swelling of the right knee, even when there is much effusion in the joint and bursa. The joints that are affected may also make a cracking sound when moved. The child may become more insecure or irritable with a flare-up of arthritis.

A common observation made about *Lycopodium* children is the **restless motion of the legs.** In the interview one notices that the legs are in constant motion, going around in circles from the knees down, not from the ankles down as is found with *Natrum muriaticum.* Parents may report that the child moves the limbs about in bed at night.

The keynote of **dry, cracked skin covering the heels** may already have developed and be observed in teenaged girls, though not as commonly as in adult *Lycopodium* women.

Some children develop **plantar warts on the right heel.** Nail biting is a frequent complaint of parents about their children; the gnawing arises out of nervousness as well as excess energy and restlessness.

Skin

The child is often plagued by **eczema from birth,** as are *Medorrhinum, Sulphur, Tuberculinum,* and *Calcarea carbonica.* The feet, fingers, and scalp (especially behind the ears) are the most affected areas. One may also elicit the history that the child was **jaundiced** at birth, had tenderness in the liver area, and had much flatulence. These children may not completely lose the yellowness of the skin, and in these cases will always maintain a golden or sallow hue.

Moles and freckles easily appear on these children.

Lycopodium is often the remedy for the child who develops **neurodermatitis.** The itching forms vesicles, which may cover a small or large portion of the body. They may ulcerate and heal slowly because the child picks at them constantly. The eruptions leave the skin with a discolored, hardened scar.

These same children may also develop a tendency for **hives** that is aggravated by anxiety and by eating foods to which they are sensitive. Both the hives and neurodermatitis are aggravated by summertime heat, or from the heat of the bed or a hot shower. The intense itching lessens by going outside into the cool air. The child may likewise develop **dry, chapped skin**, especially upon the face, buttocks, and legs. Such dryness tends to be aggravated in winter and from eating certain foods such as milk, tomatoes, and citrus fruits.

The children may develop warts on their hands and especially on the soles of their feet (plantar warts).

Physical Generals

Complaints are **right-sided** or begin on the right side and spread to the left. Respiratory diseases spread from top to bottom.

Thinness, especially in boys, is often observed. The child eats much, at times more than the parent, yet does not gain weight and even loses weight, resembling *Calcarea carbonica*, *Natrum muriaticum*, or *Tuberculinum*. However, if this tendency for gauntness is accompanied by much flatulence, *Lycopodium* is the better remedy choice.

Aggravation in the morning and from four to eight o'clock in the evening, especially when both time modalities are present, constitute guiding symptoms noted in any diseased states as well as in times of a general drop in energy.

They are often **chilly** and like to wear hats, and may sleep with their socks on and the windows closed. This is unusual as most children are warm-blooded. The only time *Lycopodium* children like coolness is when they have skin disorders and, possibly, headaches; otherwise, they feel chilly and like everything warm—the room, food, drink, and bath.

The old materia medicas often advised the prescriber not to begin treating the case by giving the remedy *Lycopodium*. They suggested beginning the case by giving *Sulphur* or *Calcarea carbonica*. This is not borne out in clinical experience and should be disregarded. Begin the case with the simillimum always.

Notes on *Lycopodium* Infants

These are very fearful babies who need to be near the mother or on a parent's lap for security. *Lycopodium* infants become especially afraid when alone and when around people other than the parents, especially loud strangers. Fear and anxiety are easy to see in the stare and in the facial expression, especially the characteristic wrinkling of the forehead.

These irritable babies frown and scream at the slightest provocation. The crying has a demanding tone to it. They are especially cranky when hungry or tired, upon awakening, during colic, and during any acute illness.

Infants may cry every time the lights are turned off or when they are left alone in bed; they wish to sleep with the parents. They awake often at night to nurse or due to colic, and are hungry and cranky in the morning.

The head seems large, but is so only in proportion to the small body or spindly extremities.

The skin cracks behind the ears. Middle ear infections are frequent and begin on the right side, and finally exude a thick, smelly discharge. Irritability continues throughout such episodes.

The nasal passages of infants are commonly obstructed by mucus, making nursing for long impossible. Infants must pull off the breast, breathe through the mouth, cry, and then attempt to nurse again. Mothers must suction the mucus out of the nose frequently. Snuffles are common in babies, especially when they lie down at night. Mucus may be thick and yellow-green or there may only be dry snuffles with swelling high inside the nostrils causing obstruction.

Nostrils flare during acute respiratory tract infections.

Colds descend into the bronchi, causing bronchitis and pneumonia.

Chest colds recur and are accompanied by mucus that rattles in the chest, wrinkling of the forehead, and flaring nostrils. Coughing fits are most common at night when the child is lying down. The right middle lobe of the lung is most often affected.

Colic and rapid weight loss are common digestive complaints. There can be a great deal of trapped gas in the intestines that begins in the afternoon or nighttime, causing fussiness, irritability, and pain. Children may scream with the pain and roll around seeking relief. They feel better with hot compresses applied to the abdomen, by being carried, occasionally by nursing, and always by passing flatus; they become very hungry after the pain is relieved.

The infant has a big appetite, waking often to nurse and not ceasing until the mother stops. Mothers have been known to call this infant a "wild nurser." Hiccoughs occur after nursing. In malabsorptive syndromes the abdomen may distend with gas, which is released just before a bowel movement.

There are many birth anomalies in the urogenital tract: too many, not enough, or malposition of tissues and organs. While these cannot be corrected by homeopathic medicine, such symptoms do point to this remedy and the side effects of surgical repair often respond to *Lycopodium*.

Boys may be born with undescended testicles or hernias, especially of the right side.

Babies have poor motor skills, such as poor sucking reflexes or not learning to crawl properly. Dyslexia or other problems may develop later in life in these infants.

Eczema occurs from birth, especially behind the ears but also on the feet, fingers, and scalp.

In infants with failure to thrive, the skin wrinkles and hangs. The child also wrinkles the face when in pain and while screaming. The facial expression alternates between a fearful gaze of apprehension and a cranky, irritated frown. The skin may be jaundiced and may never lose its yellow tinge completely.

These are characteristically thin infants with right-sided problems that are aggravated from four to eight o'clock in the evening.

Lycopodium Outline

I. Mental/Emotional Characteristics
  A. Indecisive
    1. In the interview
      a) Do not want to answer questions
      b) Look at a parent to make sure they are answering correctly
    2. If forced to make a decision
      a) May run away
      b) May cry
    3. Have the parents decide for them
    4. Appear "childish"
  B. Dictatorial
    1. Love of power
      a) Control of others
        (1) First exerted upon the family
        (2) Later grows beyond the family circle
      b) Headstrong and bossy: order others around
        (1) Especially younger siblings
        (2) Yell if not obeyed at once
      c) Parent/child relationship troubled
        (1) Power dynamics reversed
        (2) Will correct parents during the interview
      d) Intolerant of contradiction
      e) Yet fearful of strangers
    2. Irritability
      a) Seen in domineering children
      b) Used to maintain tyranny
      c) Pronounced at certain times
        (1) When contradicted
        (2) When in pain
        (3) When constipated
        (4) Upon awakening
  C. Cognitive problems
    1. Dyslexia: mistakes in writing
    2. Mistakes in motor skills
  D. Hyperactive

      1. Dyslexic

      2. Must eat often

      3. Crave sugar

      4. Sensitive to pain

      5. Irritable

  E. Fears

      1. Many fears and insecurities

      2. Fear of the unknown

         a) Strangers; the doctor in the first interview

         b) Being alone, especially in the dark

         c) New tasks

         d) Anything new

      3. Social status concerns

         a) Fear of failure, especially if in public

         b) Performance anxiety

         c) Sensitive to ridicule: fear loss of social status

         d) Compromise easily

         e) Dress appropriately

      4. Monsters

      5. Ghosts

      6. Animals that they think will attack them

      7. Fear somaticized

         a) Stomachaches

         b) Diarrhea

      8. All fears are minimized if a parent is nearby

  F. Sleep

      1. Insomnia if anxious

      2. Fear to be alone in the dark

      3. Sleep positions

         a) On the right side

         b) In the knee-to-chest position

      4. Talk or laugh during sleep

      5. Suck their thumbs when tired until late childhood or beyond

      6. Wake up unrefreshed and irritable

II. Physical Symptomatology

  A. Head Area

      1. Head

a) Eczema
- (1) On the scalp
- (2) Especially behind the ears

b) Headaches
- (1) Hypoglycemic headaches
  - (a) If a meal is missed
  - (b) Irritable in this state
  - (c) Ameliorated by eating
- (2) Nondescript headaches
  - (a) Slightly right sided
  - (b) From prolonged sleep

2. Ears

a) Skin problems behind the ears
- (1) Eruptions
- (2) Cracks
- (3) Eczema

b) Otitis
- (1) On the right side
- (2) Exudes pus
  - (a) Thick
  - (b) Yellow
  - (c) Offensive smelling
- (3) Accompanies colds

3. Nose

a) Often affected

b) Obstructed nostrils
- (1) Nursing in infants prevented
- (2) Mucus
  - (a) Thick
  - (b) Green or yellow

c) Snuffles and sniffing
- (1) Constant
- (2) Aggravations
  - (a) At night when lying down
  - (b) In the morning from accumulating mucus at night

d) Flaring nostrils
- (1) With anxiety

        (2) With respiratory tract illnesses

4. Face
   a) Common expression of anxiety on the face
   b) Jaundiced look

5. Mouth
   a) Yellowing teeth
   b) Oral fixation; often put their fingers in their mouths

6. Throat and Neck
   a) Sore throats
      (1) Recurrent
      (2) On the right side
      (3) Ameliorated by warmth
   b) Tonsils troubled
      (1) Enlarged
      (2) Exude offensive-smelling pus
   c) Mononucleosis
      (1) Right-sided
         (a) Begins on the right side of the throat
         (b) Swollen glands
         (c) Pain
      (2) Offensive-smelling pus from the throat
      (3) Nose becomes obstructed
      (4) Nausea and abdominal pains
      (5) Weight loss
      (6) Skin becomes greenish
      (7) Dark circles under the eyes
      (8) Chilliness

B. Torso
  1. Lower Respiratory System
    a) Colds descend easily into the chest
    b) Recurrent bronchitis
    c) Pneumonia
       (1) Recurrent
       (2) Respiratory tract illnesses follow poorly treated cases
  2. Alimentary System
    a) Food cravings and aversions

(1) Craving for sweets
(2) Aversions
    (a) Beans
    (b) Onions
    (c) Fat
    (d) Cabbage
    (e) Shellfish (causes hives)
(3) Thirst
    (a) Low or normal
    (b) Crave soda pop

b) Stomach
  (1) Sensitive: stomachaches
    (a) From aggravating foods
    (b) From anxiety
  (2) Appetite
    (a) Often very hungry
    (b) Do not skip meals, even breakfast

c) Infants
  (1) Hungry; voracious nursers
  (2) Hiccough after eating
  (3) Infantile colic ameliorated by warm compresses

d) Rectum
  (1) Constipation
    (a) With or without pain
    (b) Aggravation
      i) In public rest rooms
      ii) While traveling
    (c) Stools sometimes hard at the beginning and soft or loose at the end of a movement
  (2) Occasional hemorrhoids

3. Urogenital System
  a) Frequent birth anomalies
  b) Right-sided kidney stones
  c) Boys
    (1) Frequent need to urinate in the evening
    (2) Right-sided hernias

      (3) Undescended testicles
   d) Girls
      (1) Premenstrual stress
         (a) Irritability
         (b) Desire for sweets
         (c) Constipation
      (2) Menses accompanied by pain
         (a) In the abdomen
         (b) Extends down the right leg
C. Musculoskeletal System: rheumatoid arthritis
   1. Accompanied by swelling
      a) Nodular
      b) Painless, of the right knee
   2. Aggravation
      a) From first motion
      b) During cold, wet weather
   3. Amelioration
      a) From warmth
      b) From continued motion
D. Skin
   1. Dry and cracked
      a) Palms
      b) Soles, especially the heels
   2. Plantar warts
   3. Eczema from birth
      a) Scalp, especially behind the ears
      b) Feet
      c) Fingers
   4. Jaundiced
      a) At birth
      b) May not lose yellowness completely
   5. Many moles and freckles
   6. Neurodermatitis
      a) Blisters and ulcerations
      b) Scratched until bleeding
   7. Hives
      a) From eating shellfish
      b) From anxiety

8. Itching
 a) Aggravation from heat
 b) Amelioration from coolness

III. Physical Generals
 A. Respiratory illnesses that descend easily to the chest
 B. Thin children, even if they eat a great deal
 C. Chilly
 D. Right-sided problems
 E. Problems that begin on the right side and move to the left
 F. Aggravation times
  1. In the morning upon awakening
  2. From four until eight o'clock in the evening
 G. Amelioration from warmth

Lycopodium Confirmatory Picture

These children have two aspects: an anxious, insecure, indecisive side that makes them seem weak; and an irritable, bossy side that makes them seem tyrannical. It is the interplay of these two aspects that gives the major clue to this remedy. They fear strangers, failing, being in the doctor's office, being alone in the dark, ghosts, and monsters; all fears are better if an adult is nearby. Dyslexia is common.

Confirmatory Checklist

- Sleep on the right side
- Right-sided otitis
- Right-sided upper respiratory tract infections
- Snuffles and obstructed nasal passages when lying down at night
- Sore throats ameliorated by warm drinks
- Crave sweets
- Avoid beans and vegetables of the cabbage family
- Relatively thirstless
- Big appetite with poor weight gain
- Many digestive complaints, including gas and constipation
- Aggravation of complaints with missed meals
- Chilly
- Right-sided problems, or problems that begin on the right side and move to the left
- Aggravation in the morning upon awakening and from four until eight o'clock in the evening
- Amelioration from warmth

Medorrhinum

Mental/Emotional Characteristics

In his description of *Medorrhinum* in the *Materia Medica*, Kent begins by describing the children who need this remedy. One would like to believe that this is due to the **importance of miasmatic treatment in early childhood**. It is many a homeopath's dream that the most severe and debilitating illnesses afflicting our babies and toddlers could be cured early on or prevented from arising altogether. Treatment with nosodes can often accomplish this.

Medorrhinum children are among those who are frequently ill from birth, carrying as they do a **genetically determined** constitutional weakness and a propensity toward contracting certain diseases. In reviewing this chapter as well as the one describing *Tuberculinum*, a common thread running through all nosodes can be found: there is a general inability to shake acute illnesses quickly or totally.

This is because miasmatic types do not have the constitutional fortitude to end health problems thoroughly and completely as do other remedy types. Often one acute illness after another mingles with the underlying miasmatic state and leads to a more or less continuous breakdown of the individual. Understanding this process leads the perceptive prescriber to consider administering a miasmatic remedy when appropriate.

Extreme Nature

The *Medorrhinum* child has a number of distinctive characteristics in the psychological and mental spheres. **Extreme extroversion or extreme introversion may be reported, although the former is**

much more common. Most children of this type are very **extroverted and vital**, displaying much energy and life.

For some, this vitality is amplified to the point of irritating those around them. They can become loud, chattering incessantly all day long. They usually play hard and enthusiastically. These energetic entertainers have a full personality and a twinkle in their eyes; this "open" type of *Medorrhinum* makes contact with others readily. They can easily approach total strangers and begin a conversation on almost any subject. They enjoy socializing and usually have many close friends.

These children are open in the doctor's office as well, beginning conversations with equal spontaneity with the receptionist, other patients in the waiting room, and the doctor. They answer questions without hesitation, although occasionally they wander off the trail by telling stories unrelated to the question asked. For example, young Andrea would come into the office and start playing with her dolls on the floor; then she would suddenly exclaim with no preface, "Guess what I did today?" This was not done with the ingenuous, open personability of a *Phosphorus*, but rather with the degree of calculation that one might typically find in a *Lycopodium*.

Once, while taking the case of a very young boy, I asked the mother if little Eddie liked to take naps. From across the room the exploring child answered matter-of-factly for the mother without so much as glancing up at either of us, saying cooly, "No, Paul. I do not nap." This directness, at times extreme, **may first offer a clue to** the probability of a Medorrhinum layer existing in the child.

Another incident showed more nerve. An older patient in a wheelchair and wearing an eye patch was waiting in the reception area. A *Medorrhinum* child, Howard, burst into the office, and before his huffing mother could catch up, he lunged at the patient's eye and yelled, "Hey, what do you have under that thing?" and tore the patch off the astonished man's face!

Drugs

This overly exuberant, vital nature often leads to **early experimentation** with drugs and other experience-altering substances, such as model airplane glue fumes, cough medicine, pain killers, and even car exhaust.

Sexuality

There is a great deal of **sexual acting out at an early age as well**. With some embarrassment, parents report of their young children such behavior as frequent erections (including erections during sleep) and kissing and playing erotically with both adults and other children. At the age of six or seven years, **boys** masturbate or are repeatedly found naked with young neighbor girls and boys. Four- and five-year-old boys may touch and play with their mothers' breasts inappropriately. Little boys may also play role-reversal games, dressing and acting like girls or acting seductively with the father.

Medorrhinum **girls'** behavior can be just as sexually motivated. I once treated a six-year-old girl who showed violent tendencies in general and masturbated a lot. The mother noticed that the girl liked to "pick" at her vagina all the time. The child would coerce her mother to dress her in the tightest possible clothes and underwear.

Another girl became a stripper at fifteen years of age, "To earn extra money," she claimed. She also liked the atmosphere of the bar. Most probably, the excitement rather than the money lured her to take this job. The propensity to act out in this way shows that these children received not only the genetic imprint of the miasm (and with it a tendency to manifest certain illnesses), but also the tendency toward sexually promiscuous behavior.

Energy/Lassitude

Evidence of greater than normal vitality may be observed in their **hurried behavior**. During the interview, the speech patterns reflect this hurriedness with much stammering and swallowing of words. The parents confirm that the child does everything quickly, always seeming to be in a big rush.

Dan, a teenager, agreed that he was impatient and "fast-moving, rushing throughout the day, not letting anyone get in my way." He usually had a high energy level, liked to always be busy, and found it hard to relax. Like many symptoms of this remedy, the exact opposite may be true even in the same person: there may be **periodic swings** toward total, **incapacitating inertia**.

This indeed was the case for one young man. Derek was usually very energetic, but had periodic phases of no energy when he developed a negative attitude about everything and felt as if his doom lay in wait for him just around the corner. Nothing sounded good to him and he had no desire to do anything but lie about. This severe contrast in energy levels first pointed me to the remedy *Medorrhinum*, which was later confirmed by helping him greatly when administered.

Hyperactivity

Such energy sustained at a high level may lead over time to a true hyperactive state. Susceptible children are restless in the office, as if keyed up. Keep an eye on the feet of such children, which bob up and down incessantly. They just cannot sit still, becoming easily distracted by noise and by others entering the room.

At school they may become **restless to the point of wildness**. Many times, children needing the remedy *Tuberculinum* will behave well at school and only become nasty and unruly at home. On the other hand, those needing *Medorrhinum*, if nasty, are generally nasty throughout the day wherever they are. As they become more energized and hurried, they also become impatient and hard to manage.

Hyperactive *Medorrhinum* children **cannot concentrate** very well, forgetting words, concepts, and what they were about to say. These negative aspects of hyperactivity are especially noticeable if the children do not nap and therefore become overly tired.

Hyperactive *Medorrhinum* children are **messy** by nature and may be confused with hyperactive *Sulphur* children because of this. This is a common mistake, as the two remedies have many physical general symptoms in common. The extreme nature of the *Medorrhinum* youngster and the more constant energy level of the *Sulphur* may help one to find the correct remedy.

Meanness

Another negative attribute commonly found in these children is meanness and cruelty; coupled with high energy, it can lead to frequent quarrels, screaming matches, and out-and-out **fighting**. Impatience and irritability are much worse when the child is contradicted. When this happens, the child wants things his own way even more than usual and seems to develop superhuman strength. In this state, he can fight with everyone around him with great tenacity. The child becomes **implacable**, throwing things at the wall or even at his parents.

They **strike** their parents, siblings, and friends without remorse. In their hardened state, they may relish torturing and killing animals. The parents may complain that their child was forced to change schools several times due to behavior problems such as fighting with other children.

Mitchell, a boy with asthma, was particularly difficult to help. He had many fears that corresponded to a *Lycopodium* picture but had the physical general symptoms of a *Sulphur* picture. Finally one day, the parents shared with me just how mean the child could actually be. He was mean to absolute strangers and would even hit his older, stronger siblings. The fact that he hit both his stronger siblings, who possessed a known quantity of strength, and strangers, who represented an unknown quantity, ruled out the remedy *Lycopodium*, as in both situations the *Lycopodium* child would be fearful and not aggressive. The remaining physical general symptoms plus the cruelty described fit only *Medorrhinum*, a remedy that greatly ameliorated his fits of anger and his bouts of asthma.

In some, **orange juice** may aggravate this trait of meanness as if in response to a food allergy. Yet in others, orange juice has a good effect by acting as a sedative. The *Tuberculinum* child exhibits similar reactions when drinking milk; some problems are aggravated and some are ameliorated.

This mean streak follows the pattern of other physical generals of *Medorrhinum*; that is, it is worse throughout the day rather than at night.

Parents state that during these "mean" times they cannot reprimand the child for fear of **reprisals**. The parents also know that at this time the child will not learn anything from the reprimand and will only feel the power struggle and react to it with violence. One particular case in point involved ten-year-old Tyrone, who was locked in his room for a "time out" after having been abusive to a sibling. The child broke a panel on the door and escaped, becoming totally out of control and forcefully pummeling one and then the other parent who attempted to confine him.

As these parents pointed out, during such times it is impossible to establish any rules of discipline or to mete out punishment. The situation can quickly degenerate into a struggle for control in which the parents basically overpower the child in order to get him or her to stop a tantrum or other violent behavior. For many parents, the desire to avoid such all-out power struggles leads them to give in to the child just to keep some semblance of peace in the home.

Episodic Nature

The emotional nature of the child, be it expressed in anger, cruelty, or sweetness, may manifest in fits. This **episodic cruelty or rudeness**, the fitful, changeable nature of the child, when times of great aggressiveness alternate with times of introversion and playful coyness, most often indicates a need for this remedy. The parents report that the child acts fine one minute and then throws a fit of intense passion and anger the next, without apparent cause.

Often the chief complaint includes fits of **violence**. I recall four-year-old Amelia, who was brought in by her adoptive mother because she hit people in the stomach. The mother thought her daughter was "actually two different beings" in her estimation. The girl would be well behaved and quiet at school, perhaps even shy. In my office, in fact, she whispered all her answers. The mother reported that she did all of her homework and was attentive, but that suddenly her personality "switched" and she proceeded to hit her parents and bystanders in the stomach and put her fingers in other children's eyes. She became very loud and had a great deal of excess energy that she expended by running all over the playground. This dual nature plus the physical general symptoms led to the prescription of *Medorrhinum*, which brought emotional balance into this young girl's life.

Extreme polarity of behavior, swinging from very sweet and charming to very nasty and destructive, may indicate a need for this remedy. Such reflexive forays into violence are often carried out without thought of the pain it might impose on the child himself. One troubled teenager who suddenly became angry punched his fist through a door, breaking three bones in his hand. **Self-destructive** tendencies born of hot tempers and mindless fitfulness are characteristic of this remedy as well as of *Nux vomica*, *Tarentula hispanica*, and *Tuberculinum*.

This extreme nature may also be evidenced by sudden flips into emotionally **regressive behavior**. The child begins to suck the thumb, talk like a baby, and crawl around on the floor. She may want to be carried, held, or rocked, and calls for "Ma-Ma" and "Da-Da." She may demand to sleep with her parents. This can even be observed in a child of six or seven years. While in this state, the cuteness and regression displayed may resonate of *Pulsatilla*. By eliciting all the facts of the case—finding out that perhaps this is only one phase of many, really just one charming period among many terrifying ones—the practitioner comes to understand the entire *Medorrhinum* picture.

Obstinacy

These fitful children may become very obstinate. The *Medorrhinum* child likes to be **bossy**, like *Lycopodium*, and tell the parents what to do and how to act. The parents feel discord from the very beginning, and although they love their child, the relationship is extremely challenging. They bemoan the constant struggle to determine who is in control, even in the case of a three-year-old.

While the family is in the office, one may observe the obstinacy of such a child, who yells, "I want this!" while tugging at the doctor's stethoscope and screams and carries on until the object is handed over, as in *Calcarea carbonica* and *Tuberculinum*. The parents assert that it is of no use to try and reason with the child once his mind is made up. Parents will often not dare to punish the child in this state even if they wish to because the punishment has a deleterious or negligible effect. From the very beginning the parents realize that "the child has a mind of his own; once he wants something, he gets it."

Another way to gauge the depth of the obstinacy is to see how long children hold **grudges**. The length of time can be amazing, even in small children, for harboring deep resentments against people who offended them for some insignificant reason. They blurt out angrily, "I was right, you were wrong, admit it!" or perhaps, "I'm gonna get back at him, I'm gonna beat him up next time I see him!" It is astounding how well the little ones remember everyone else's perceived transgressions and how they desire to mete out appropriate retribution while forgetting their own substantial meanness and trespasses against others.

Violence

Medorrhinum children exhibit **temper tantrums,** as do the other remedy types just mentioned: *Calcarea carbonica* and *Tuberculinum*. One precipitating cause for tantrums stems from a flaw in the thinking process. Even though the children have the language skills to ask for what they want, a mental confusion occasionally hampers their ability to request clearly what exactly they desire. Instead, they become frustrated and revert to crying. The uncontrollable crying may drive the parents mad with frustration because they have to guess what specifically the child wants. Often a small thing turns out to have begun the attack, like needing help with tying a shoe. Unlike the *Tuberculinum* child, who may continue to cry and even throw away the object requested, the *Medorrhinum* child is mollified if given what was wished.

Also at the root of many of these tantrums is a great **intolerance to contradiction.** The child seems to become almost demonic upon the slightest contradiction, exploding with violent behavior.

Fighting with the parents is graphically demonstrated in the doctor's office. It is interesting that both *Medorrhinum* and *Tuberculinum* types may both hit their poor parents with considerable force during the interview because of what appear to be insignificant causal factors.

A great deal of biting, kicking, punching, and other generally **antisocial behavior** is reported. *Medorrhinum* children may curse, break things, throw objects at a parent's face, or even tear the wallpaper off the wall! In their anger they may shout threats such as "When I get older, I'm going to kill you!" The violent anger that this child exhibits should be added to the appropriate rubrics in the *Repertory*, such as Mind; Anger, contradiction, and Mind; Anger, violent, and Mind; Violent.

Punishment

The child nags and confronts a parent until getting an emotional rise out of him or her. It is as if she wants, needs, and almost **longs for reprimand** and punishment. Parents often wonder if punishment is a language with which the child is more conversant than reward, and therefore likes it just because she understands it better than she does praise. The sweet, loving attention given by a parent may go unheeded or may even be rejected by such a child.

I remember nine-year-old Sally, who would at times become as violent as here described. As soon as the violent fit was finished, or as soon as the parents became angry with her, she would become cooperative and sweet. She would provoke a fight whenever possible. If the mother told her not to make noise at the theater, it was guaranteed that she would yell so her mother would be moved to swat her. It was as if the contact that she made with her parent in that fashion was desirable.

It is important to note that cases where verbal or physical punishment are the primary sources of contact the child has with the parents are not what is being described here. What I am referring to may be found in very nurturing, loving households where there is ample opportunity for the child to receive and respond to positive attention, yet this angry sort of interchange is a style of communication upon which the child seems to thrive.

In the same fashion, these children may **throw things at people they like**. It is their way of opening up a line of communication in lieu of creating a more conventional dialogue.

In addition to behaving violently themselves, these children **love to observe violence** as well. Perhaps, like a tourist traveling in a foreign land becoming captivated by a television broadcast delivered in his native tongue, these children love to watch scary or violent movies with lots of blood, guts, and gore as if it were being presented in their own language. They thrill to watch the projected violence and somehow "connect" with it, experiencing it vicariously.

Lying

Medorrhinum children are often caught lying. Because of the child's discontinuous reality (discussed later), telling falsehoods comes easily. An aspect of morality dies at an early age, or perhaps never develops normally in the first place. Lying often begins with the relatively innocuous and common excuse, **"It's not my fault."**

In the office a careful listener will frequently hear this type of lying: the parent describes a negative trait, like temper tantrums or cursing, and the child will exclaim over and over again with the utmost conviction, "No I don't! No I don't!" in response to every point. As the parent recounts anecdotes, the child categorically denies everything that paints him or her in a less than favorable light. If the doctor finally turns to the child and asks point blank, "What didn't happen?" the child will pout, "That didn't happen *lately*," or, "That didn't happen on *Thursday* like Mom said." It is as if the child thinks that by exposing the little mistake the parent made during the recounting the doctor could be lead to assume something else and thereby vindicate the child from blame in the situation.

This **lying by omission** in children can evolve in the adult into the classic *Thuja* symptom of not finishing sentences, merely trailing off at the end instead; or in the *Medorrhinum* individual, rambling from sentence to sentence, never finishing a whole thought. By not completing ideas, much responsibility can be evaded and truth perverted.

Another form of lying by omission is noted in children who have a **great wish not to have anything "bad" said about them.** No one does, but their reactions speak loudly of the remedy itself. They scream, "No! No! Stop!" at the parents as they describe the symptoms to the doctor. Some even raise their fists and demand the parents to stop or threaten to strike them. Others hide behind a parent's chair or behind a plant or bookshelf and yell, "I am not telling!" in answer to any question asked of them. This last group, the ones who hide, will slip most easily into the shy states described later in this chapter and may eventually need *Thuja* as a complementary remedy after the administration of *Medorrhinum*.

Some lying is evoked by **jealousy of siblings**. Since they do not comprehend parental love, they may measure love by getting equal shares of objects, toys, and food. I know a boy who wanted to have a duplicate of everything that his brother had. He would lie, cheat, and steal to get the parents to buy him the same toys. He would steal and hide his brother's favorite toy because he did not get one also. He would even hide his own toys and blame his brother for stealing them just to get him into trouble, like a *Tuberculinum* or *Tarentula hispanica* child might also do. A strong impression of just how skewed this boy's values had become was gained from his lack of desire for the love and warmth that others normally seek. He seemed not to be interested in or know of affection at all, desiring only the outer manifestations, the physical trappings, of love.

Selfishness

The mean children have broad streaks of selfishness as well. The following scene describes its subtle nature. Young Bruno, who was being seen for asthma, would come into the clinic and begin to play with cars while lying on the floor in the knee-to-chest position. He would interrupt the interview countless times by asking for more cars or other toys, or disturb the flow of conversation by trying to open all the cabinets or endeavoring to take all the objects off my desk. He would ask or do anything as long as it hindered the interview process. The **thoughtlessness** with which the child behaved reflected a complete disregard for the wishes of the adults in the room.

The subject may also spy or tattle on other siblings' behavior to the parents so that he will receive more attention, even lying to get a sibling into trouble with the parents. This **manipulativeness** shows the complete selfishness and disregard for the welfare of others.

Such selfishness can also lead to strong feelings of **possessiveness** about one of the parents and therefore jealousy of another's claim on that parent's attention. The child may become upset when the father is alone with the mother and so try to be included in all the parents' activities. He may yell at the mother, "Don't talk to Daddy!" or vice versa, or monopolize the conversation so that no one else can get a word in. This is normal behavior for most children of all types when intermittent and during especially stressful times such as after the birth of a sibling, but when protracted and constant it becomes pathological and needs to be treated.

The incident previously cited of the miasmatic boy and the wheelchair-bound man with the eye patch also illustrates the characteristic total disregard for other human beings. Another example is the selfish child who yells at her father who wants to lovingly share food, "This is my yogurt!" and begins to scream and pull the container away from him. Similar possessiveness with toys will be found.

They are usually **critical of others** and disregard the feelings and wishes of those around them. Their complaining is of a characteristically self-centered nature, and even as adolescents they are unaware of how much others are negatively affected by it. Self-centeredness combined with not being aware of or caring about the consequences of their actions allows them to be impolite and insolent with impunity.

Cognitive Difficulties

The child needing the remedy *Medorrhinum* may have one of two main problems in the ability to think clearly. The first problem is an **inborn mental and physical dwarfing**, as though from a minor chromosomal aberration. The second is only a **functional problem with the ability to concentrate**.

The former difficulties include a **memory weak from babyhood on**, especially for conceptual thought. They are usually poor spellers and forget the meaning of common words, names in particular. A cloud of confusion comes upon the child during which he is unable to speak clearly. It is as if the circuits of the brain are not connected correctly or that there are too many nerve impulses firing simultaneously in the brain. The child is left tongue-tied and unable to communicate.

One way in which this problem can manifest is as an inability to judge the passage of time accurately, leading to the famous symptom described as the sensation that **time passes too slowly**. With this error, things that took place today seem as though they happened a few days before. It is more common to find this complaint in the adult, but the teenager needing *Medorrhinum* may also be troubled by it.

Anomalies in the development of gross or fine motor skills abound. A child may not be able to pick up small objects, color in pictures, or demonstrate good penmanship. He may also walk with a jerky gait, as if his entire body is twitching forward instead of advancing with a more fluid motion.

For the second type of child with concentration problems, the **short attention span** often leads other doctors to diagnose an attention deficit disorder. Parents are often told that the child requires Ritalin and may in fact come to the first interview with the patient taking it already.

This type of child begins to **lose the thread of conversations**, as also observed in those patients needing the remedy *Thuja*. When asked a question, the *Medorrhinum* child with this problem either ends the answer in the middle of a thought or answers inappropriately. One may perceive this more easily in adults because they are expected to follow through on thoughts, but it can be present in children as well. The occasional "spacing out" that we all experience is a way of life for the *Medorrhinum* youngster with concentration problems.

In **teenagers, confusion** takes on many forms and may be described in many ways. In lesser states of illness it is described as a lack of the ability to concentrate, seen most commonly with school-related learning. In the more seriously ill, the feeling of a lack of connection to others in particular and society and life in general is a much more deep-seated problem of concentration.

Sufferers describe this deeply pathological state as the feeling as though they are **living in a dream world**. As with *Cannabis indica* and *Thuja* types, they feel isolated from others. The mind and body may feel numb, as if one or both were fading away. This can be especially sensed while lying in bed—a panic attack may ensue because of it, causing them to get up again.

When they feel as if they are about to "space out," that their thought processes are on the verge of disintegrating, they **panic** and desperately force themselves to focus on anything that comes to mind in order to prevent their mental state from slipping away any further. While this specific example may fit other remedy types such as *Cannabis indica* and *Platina*, the important point is the chronic mental disconnectedness symptomatic of both the remedy and the miasm, the slow dissipation of attention that takes place over a period of months or years and is replaced by growing confusion.

While in other remedies this disassociation may be, even if episodic, the central focus of the pathology, in *Medorrhinum* it is only a small part of the problem and usually **not the chief complaint**. For this reason one must be sure to focus on the logical totality of the case and not on the peripheral symptoms.

This syndrome is only rarely seen in children, but is more commonly found in adolescents.

Confusion manifests in other ways as well. Slow answers to the doctor's questions and visible confusion on the youth's face provide evidence of the **inability to focus or make sense of the words spoken**. Some cannot link together the ideas conveyed by speech to make cogent thoughts. These children become irritable and yell or strike a sibling who makes noise because it breaks their fragile concentration. They also cannot manage to do homework if the radio or television is on because they need absolute silence to focus on their work.

Mental confusion may lead to **dyslexia**, with mistakes then being made in reading, writing, and arithmetic, and sometimes in hearing or even aesthetics, as evidenced by painting or drawing subjects upside down. Spelling mistakes may also occur when the child is in a rush to finish quickly, even if she does know how to spell the word correctly, as is also the case with *Lycopodium*.

Mistakes in speech occur when the child says words that are slightly similar, as exemplified by a child wanting to say "I am leaving," but instead saying "I am needing." With many of the children a portion of a word is left out. For example, instead of saying "nothing," they say "nuh-ing." One child who responded well to treatment with the nosode *Medorrhinum* constantly exchanged consonants. For instance, he would say "I want to lie down on the soda" instead of "I want to lie down on the sofa."

The **mistakes of speech are not predictable or fixed** and repeated but may happen only once. The next instance will involve a different word or phrase. The constant changing of the objects of such mistakes shows that the children have not learned the word incorrectly; rather, their mental recall during conversation is either slower than normal or somehow slightly scrambled. As they speak they become confused; unable to pull the proper word from their minds, they substitute an incorrect but perhaps similar one.

This is not due to mental dullness so much as to confusion. Part of this problem, in the words of a parent, is that "the mind is ahead of the mouth," causing confused and garbled speech.

Confusion may also be heard in sentence structure. The sentences may be choppy and mechanized, with the words sounding as if the child had a foreign accent, reflecting a lack of coordinated communication between the brain and the tongue.

Ted had recurrent upper respiratory tract infections. Every time he developed one he began to stutter, sleep in the knee-to-chest position, confuse words, and act shy until the infection cleared up. These four points alone pointed to the remedy *Medorrhinum*, which stopped his sensitivity to colds.

While one may hear these mistakes in speech during the office visit, it is more likely that any mention of them has to be elicited from the parents. Some parents deny that such errors happen, either because they are so used to them that they no longer perceive their occurrence, or, as is more often the case, because they need the same remedy and make the same mistakes themselves!

As **memory declines** over time, abstract theoretical knowledge is easily lost. While the child may forget with ease what was heard or read, she can still remember concepts that have visual, experiential clues. For example, when ten-year-old Mary, a mentally handicapped girl, was driven past a certain street, she would blurt out, "There is the store you and Grandma went to last year." What makes this recollection perplexing is that Mary cannot add two numbers together, write, or perform any other abstract learning tasks.

Many children who require the remedy *Medorrhinum* are **pseudoambidextrous**. In these children, it is not that they are equally able to use either hand as a true ambidextrous person can, but rather that they cannot decide which hand to use as neither feels quite right. In this confused state they are no longer

105

sure which hand is their dominant one; because of this, they may switch hands during activities and never quite master a skill with either one.

Initially, the *Medorrhinum* child who is a slow learner is perfectionistic, spending a long time trying to fashion the letters correctly when learning to write. As the confused state worsens over months and years, the child **begins to procrastinate** and to hate being pushed to read, write, or do homework. He becomes increasingly irritated if the parent prods him and he expresses intense frustration in response. As a consequence, it appears that the child is lazy, just moping about the house and not finishing tasks or projects. He may become reluctant to go to school.

The shy, introverted *Medorrhinum* type described below can become mentally dull and develop **increased anxiety about upcoming events,** especially those revolving around school projects. This is due to **decreased confidence in his own mental capabilities.** Teenagers who experience this mental dullness cannot speak before a group without losing their way verbally and becoming confused and tongue-tied.

Introversion

There is one subgroup of *Medorrhinum* children that is either intermittently or consistently very shy and timid. An inferiority complex is observed in their demeanor during the interview. These children are very bashful and introverted, looking at the mother during the entire session and whispering their responses during the interview. They have an aversion to being looked at and will not look back at the doctor as he or she gazes at them.

The **boys** of this subgroup are **softhearted and sensitive** to an extreme degree. Sensitive boys play easily with girls living nearby, amusing themselves with dolls and other "soft" games. These sensitive children become sad and cry easily. Weeping ameliorates the *Medorrhinum* child's sadness. Extremity of this nature grabs the doctor's attention; the intensity of the child's sensitivity is unusual. While one may confuse this type of boy with a *Natrum muriaticum,* one will not feel the same level of compassion toward the child as one does toward the average *Natrum muriaticum* patient. *Medorrhinum* feels, and is, distant from the rest of humanity, a distance that makes the child increasingly a loner and less emotionally attached to others.

The mother may state that the child has been psychologically tested and found to have very low self-esteem. These unfortunates have **no confidence or pride** in themselves. In some members of this group, the sensitivity is seen only during fitful states during which the child is shy and which alternate with fits of anger and contradictory behavior. Teenaged Rachel, being treated for bronchitis, was usually quite shy; occasionally, though, she became contrary, doing just the opposite of what she was told. She was dictatorial and deceitful and wanted everything her own way when she got into this state, and was, all in all, very difficult to manage. The remedy *Medorrhinum* greatly helped her respiratory infection and resolved these horrible mood swings.

The **love of animals** may be quite keen in some of the shy *Medorrhinum* children. They become very emotionally attached to pets, spending much time with them, especially when upset or sad. Since these children feel distant from humanity, when they are upset they cannot talk to other people very easily and so go instead to talk to the family dog. One father told me that his son loved dogs and that the first word his son spoke was "dog." This same boy was later mean to dogs, kicking them and pulling them by their tails if they did not do immediately as he bid them. It should be mentioned that this love of pets is not always seen in practice, as some materia medicas infer, although when it does occur the affection is quite strong.

As these timid children grow up they become increasingly more introverted, feeling the distance grow between themselves and the outside world. Many become **depressed** at some point due to this isolating interpersonal gap. In their depression they begin to act out, just as more extroverted *Medorrhinum* children do. They start to take drugs and smoke cigarettes.

This **taking of drugs** is not done with the relish and enjoyment found in their outgoing counterparts, but instead with a sense of despondency. They have given up hope and harbor an "I no longer care" attitude. They become gloomy, feeling that all around them is blackness and depression. Before they reach this deeply despondent stage where all that is left is a feeling that they are separated from all others, they try to resist, fighting against giving in to this feeling. In this more profound state, however, they cannot fight any longer and surrender to the abyss. It is at this point that these youngsters start to desire to disappear, **to die**.

In such a severe emotional condition, some girls may develop **anorexic or bulimic** behavior. This disordered state may frequently be mistaken for that found in *Ignatia amara*, with the common symptoms of depression, blocked feelings, anorexia, and the desire for death.

If at no other time, there should be one major clue found that will make one consider the remedy *Medorrhinum* for the anorexia: the adolescent may not eat for days, starving herself so that she emaciates, but **when she finally forces herself to eat, she will eat mainly fruit**. While one may falsely think of this as just another way of attempting to not gain weight, it is nevertheless a major indication for the nosode. The food preferences of these girls should always be carefully explored, as many times the food truly craved will be the food binged upon as well. For instance, the *Cinchona* girl will not usually eat fruit, and the *Ignatia amara* in this state will definitely not put a piece of fruit in her mouth.

A *Medorrhinum* girl becomes even more introverted and closed in an anorexic or bulimic state. She blames herself for anything that goes wrong in her life as a way of justifying her self-destructive behavior, thus feeding her desire for death. This **self-blame** leads to more extreme **self-destructive** behavior as she begins to physically punish herself. Some girls cut their bodies—often their arms and forearms—with razors. Others constantly dwell on suicide, repeating to themselves in essence, "I am a bad person."

Anything that increases emotional stress for these anorexic, introverted children also increases their depression. The two most common stressors are drugs and the menses. Whenever they take drugs it increases their suicidal thoughts and the intensity of depression as well as their paranoid feelings. The increase of depression and of suicidal sentiments also often coincides with premenstrual tension.

One final comment on **eating disorders**: while homeopathic remedies can be very effective in helping to rebuild the body as well as the mind, they should never be the sole treatment. A doctor's success rate with these disorders will rise dramatically if the homeopathic treatment is combined with counseling, especially family-centered and skill-oriented therapies that work on developing new methods of relating to food.

In general, *Medorrhinum* children who are introverted and shy have one big, constant conflict looming over their lives: their fathers. More than likely, the reason the child needs the remedy *Medorrhinum* in the first place is that the father (or his father before him) was very outgoing or promiscuous and contracted the miasm from others through intimate contact. These fathers, then, tend to behave like the outgoing, vital, hyperactive *Medorrhinum* or *Nux vomica* types. The conflict between these two divergent personalities—the shy child and the **overbearing father**—wreaks havoc with the sensitive child, who **withdraws** more with every interaction with his father.

This scenario may confuse the prescriber into thinking that the child needs the remedy *Staphysagria* because the child becomes so tremendously withdrawn and inhibited. In fact, there are times when only the physical generals and the family history will help to differentiate between the two and lead to the correct remedy. The two similar mental pictures that these remedies accommodate, usually more applicable to boys than to girls, can seem indistinguishable in these cases.

Fears

A common fear of *Medorrhinum* children is the fear of **being alone, especially in the dark**; this is also found with *Lycopodium*, *Phosphorus*, and *Pulsatilla*. The reason behind this fear is really a deeper fear; *Medorrhinum* should be one of the first remedies thought of for a child who fears an **unseen "presence"** in the environment. Some children describe this as a fear of ghosts, monsters, burglars, or just an indescribable "something" in the house. More to the point, teenagers may describe the fear that there is something eerie in the house lurking in the dark.

The child may be glued to his parents until they look under the bed or walk with him to search the room for monsters. The fear of the dark may make the child sleep with the lights on or with the parents. The father reports that his child fears shadows while lying in bed and sees monsters when the lights are turned off to go to sleep, as do *Calcarea carbonica* and *Phosphorus* children. While these fears may seem similar to that of other remedy types, the central fear of an outside influence in the house combined with the nasty behavior previously described should lead one to the remedy *Medorrhinum*.

Fear of **water** is the other well-known fear of this remedy type. While in *Stramonium* the fear is of running water or of water poured on the head, in *Medorrhinum* the fear is mainly of large bodies of water. The child may not be able to force himself to swim in the ocean or even in a large lake, although swimming in a pool can be very enjoyable for him.

This fear is connected to the fear of **eerie, unseen things**. While some talk of sharks and snakes, others fear something scary under the water that may come up and snatch them, as did a poor girl who was taunted by other swimmers about there being snakes in the lake where she was swimming. She screamed and swam for dear life to shore in response.

Such a fear is deeply rooted in the child and becomes stronger as she grows older. Some *Medorrhinum* adults may actually get to the point where they cannot even look at photographs of the ocean without experiencing chills and becoming fearful. This is not seen throughout the remedy, however, as *Medorrhinum* is also the main remedy to contemplate giving to the child or adult who loves to bathe in the ocean and must be coaxed out of the sea at the end of a day at the beach.

A number of these children have a distinct fear of **animals**, especially of **dogs**. Some have nightmares about them. As this is not spoken of in the older materia medicas, it may be one reason why there has been such confusion in the past between *Tuberculinum* and *Medorrhinum*, with doctors often prescribing the remedy *Tuberculinum* incorrectly for *Medorrhinum* cases.

Some *Medorrhinum* children have a fear of **slimy creatures** such as toads and jellyfish.

Another fear that about one in five *Medorrhinum* children has is the fear of **closed-in places**. Any time the child wrestles and becomes pinned down, he aggressively punches his way out, completely losing all reason in doing so. One such teenager lost all composure while playing football when he was tackled and a few others fell on top of him; he hit the other players ferociously until they let him up and ran away.

The **hyperactive** child or the child with an attention deficit disorder has fears that relate to being **startled**. These fears are mostly of any sudden intrusion into the personal sensory spheres, especially auditory. When a car horn blasts, or even when someone across the room drops a pencil on the floor, the *Medorrhinum* child involuntarily starts.

Shy **adolescent** children become **apprehensive** before any upcoming event in which they have to perform. This fear of being observed may be one of the first transition points showing that the child is going into a *Thuja* state.

Often one state of health or remedy picture flows into another **complementary remedy type**. This commonly happens when the correct homeopathic remedy is given and the case improves; certain symptoms disappear but the symptoms that are left or any new symptoms that appear belong to the complementary remedy. The progression of symptoms can also occur in the opposite direction.

If a patient becomes increasingly ill over time, the disease picture may change and require another remedy to cure the more serious symptoms now emerging. Often the *Thuja* picture and the *Medorrhinum* picture change from one into the other. After prescribing one, the symptoms that remain after this initial remedy has acted often belong to the other remedy and can be treated with that second remedy.

One final note on the mind: if the doctor is very attentive to his or her own feelings about and reactions to the patient, this alone may provide a very strong clue as to whether or not this remedy is needed. Some of these children **elicit a feeling of disgust in others**. It is not that they do or say anything in particular that could be considered repulsive; it is just a general feeling in the observer of something repellent that seems to exude from the child when first encountered. This same feeling may continually resurface every time the child comes in for a visit. This feeling of repulsion may also be mentioned by one of the parents: the one who married into the miasm.

Sleep

The *Medorrhinum* child tends to be a **"night person,"** finding it difficult to fall asleep until late at night. Some children regularly spend one or two hours tossing about until they finally fall asleep. Younger children may be able to sleep more easily if the mother lies down with them. Their sleep from the beginning of the night on through to the morning is very restless as they toss and turn all over the bed. Most especially commented upon is the thrashing of the legs throughout the night. Babies may wake up every couple of hours crying due to colic.

The child is very **hot** and will often sleep naked and uncovered, especially the feet, as they roast while the night progresses. They may in fact be so warm as to desire a fan on during the night. With this warmth they may perspire on the face. The perspiration has an offensive odor, which is best described as being a combination of pungent, sweet, and sour.

Even though their sleep is **restless**, they favor sleeping on the **abdomen** or in the **knee-to-chest** position with the buttocks in the air. While this is common in many infants, it will be seen in older children too. As the children age they eventually favor the abdominal position. Occasionally they may sleep on the back with the hands above the head, as is often seen in *Pulsatilla* children.

Many *Medorrhinum* children have **nightmares**, a point not often described. These nightmares are sometimes caused by eating sweets before bedtime and usually involve things they consciously fear. Being chased or bitten by dogs is a common theme. Other animals are also represented, such as snakes and insects. Their dreams may resemble those of *Calcarea carbonica*, in which they envision monsters, ghosts, and goblins chasing them. Others may have more violent themes such as being chased by someone brandishing a knife. They may wake up at night screaming that someone is trying to kill them. Due to these dreams, as well as the feeling that there are frightful things in the dark, the child may sleep with the light on or go into the parents' room when frightened.

The child may either **wake up** with much **frantic energy** and not be inclined to slow down until nighttime, or wake up **unre-**

freshed. Although in the latter case the child is fatigued in the morning, it will not be to the same degree or frequency as that found in the adult.

Physical Symptomatology

Head

The head in general does **not** give **many clues** to this remedy.

The scalp lacks oils in an inverse proportion to that which the face produces. The hair may be so dry that it stands in whatever position it is pulled. This dryness may exist to the same extent as that found with *Thuja* or *Sulphur* types, and may lead to the production of dandruff and flaking skin. There can be so much desquamation that the scalp bleeds, even in a very young child.

The *Medorrhinum* teenager may complain of **headaches**, especially those that are **sinus related**, frontal, and aggravated by motion, cold, and the eating of citrus fruit or pineapple.

Eyes

The eyes are affected in a manner similar to the way that the disease **gonorrhea** affects a newborn's eyes. Such an infant develops conjunctivitis or blepharitis with much swelling and redness. The pus that is exuded is thick, green, and excoriates the entire area of the eye. The eyelids are glued together in the morning with dried pus. A four-month-old baby boy developed recurrent pinkeye with the chief problem of much pus and matter accumulating in the eyes all day long. This symptom, along with a sycotic family history, a diaper rash, and a knee-to-chest sleeping position, pointed to the correct remedy: *Medorrhinum*.

Older children may report these eye inflammations as something that has occurred in the past, or complain of low-level **chronic blepharitis** as the chief complaint. The symptoms that they mention—eyelashes falling out and a sensation of sand in the eyes—may seem to point to the remedy *Sulphur*. Since the child will probably have other keynotes that are shared with *Sulphur*, a careful differentiation should be made by the doctor, basing the prescription on the physical generals and on the differing mental states of the two remedy types under consideration.

Some teenagers describe upon careful questioning that they occasionally **perceive quick motions** peripherally, as if an insect or other small creature had whizzed by. This always seems to take place at the edge of the visual field so that they never fully recognize what it might be. While this is mentioned often in older materia medicas, it is not commonly found in practice today with adults and even less so with children.

A similar complaint commonly mentioned by *Medorrhinum* children is that during fevers they develop visual distortions, such as objects appearing larger or smaller than they actually are.

Ears

Some *Medorrhinum* children develop **frequent colds.** Should these children and infants develop colds that are repeatedly treated with antibiotics, sequelae develop in the ears. The most common sequela is a great amount of fluid in the middle ear that causes partial or total deafness, demonstrable by a flattened tympanogram reading. The buildup of fluid and pressure in the middle ear may also lead to a rupture of the eardrum or a history of myringotomies: incisions of the eardrum that release the fluid that makes the eardrum bulge and hurt. In *Medorrhinum* children one finds that the fluid pours out of the ear for a long time, not easily resolving as it does in children of other types.

The ears can itch greatly, particularly those of children who complain of a dry scalp. The sensation, similar to that experienced by *Pulsatilla* and *Silicea* children, is that there are worms in the ear trying to push their way out. This feeling causes them to scratch and scratch with little or no relief.

Nose

Since the immune system is damaged from birth, problems such as **eczema, asthma, and hay fever abound.** At first, the parents only notice the baby's snuffles. The infant or child will **catch colds** very easily and it may seem as if he always has mucus either running from or stuffing up the nose. The parents remember that from the first few months of life the child sneezed often and developed crusts surrounding the outside of the nostrils and was plagued by thick, yellow-green mucus that had to be suctioned out of the nose.

This condition may be quite intractable and obstinate, not yielding to orthodox treatment or more common homeopathic remedies such as *Lycopodium*, *Pulsatilla*, or *Tuberculinum*. As this state often establishes itself at birth, it shows that the nasal area is a weak point in the defense system of the individual and will likely remain susceptible to future problems there. This state of the nose should be considered a major confirmatory clue in the diagnosis of *Medorrhinum*, as in many cases the child has only a few confirmatory symptoms that might lead to this prescription.

Colds may worsen as the infection works its way more deeply into the body and develops into such illnesses as **sinusitis, bronchitis, or asthma.** Parents may mention the repeated use of antibiotics for these more serious conditions, stating that the antibiotics drive the illness back to the nose and cure the bronchitis, but never eradicate the mucous condition in the nose.

The children may also develop nosebleeds along with the infections or in between these bouts.

Older teenagers tend to contract **staphylococcal infections** that resemble those common to *Sulphur* with their red, painful sores.

One should also note that every time some of these children eat **citrus fruit** the nose begins to itch and allergic or asthmatic attacks are set off.

Lastly, there may be problems with hay fever, the main symptoms of which are sneezing and itching of the nose.

Mouth

The mouth, in general, is not greatly affected in *Medorrhinum* children. Occasionally a child complains of **tiny blisters** in the mouth that recur, especially after drinking citrus juice. The blisters may appear either on the tongue or on the inner cheek (the buccal mucosa), as found in *Natrum muriaticum*. The child may also develop fever blisters and herpes as readily as would a *Natrum muriaticum*.

The lips may be **dry, cracked, and peeling.** Mothers may constantly chastise their children for picking at these dry lips. The only time there is a lot of saliva found in the mouth is when they drool in their sleep.

The **teeth** can be identical to *Tuberculinum* teeth in that they are often **serrated and soft**, promoting the easy formation and growth of cavities.

It should be noted that it is impossible to distinguish the remedy *Medorrhinum* from *Tuberculinum* based on the characteristics of the teeth, even though these dental conditions are mentioned as a specific guide to *Tuberculinum* in other materia medicas. The teeth do not differ enough between the two remedies to be able to differentiate one from the other. The only clue that may lead one to prescribe the remedy *Tuberculinum* and not *Medorrhinum* is that the teeth of *Tuberculinum* will not line up correctly, and even after years of orthodontic work may revert to their old crooked lineup, especially in a child with allergies.

The teeth also **discolor** early in life, just as they do in *Lycopodium* children.

Face -

The faces of these children are often graced with very **distinctive features**. The skin may be **pale or gray toned**, as is found with *Tuberculinum* and *Silicea*. The differentiating point is that *Medorrhinum* children often have a **greenish, shiny** look to their skin. The skin looks as if it were polished with wax.

While the **excess oil** produced by overzealous sebaceous glands may be obvious to you, it may not be to the parents. A mother once came to my clinic for the treatment of her little girl, who had earaches. After eliciting the child's medical history, I decided upon the remedy *Medorrhinum*. When asked what the remedy would do for the child, I responded that among other things, one might expect it to normalize the oiliness of her skin. The mother asked, "What oiliness?" I explained, "The oiliness of her face. Don't you see how the light shines off her face, how everything is reflected on the surface of her skin?" The mother still did not understand to what I was alluding. Exasperated, I looked up at the mother—and smiled, as I saw my reflection crudely mirrored on the oily surface of her own face! I eventually treated the entire family of nine people, all but one of whom needed the remedy *Medorrhinum*. One by one, the family members lost the oily condition of their skin. In the end, they all felt quite well, although they still did not seem to understand what I had meant by "oily skin."

The amount of **facial hair is minimal.** This may be noted as a thinness of the beard of teenaged boys. What may be observed in many *Medorrhinum* children is pencil-thin, narrow eyebrows.

Occasionally, the face bears a keynote of this remedy and of this miasmatic inherited tendency in general: **spider hemangiomas.** While these lesions are recognized to be a keynote of *Thuja*, the remedy most closely related to *Medorrhinum*, they should also be thought of as a symptom of *Medorrhinum*. The reddish-blue, spidery-looking spots made up of dilated capillaries under the surface of the skin can be seen in infants as well as children and adults.

Girls may develop **acne** before the onset of the monthly menstrual flow, but this outbreak is much less severe than can be seen in many other remedy types such as *Natrum muriaticum* and *Tuberculinum*.

Younger children develop **fever blisters** easily, especially on and around the lips. Older children may develop other herpetic eruptions on the cheeks that are activated by fevers or by exposure to the sun.

Throat and Neck

As mentioned earlier, the child tends to get colds that lead to a postnasal drip with copious, thick, yellowish mucus. The child snores, hawks, or coughs up phlegm, almost choking on it at times. Colds often drop into the throat, causing painfully swollen tonsils and a raw pain in the throat. The glands of the neck may likewise be swollen and tender during such infections.

Lower Respiratory System

The *Medorrhinum* child is susceptible to **chest colds and/or asthma** from birth. The more severe outcome of these possibilities is that the child is born with asthma.

Asthma

The asthma, described as "tightness," may be felt high up in the chest as opposed to lower in the chest, where most other asthmatics describe the location of this sensation. The cough that accompanies the asthma as well as shortness of breath are both aggravated by dampness, the cold, drafts, drinking orange juice, running, and the season of spring. These conditions are **ameliorated by lying down**, especially on the abdomen. Some children exhibit the keynote that when they begin to cough, they throw themselves onto the bed and bury their heads in the pillows. They either lie in the knee-to-chest position, on their knees at the side of the bed with the abdomen and head pressed on the bed, or on the abdomen. The remedy *Medorrhinum* may at times be prescribed on these signs alone. I treated two-year-old Amanda for a chronic cough. She developed an asthmatic cough at night and had to lie down on her abdomen and bury her face in the pillow in order to fall asleep.

Vomiting may ameliorate an asthmatic attack. Adolescent boys may put their hands in cold water to obtain great relief of their asthma.

The asthma may be worse during the day or from one to five o'clock in the early morning, resembling the *Kali* group in time aggravation.

With asthma, the afflicted may also complain of a **wheezy cough** that arises from high up in the chest. Occasionally, while treating a patient for asthma, one finds that after the first correct remedy is prescribed the asthma stops being low in the chest and is now felt higher up, closer to the throat. Now the child needs to bury his face in the pillows to stop the cough or asthma. This is a time when *Medorrhinum* may be used as the second remedy, complementing the action of the first remedy.

Chest Colds

Chronic chest colds also plague *Medorrhinum* children. The postnasal drip and attendant pharyngitis often drop into the chest and manifest as a **deep, rattling cough**. No matter how hard they try, they cannot dislodge the mucus. The constant, dry cough is severe and seems to tear the throat apart. I have found that if the constitutional remedy *Medorrhinum* does not work, *Spongia tosta* often will. *Spongia tosta* should be added as a complementary remedy to *Medorrhinum* for these coughs.

118

While the cough is aggravated in hot and humid weather, it may originate from exposure to cold, dry air. As with asthma, the cough may be ameliorated by lying on the abdomen. The expectoration tends to be yellow-green and form clumps of mucus that are difficult to dislodge.

A one-year-old girl was brought in for chronic upper respiratory tract infections. The worst complaint for the mother was the child's incessant wet cough. It was most noticeable at night when the child was lying down. The child's chest would tighten up and she would cough and retch on the mucus. As an infant she had spit up mucus along with milk. She would wake up between two and four o'clock in the morning coughing with all her might. While all this pointed to the remedy, I correctly guessed what it would be before the mother ever uttered a word, for she had carried the sleeping child into the office and put her down on the floor and the child promptly rolled up into the knee-to-chest position, burying her face in the carpet and thrusting her seat up into the air. This was the first clue to the remedy. However, after the mother gave the whole case history, an hour had passed and the child remained unmoved in the same position, thereby confirming *Medorrhinum*, which was given to the great benefit of the tiny patient.

Alimentary System

Food Cravings and Aversions

The food **cravings** are quite **unique** and point directly to this remedy. The strongest food cravings are for **salt, sweets, and unripe fruit**, especially the **sour, tart,** or green varieties of plums, bananas, apples, raspberries and others. Many times the favorite is **citrus**: oranges, grapefruits, and even lemons. They may even relish the bitter rind of these fruits. Some children develop canker sores from eating too many of these acid fruits but crave them anyway. Babies often like **juice** in general and orange juice in particular.

They can eat many pieces of citrus fruit at one sitting: "As many as there are in the house," tells one mother. They crave citrus fruit so intensely that they may devour the undiluted frozen fruit juice concentrate if they can get their hands on it.

Some say that they are not hungry in the morning and only wish to drink their orange juice. Occasionally, when a parent becomes a vegetarian and eats many pieces of fruit a day, he or she reports that the *Medorrhinum* child was the most easily convinced member of the household to eat a substantially fruit-filled diet and that it was not a difficult transition.

Besides these sour, acid fruits, they also crave **fat**, especially that which can be found on peppered meats. Only rarely does a patient state that he or she does not crave fat.

While most crave **ice cream** like *Sulphur* children do, at least half the children will also like fish, a symptom that may help to differentiate *Medorrhinum* from *Sulphur* individuals, who hate fish.

These children strongly dislike any foods that tend to be **slimy** such as **eggplant, okra,** and **soft-boiled eggs,** as well as **onions, beans,** and **peas.**

They have a **great thirst for cold drinks** and especially crave to **chew on ice.** The parent may remark that the child drinks the glass down quickly and then loves to chew on any remaining ice. This point is yet another keynote of the remedy *Medorrhinum.*

While Boericke states in his *Materia Medica* that the *Medorrhinum* type craves warm drinks, this finding has not been borne out in my pediatric practice.

Stomach

Medorrhinum is one of the main remedies for the infantile condition commonly known as **failure to thrive** or marasmus. The appetite in this case is great enough to awaken the infant or child to demand food in the middle of the night. At these times the infant becomes restless and irritable, crying or screaming for food. But although the child has a large appetite, due to the vomiting and diarrhea that constantly arise he will be slow to develop. Mothers notice that after the baby nurses he vomits not only milk but also yellow mucus along with the milk.

In older children, this state may also be seen in shy boys; they eat but do not gain weight as they should. After the remedy is given the children usually quickly begin to put on weight and height. Those suffering from this condition will generally also be susceptible to food allergies that cause gastrointestinal or respiratory symptoms.

In **older girls,** anxiety and **tension may lead to nausea** and a tight feeling in the stomach. Teenaged girls, if shy, may develop anorexia or bulimia as discussed in the Mind section. And a point seldom mentioned in older materia medicas is that many *Medorrhinum* teenagers complain of bloated, distended abdomens after eating.

Rectum

The infants usually have a characteristic rash around the genitals, perineum, and anus. This may be in one instance a yeast infection; in another, eczema; and yet in another, psoriasis.

The factor that all these rashes have in common is the intensity of the inflammation. The parents and doctor all worry about this fiery red rash. It may be moist and itchy and in its worst state form vesicles. These more vesicular rashes may resemble a burn.

This is such a persistent eruption that it is remembered by the parents and reported even when the child is seen much later in life after the rash has disappeared. The parents report that they went from one doctor to another trying to find a cure for this rash, yet no matter what treatment was tried, the rash would not disappear.

Colicky infants who have mucus in the stool and must lie on their bellies in a knee-to-chest position may need this remedy. The child may have diarrhea from birth along with the other symptoms of marasmus previously described. This diarrhea in infants is yellow-green and excoriates the anus and surrounding area. It will have an offensive odor. These last two points will aid in differentiating *Medorrhinum* from the more common *Tuberculinum* diarrhea, which, though it may have the same color, typically does not excoriate the skin or have as strong an odor.

Although infantile diarrhea may be present in some cases, many more of the children have chronic constipation from birth; some have a bowel movement only once every five days. The child strains and strains, only to pass very hard, round pellets. Materia medicas give the keynote that the patients strain and pass stool only if leaning backward while on the toilet. This is actually rare in adults and even rarer in children; one should not wait for this confirmation before prescribing the remedy.

Hyperactive boys may not be easily toilet trained; some boys will actually soil their pants whenever they are mad, thereby forcing parents to take the time to clean them and the pants.

Urogenital System

Enuresis

Medorrhinum children, like *Tuberculinum* children, are plagued by nocturnal enuresis, though they usually wet the bed only after they have played very vigorously that day. And, just as in *Tuberculinum*, the urine has a very strong odor. This strong, acrid urine may in fact cause or at least exacerbate the fiery red rash just described. Little girls with such a rash around the perineum may scream and cry when the urine touches the area, as it causes painful burning. Girls may also at an early age develop frequent **cystitis** accompanied by extremely painful urination.

Boys

The **sex organs are adversely affected early in both sexes.** Boys may develop of acute **phimosis** (inflammation of the foreskin of the penis). They may also develop **rashes and warts on the penis.** In an infant or young child such a history reveals the indiscretions of a parent or grandparent. Many boys awaken with **erections** and, if in the same bed, like to rub against the parents or siblings or masturbate, as do *Tuberculinum* boys.

Girls

Girls may develop a variety of **vaginal infections** very early. Even infant girls may develop a vaginal discharge that ranges from a constant, mild yellow stain on the diapers to a full-blown case of vaginitis with an offensive leukorrhea that makes the perineum bright red and blistered. It may itch and discharge a thin, greenish, offensive mucus that excoriates the surrounding tissue.

Older girls may likewise develop vaginitis and, what is more unusual in sexually inactive girls, **pelvic inflammatory disease.** This may also be found later on in life in a woman who constantly complains of ovarian pains or repeated cramping with the menses or ovulation. During laparoscopy it will be discovered that as a child she must have had a pelvic inflammatory infection and now has ovarian cysts and scarring of the fallopian tubes. This sort of history is commonly indicative of this remedy, as the early attack on these organs points to an inherited weakness.

The **menstrual flow** in adolescents is also often affected. The cycle tends to be irregular. The blood may have an unhealthy color, usually being dark and clotted, and gives off an offensive odor.

The flow may arrive with ovarian pains so intense that the girl doubles over with them. An accurate keynote, if one can ask and confirm it, is that the adolescent feels chilly before the flow, especially in the breast area. Also before the menstrual flow, girls may become sad, weepy, and occasionally suicidal.

Both sexes engage in **early sexual experimentation**, and both tend to masturbate as children to release their pent-up sexual energy.

Musculoskeletal System

Extremities

One clue to the prescription of *Medorrhinum* is to watch the children's feet in the office. They persistently **move their feet up and down quickly**. This nervous habit is done unconsciously, and the parents may describe this motion of the feet as one that they see more often at night before the child falls asleep or in the morning when the child first wakes up.

Uncommon **warmth of the feet** is a keynote for these children, sometimes experienced as a burning sensation of the soles. During the day the child wants her shoes and socks off and often **walks barefoot** through the house. This is true even in the wintertime or on cold cement.

In the evening the two characteristics mentioned combine, and fidgety, hot feet can be seen protruding from the covers during sleep.

Along with fidgety feet, children or adolescents may describe the feeling that all their joints (in some, only the furthest joints of the extremities) feel as if they are tightening up and that they must "pop" them to loosen them up and get relief. They may in fact **pop their joints** many times during the interview, especially their knuckles and ankles.

Other distinctive keynotes are **pain and swelling of the soles and ankles.** *Medorrhinum* should be the first remedy considered for the child who complains of painful soles. While this symptom is more common in the adult, a child or teenager occasionally complains of this. They often describe the sensation as needles or sharp pains shooting into the feet and up the ankles. Others say that they feel a pinching in the soles and arches of the feet when they walk, making them favor the sides or edges of the feet as a walking surface. The arches of the feet may ache as well.

Other bones and joints may also suffer discomfort in wet weather. The most common of these complaints is a painful tenderness of the heels or a burning tenderness of the soles of the feet. The soles may also itch and perspire.

Teens may complain of a **painful stiffness in the joints**. As is also found in children needing *Tuberculinum*, *Medorrhinum* can be a remedy for arthritis in youth, especially if it exhibits *Rhus toxicodendron* modalities. Arthritis is aggravated at night and by cold, wet weather, and ameliorated by motion. A strong feature of this miasm is the development of acute rheumatism with pain and swelling in the extremities. The ankles are often the primary seat of the trouble, but the knees are affected also, just as they are in *Thuja* and *Lycopodium* types. Sometimes, not only are the joints affected, as is also found in *Thuja*, but also the bones themselves may hurt—a symptom that is definitely aggravated by touch, or even pressure applied by the body's own weight bearing down on the sufferer's limbs. A slight difference between the two remedies is that *Thuja* bone conditions are very aggravated by the cold, whereas *Medorrhinum* conditions are not nearly so bothered by cold as much as by dampness.

What stands out most in *Medorrhinum* cases is the degree of **swelling of the joints**, most especially of the **ankles**. The swelling is more marked in *Medorrhinum* than in any of the other polychrest remedies. In some teenagers one may find swelling of the ankles without any apparent physiological reason. This swelling is a good guiding symptom for *Medorrhinum*, and if pronounced, should be considered a confirmation of the remedy. This is seen more frequenty in adult women but may also be found in some teenagers.

The child may turn his ankle easily, like other remedy types that have a basically weak constitution.

124

Another common keynote of *Medorrhinum* is that many times the children **bite their nails** and even their cuticles. The nails may split easily, as they do in the related remedy *Thuja*. With *Medorrhinum*, however, the nails will not deform as much as they do with *Thuja* when they grow out.

Skin

The skin of *Medorrhinum* children is susceptible to **growths such as moles and warts**. Children may be covered with many skin tags or warts from birth. They may also develop warts many times during their lives. After giving the remedy *Medorrhinum*, one of the following comments may be heard from the parents: "My son developed warts after taking that remedy." "My daughter developed warts that appeared and then disappeared within a month." "My child's warts started to become painful, especially on the hands and fingers, after taking the remedy." "All the warts have fallen off since the remedy was taken."

While some may fear that these warts are symptoms of a proving, they are actually part of the curative response on the part of the child. One should not change the remedy because of these growths. If one delves into the case more deeply, many times one finds that the child has had these warts before and had them removed. If asked, the children may say that since the remedy was given and the warts appeared, they feel great!

The **infants** often have very **bad rashes in the genital area**, either around the pubic or the perineal area. *Medorrhinum* should be one of the first remedies considered for infants who have eczema from birth, especially if the eczema alternates with bouts of asthma. The *Medorrhinum* eczema has periods when the skin becomes bright red and blistery. The eruption itches severely and oozes a yellow, serous fluid. It may also crack and bleed. The rash may not only be on the perineal area but on the penis or vagina as well.

Frequently after a remedy is given, be it *Medorrhinum* or another, and the complaints disappear, this perineal rash appears. The parent may describe in wonder how this rash used to bother the child years ago, but had finally disappeared with strong medication only to be replaced by the currently presenting chief complaint. When this rash reappears, the other illness will disappear. It is wise to wait and not give the remedy *Medorrhinum* right away. If *Medorrhinum* was the original remedy given, this is a clear sign that it is working and that one should wait; but if another remedy was given, the appearance of the rash heralds the child's reentry into the *Medorrhinum* picture exhibited at birth. One should wait to prescribe this remedy, however, until the *Medorrhinum* picture develops more fully, and more importantly, until the child develops problems that need to be treated. Quite often, if one waits long enough in the cases that do not develop other illnesses, the rash will disappear and the child will become well even without taking the remedy *Medorrhinum*.

A keynote of skin problems that lead to this remedy is the location: the fingertips and the soles of the feet, both of which are peculiar to *Medorrhinum*.

The **alternation of eczema and asthma or eczema and allergies** is very consistent with this remedy type. Also consistent is the ease with which the eczema is suppressed and the child develops respiratory problems or bone disease in response.

The child may also develop **neurodermatitis and urticaria from drinking citrus juice or eating strawberries.** Along with the remedy *Dulcamara, Medorrhinum* may be thought of for the treatment of hives that appear along with upper respiratory tract infections.

Occasionally a child presents with **lipomas, fat cysts, or wens.** *Medorrhinum* should be among the first remedies contemplated, as well as *Calcarea carbonica* and *Thuja*.

Quite a few *Medorrhinum* children have **vitiligo,** consisting of large, circular patches of pale discoloration on the face and abdomen. After the remedy is given, one may find the patches becoming pigmented and fading away.

The skin may appear **oily** all over the body, especially on the face.

It is peculiar, but these children also tend to get many insect bites and allergic reactions to these bites, all over the extremities. These bites are itchy, causing the bitten to scratch them frequently and therefore make them bleed. A neurodermatitis may begin with these reactions to insect stings.

Physical Generals

A frequent time to prescribe the remedy *Medorrhinum* is after the case has been treated first with another remedy. A common scenario follows.

After prescribing the first correct non-*Medorrhinum* remedy, the child does very well. Yet after a certain period of time the case stalls. Simultaneously, a few *Medorrhinum* keynotes arise. The remedy is prescribed and the child progresses nicely again, sometimes requiring yet another "next remedy" at a future time.

Throughout the history of our profession this has been noticed to occur, and from it a persistent misunderstanding developed. The doctor of the past assumed that if the child presented symptoms of the sycotic miasm, the remedy *Medorrhinum* should be prescribed. *Medorrhinum* was then prescribed for anyone who fit the miasm, for anyone who had taken another sycotic remedy, and for anyone who did not improve when given what the doctor had mistakenly thought was the most accurate homeopathic remedy. This program only worked for a certain percentage of patients but not for most.

A more correct analysis follows. The child is given a remedy other than *Medorrhinum*. The remedy acts and progress is made, but then the case grinds to a halt and keynotes of the sycotic miasm arise. It is the nature of the sycotic and tubercular miasms that, if the miasm is actually playing a role in the current disease process, a cure is not easily achieved. It is as if there is a genetic flaw that induces a break in the defenses of the body and makes it too weak to reestablish homeostasis.

At the time subsequent to a remedy's administration, the human organism is usually stimulated to effect a cure. The response of a patient with a miasmatic flaw is to show the genetic weakness by displaying clearly the symptoms of the miasm involved. Many remedies may be called for to treat this miasm, based on differing symptoms. Many times, but not always, when the sycotic patient responds in such a fashion, symptoms indicative of *Medorrhinum* then arise. Properly prescribed, the remedy should only be given when the keynotes begin to show themselves and thus is truly indicated. In these situations one should not expect a full picture of the remedy to emerge because it generally will not. Prescribing with this in mind, the percentage of cases that respond to the remedy *Medorrhinum* will be greatly increased.

Medorrhinum should be considered for children who appear stunted in physical, emotional, or mental development. These children do not develop at a normal rate; it is as if they cannot properly assimilate the nutrients of the food they eat. They often appear emaciated. As with *Natrum muriaticum*, *Lycopodium*, and *Calcarea carbonica*, such thinness disappears as they sprout up and gain weight and height almost as soon as the remedy is given.

The remedy *Medorrhinum* may eventually be needed for the child who is born into a sycotic family. The family history contains diseases common to the miasm such as gonorrhea, asthma, arthritis, angina, and heart attacks. The family tree may begin with diseases of the skin, which progress from there to the respiratory tract, then to the bones or joints, and then to the heart. What one observes and what is important is the progression of these diseases, whether in one person or across a family lineage. In a child such as this, when another well-chosen remedy does not act as it should, **consider *Medorrhinum*—but only if there are strong keynotes of the remedy present.**

These are **hot-blooded** children who like the cool, open air and dislike heat. As a result, they like to uncover and to walk barefoot in any temperature. In differentiating between other "hot" remedies such as *Sulphur* or *Pulsatilla*, it should be noted that *Medorrhinum* may be more sensitive to drafts.

All their discharges are offensive smelling, acrid, and profuse.

They may desire to bathe in cool water, as do *Natrum muriaticum* children. Many materia medicas list the conditions of these children as being ameliorated by dampness, but in practice they often are not. While their health problems are actually aggravated by dampnesss, they are ameliorated by bathing in the sea, which is effective both for specific physical complaints and for general health.

Health complaints are ameliorated by lying on the abdomen, especially respiratory symptoms. Physical, mental, and emotional problems are better in the evening and aggravated in the morning.

Notes on *Medorrhinum* Infants

Serious illnesses that begin from birth help point to this remedy. *Medorrhinum* infants may have difficulty falling asleep, being too restless to relax. Babies wake up often from the abdominal pains of colic. This is especially seen in infants with other characteristic digestive symptoms. Toddlers sleep very warmly and roll out from under the covers. They favor sleeping on their stomachs with their knees tucked under their chests and their buttocks in the air.

Eyes are susceptible to conjunctivitis (recurrent pinkeye) accompanied by swelling, redness, and an excoriating, thick, green discharge.

Frequent colds extend to the ears. Babies have frequent snuffles and colds with thick, yellow-green mucus that crusts outside the nostrils.

Faces may have spider hemangiomas.

Chest colds may occur from birth. These are especially brought on by dampness. The coughs that accompany these colds are wet sounding, noted especially at night. During chest colds toddlers may lie in the knee-to-chest position, which helps prevent coughing. Infants and toddlers may also develop chronic chest colds that eventually lead to asthma, which is ameliorated by the same position.

They may be classified as having failure to thrive with a big appetite. Babies vomit milk just swallowed; such milk often has yellow mucus in it. Babies will like juice, especially orange juice.

The perineum of boys and girls may show characteristic redness and blistering, which can be due to various conditions.

Diarrhea from birth can be found in children who have failure to thrive. The stool is a mucous yellow-green and excoriates the anus.

The urine can be very acidic and cause a recurrent, persistent red rash of the surrounding tissue. Boys may also develop recurrent phimosis.

Vaginal infections can occur in infants and toddlers. The discharge stains the diapers yellow and may be offensive in odor and very excoriating, making the surrounding area red and raw.

Toddlers bite their nails, including their toenails.

Eczema can develop from birth. The rash may begin or be worst in the perineal area. Eczema may alternate with bouts of asthma.

Toddlers are warm and like to wear as little clothing as possible.

Infants have a family history of this miasm.

Infants often appear stunted physically, emotionally, and/or mentally.

Medorrhinum Outline

I. Mental/Emotional Characteristics
  A. Extremes of personality
    1. Extreme extroversion
      a) Very vital
      b) Loud
      c) Abundant energy
      d) Very open
        (1) Meet others easily
        (2) Talk spontaneously during the interview
      e) May lead to early experimentation with drugs and sex
      f) Energy may alternate with total inertia
      g) Hyperactivity
        (1) Great amount of energy
        (2) Cannot sit still
        (3) Nasty
        (4) Cannot concentrate, especially after eating citrus fruit
    2. Extreme introversion
      a) Very shy and timid
      b) Loners
      c) Feel very distant from other people
      d) Love animals
      e) Whisper in the interview
      f) Become sad and cry easily
      g) Become despondent
        (1) Lonely
        (2) May become suicidal
      h) Self-punishing; may mutilate themselves with razors
      i) Anorexic
    3. Oscillating behavioral extremes
      a) From extroverted cruelty may become coy and introverted
      b) Fitful emotions
        (1) Jekyll and Hyde personality; extreme

polarity of behavior
(2) May be serene one moment and throw a
temper tantrum the next
B. Meanness and cruelty
1. High energy
2. Much fighting and hitting
3. Cannot be reasoned with during rages
4. Strike parents in the interview
5. Like to hit and be hit
6. Like to watch frightening, violent movies
a) As if violence were their native language
b) As if they cannot comprehend love
7. May become obstinate
C. Lying
1. Attempt to deceive others by omission of information
2. Disregard for the feelings of others
D. Confusion
1. Difficulty concentrating
a) Writing
b) Forget words
2. Difficulty judging the passage of time
3. Short attention span; "space out" often
4. May lead to feeling very alienated from others
5. May feel "out of body"
a) As though disintegrating
b) Leads to panic
6. Answer slowly in the interview
7. May lead to dyslexia; all types of mistakes in writing
8. Mistakes in speech
H. Fears
1. Being alone in the dark
a) Ghosts
b) An ominous "something" out to "get" them
2. Large bodies of water
3. Animals
a) Sometimes feared
b) Especially "slimy" ones
(1) Toads

  (2) Snakes

  (3) Jellyfish

I. Sleep

 1. "Night people"; hard to put to bed at night

 2. Thrash about during sleep, especially the feet

 3. Very warm and may uncover

  a) Whole body

  b) Feet only

 4. Sleep positions

  a) On the abdomen

  b) Knee-to-chest

 5. Nightmares of being chased

 6. Awaken unrefreshed

II. Physical Symptomatology

 A. Head area

  1. Head

   a) Hair may be very dry and brittle

   b) Flaking of the scalp

  2. Eyes

   a) Inflammations with intense signs

    (1) Redness

    (2) Swelling

    (3) Pus

   b) Hallucinations

    (1) Peripheral

    (2) Of the quick motions of animals

  3. Ears

   a) Fluid in the middle ear due to coryza

   b) Itchy ears

  4. Nose

   a) Chronic snuffles in babies

   b) Repeated coryzas; crusts of mucus develop
    around the nasal alae

  5. Face

   a) Skin tone

    (1) Pale

    (2) Gray

    (3) Greenish

      b) Oily skin; reflects light well

      c) Facial hair is minimal; thin eyebrows

      d) Spider hemangiomas

      e) Herpetic eruptions develop easily

6. Mouth

      a) Fever blisters

         (1) In the mouth

         (2) On the tongue

         (3) Worse after eating citrus fruit

      b) Deeply serrated teeth

7. Throat and Neck: colds become chronic postnasal catarrh

      a) Phlegm

         (1) Thick

         (2) Yellowish

      b) Much hawking up to clear passages

B. Torso

1. Lower Respiratory System

      a) Bronchitis from birth

      b) Colds that drop into the lungs

         (1) Rattling cough

         (2) Amelioration from lying on the abdomen

      c) Asthma from birth

         (1) Tightness in the upper chest

         (2) Cough

         (3) Aggravations

            (a) Dampness

            (b) Cold

            (c) Drafts

         (4) Amelioration from lying on the abdomen

2. Alimentary System

      a) Food cravings and aversions

         (1) Cravings

            (a) Sour fruit

               i) Unripe

               ii) Juicy

               iii) Citrus (oranges)

               iv) Granny Smith apples

        (b) Salt

        (c) Sweets

        (d) Fat

        (e) Meat

    (2) Aversions: slimy foods

        (a) Runny eggs

        (b) Oysters

        (c) Okra

        (d) Eggplant

        (e) Onions

    (3) Thirst

        (a) For cold drinks

        (b) Chew on ice

b) Stomach: failure to thrive

    (1) With a big appetite

    (2) In infants

c) Rectum

    (1) Perineal rash

        (a) Characteristic and common

        (b) In infants

        (c) May accompany any disease

        (d) Bright red

        (e) Blistery

        (f) May be resistant to treatment with ointments

    (2) Diarrhea in infants

        (a) With marasmus

        (b) Red rash of the buttocks

    (3) Difficult to toilet train when hyperactive

    (4) Usually tend toward constipation

3. Urogenital System

  a) Bed-wetting after vigorous exertion during the day

  b) Boys

    (1) Inflammations such as phimosis

    (2) Growths on the penis such as warts

    (3) Frequent erections and masturbation from an early age

        (4) Fiery red rash of the genital area

    c) Girls

        (1) Vaginitis from an early age

           (a) Yellowish-green discharge

           (b) Excoriating discharge

        (2) Pelvic inflammatory disease in the sexually inactive

        (3) Sexually active; masturbation from an early age

        (4) Fiery red rash of the labia

        (5) Menstruation problems

           (a) Premenstrual syndrome

              i) Sad and weepy

              ii) Suicidal

           (b) Menstrual pains

              i) Severe

              ii) During the flow

C. Musculoskeletal System: extremities

    1. Feet

        a) Move them up and down

        (1) Continuously

        (2) Observed in the office

        b) Very warm

        (1) Uncover during sleep

        (2) Walk barefoot in the wintertime

        c) Very painful soles

    2. Swollen ankles

    3. Joints

        a) Stiff joints that need to be "popped"

        b) Arthritis that begins in the feet or ankles

        (1) Aggravation from first motion

        (2) Amelioration

           (a) From continued motion

           (b) Sometimes from bathing in the ocean

           (c) Acute rheumatism with swelling of the joints

    4. Bite their fingernails and toenails to the quick

D. Skin

1. Many growths
   a) Moles
   b) Warts
   c) Skin tags
   d) Anywhere on the body
2. Genital skin problems
   a) Rashes
   b) Inflammations
   c) Eczema
3. Eczema from birth
4. Lipomas
5. Vitiligo
6. Oily appearance
7. Insect bites on the extremities
   a) Itch greatly
   b) Become inflamed

III. Physical Generals
   A. Very warm-blooded
   B. All discharges are offensive and acrid
   C. History of gonorrhea in the parents
   D. Parent who died of a heart attack
      1. Apparently healthy
      2. In his thirties or forties
   E. A strong family history of the above symptoms
   F. Aggravation from dampness
   G. Amelioration by lying on the abdomen
   H. Amelioration at the seaside

Medorrhinum Confirmatory Picture

This type has a volatile personality that flips between extremes of extroversion and shyness. These children are immensely vital; they experiment early with sex and drugs and make contact with others easily. They may become mean. The same children may become very introverted, shy, and sad; they may love and talk to animals to the exclusion of people. They have periods of confusion and short attention spans. They fear that "something out there" will come to "get" them.

Confirmatory Checklist

- Night people; awaken unrefreshed in the morning
- Repeated colds, bronchitis, and asthma from birth that are aggravated by dampness
- Postnasal catarrh, forcing frequent clearing of the throat
- Pale, greenish, greasy face with little hair and spider hemangiomas
- Crave unripe fruit, sweets, salt, and fat
- Avoid eggplant and slimy foods
- Thirsty for ice-cold drinks and chew on ice
- Intense, chronic perineal rash
- High sex drive; masturbate early
- Very warm-blooded
- Hot feet; walk barefoot and uncover
- Painful soles and swollen ankles
- Often bite the nails
- Skin growths
- A strong family history of the above symptoms
- History of gonorrhea in the family
- Aggravation from dampness
- Amelioration at the seaside
- Amelioration from lying on the abdomen

Natrum muriaticum

Mental/Emotional Characteristics

"Youth is wasted on the young" is a saying that adults, observing young ones at play, often repeat. How sad, then, to find a child who has the seriousness and the heavy burden of the aged upon his young shoulders. And yet this is exactly what one finds in a *Natrum muriaticum* child.

Reserved in the Interview

As a group, *Natrum muriaticum* children are very **well behaved and obedient**. Their behavior and neatness may make some of these youths appear sharp-featured and severe, in contrast to their sensitive eyes and gentle manner. Their behavior is reserved in public, even if among siblings in the doctor's office. In the waiting room they either sit patiently and play quiet games or act as though they were the parents, picking up after younger siblings.

One may find a young *Natrum muriaticum* scholar sitting in a chair doing homework or hidden in a corner seat with his bookish, bespectacled face buried in the latest science fiction adventure or novel. He may be shy or boisterous in a small crowd, but if the parent intimates that what he is doing is not proper, he snaps into shape.

Teenaged Nina, helped by the remedy *Natrum muriaticum*, was too reserved, shy, and sensitive to wait in the office and preferred to sit outside on the the trunk of her car playing woeful ballads on her guitar. She showed us the contents of her trunk, which was filled with emotionally charged mementos. In it were original paintings, special books, and songs she had written; precious sentimental objects she carried around with her wherever she went.

139

In the examination room the doctor may find several different behaviors. One child sits up straight with her legs crossed, her hands folded, and all her muscles tensed. Another child, perhaps adolescent, exhibits how physical distancing can be manifested by slouching with his legs up on the seat, putting those legs and his entire body between the doctor's intrusive questions and himself. Yet another child sprawls on the floor behind his parent's chair, apparently relaxed while reading a book. While this may seem to show a nonchalant attitude as may be found in a more carefree remedy type such as *Sulphur*, the *Natrum muriaticum* child acts this way to **avoid emotional communication with the doctor.**

Some children may constantly look to the parent to answer for them, never wishing to answer for themselves. However, other *Natrum muriaticum* children respond to questions very maturely and resent it if a parent interrupts or interferes in any way. One may also find, especially in **teenaged boys**, that they **respond grudgingly yet completely.** In these boys, disgust is easily observed on the face; the mouth grimaces as if eating a rotten cherry with every answer. The monosyllabic yes or no answer to each question is but a thin veneer that does not hide the facial expression, which conveys another message. It is as if one can clearly observe the thought processes leading to this mask of repulsion: "I do not want to be here. I was brought here against my will by my parents. Okay, one day I may forgive them for that, but why all these stupid questions? I was brought in for my headaches; why am I being grilled about my friends, my fears, my schoolwork?"

A child may wear too much clothing and refuse to take off her coat during the interview. She sits with her hands stuffed deep into her pockets, her body shifted away from the doctor. With stooped shoulders and a narrowed chest, she acts shy and reticent, answering almost in a whisper. Such patients close off their chests to any possible emotional connection that may occur at this new office with this new doctor.

Others seem very **nervous**, as if they are about to faint from the sheer trauma of the initial interview. They may try to act in a mature manner and offer appropriate answers, yet the responses are followed by a nervous giggle. They may attempt to not appear nervous—for instance, by slouching in their chairs—but as always, their body language betrays them. The whole body may be turned away from the doctor and they may never make any significant eye contact. Even in their most relaxed posture they appear tense. By taking a step back and observing the child's whole demeanor, it can be seen that only the mouth is moving: the rest of the body seems very stiff, as if frozen.

Natrum muriaticum **girls** often **cross their legs and ceaselessly move an ankle in a circle**, round and round, as if they are releasing the tension brought on by the interview. The foot moves more and more slowly as one delves into touchier emotional issues and speeds up during lighter, more enjoyable questions.

Occasionally it is felt by all in the room that a child is baring his or her soul to the interviewer. Suddenly the mood in the room changes and a very intimate bond begins to form; all joking disappears and the child begins to reveal what becomes the central focus of the case—the true **sensitive, grieved, emotional state.**

It is not uncommon to have a *Natrum muriaticum* patient who is extremely **attentive and proper,** asking, "Pardon?" or "Excuse me?" if he did not hear what was asked of him.

Perfectionism

The first thing that strikes one about a *Natrum muriaticum* child is how **well-groomed** he or she is. Clean clothes and meticulously combed hair are the rule. The great attention paid to physical appearance complements the fine features and sensitive eyes. At a very early age these children may pick out coordinated outfits and demand to dress themselves. Hair barrettes match the skirt and the socks, which are folded neatly right above the ankle. The boys' shirts are tucked in tightly and the hair is parted perfectly. The doctor himself is impressed and may look at these clean, handsome boys and think, "This is the type I want my daughter to marry."

Almost all *Natrum muriaticum* children tend toward perfectionism, which **may manifest at a very tender age.** Toddlers may become toilet trained at seventeen or eighteen months. By nineteen months they may walk up to the mother with a diaper and demand to be changed. At two years of age they may ask to have their hands washed several times throughout the day. At the age of four they may dust their furniture. They **like their rooms neat,** their beds made, and their books and toys put away. They become irritated if a sibling is messy. If a room is shared with a sibling, they may ask for clear borders to be placed in the room, demanding such an arrangement especially if they share a space with a *Sulphur* youth. Their side of the room stays clean! One boy would sleep on the living room couch in protest if his sister, who shared his room, would not pick up after herself.

They **may seem possessive** by not letting their friends or siblings touch their special objects, but this is not out of true possessiveness; rather, it is out of the desire to keep their things clean, in order, and unbroken. These children never lose any items of personal value and will **categorize, organize, and clean** them with enjoyment and great care. Their things are kept neat and in place, from books to baseball cards, toy cars to dolls.

Perfectionism is noted out of the house as well. One may find them to be as **neat at school** as at home; their lockers and cubbyholes are far neater than those of their classmates. The **drive for perfection and success** often finds a *Natrum muriaticum* youngster the school paper editor or running for a post in student government.

They become depressed or hysterical if they do not receive good grades on exams or report cards. They cry or tear up the offending page if they make a mistake while writing. They often work on homework assignments until they are absolutely sure there are no mistakes, especially if it is to be graded. While coloring, they may tear up the picture if they accidentally cross over the black line. They may weep and pound the bed when frustrated; if, for instance, they cannot figure out a math problem. If they do make a mistake, they often do not ask for help because they **think that they are "bad" people for having made the mistake** and so stop trying.

It is interesting to note that in perfectionistic *Natrum muriaticum* children who are sycotic in miasm, such fastidiousness does not win respect or approbation; instead it makes those around them absolutely nauseated by this "nit-picky" behavior. Instead of being scolded for making mistakes, the child is disliked for being too good: a "goody two-shoes."

Some children may honestly say that they do not care much about preserving their things or the organization of possessions, remaining unconcerned if their rooms become a mess. The one fussiness that does remain in these cases is that they take great pains to comb their hair and dress neatly and appropriately.

It is interesting to note that after the remedy has acted, the perfectionism that made the child's world an impenetrable sphere disintegrates and they begin to blossom and change. Often after taking the remedy the child becomes outgoing, friendly, somewhat messy, and occasionally boisterous. Even if the physical problem that brought the child in to the doctor has not been greatly ameliorated by the remedy, the prescription should not be changed too quickly, for this strong and dramatic change in the emotional sphere shows that the remedy has acted deeply and should be allowed to continue its action until otherwise indicated.

Self-Consciousness

Natrum muriaticum children are very self-conscious, asking themselves, "What do they think of my haircut, my pimples, my clothes, my parents' car?" They are very **concerned with others' opinions about them.** This is one of the reasons why they are such perfectionists. They feel strong emotions and are offended easily, so that if they are laughed at or ridiculed in any way their entire self-concept falls apart. It reinforces the **negative self-image** that dwells inside.

This degraded self-image mingled with social insecurities is the basis for many **obsessive, perfectionistic behaviors.** One way to escape the ridicules of childhood is to appear invulnerable or perfect. "I won't give anybody a chance to pick on me." This "siege mentality" creates great anxiety in the child as he strives to achieve the unachievable—perfection.

Self-consciousness shows up in other ways as well. The child may be fine while playing or talking to one or two other children. Groups, however, are a different story. The child may be **terrified of parties** and refuse to go to any, be it a friend's birthday party or a school function. If a **physical problem** of his is on the surface and noticeable, this self-conscious attitude becomes acute. If there is a scar, rash, or arthritic node, the child sidesteps public questioning and scrutiny by avoiding having to take off any clothes. It is this type of child who refuses to go swimming with other children, or is terribly embarrassed by having to change clothes in the locker room.

Fear of Ridicule

Emotionally, *Natrum muriaticum* youngsters are very **sensitive.** They become embarrassed easily. They seem tense because they do not want to make any mistakes. Many do not try anything new if they fear that they might fail. This resistance may range from that of the child who refuses to play due to poor physical coordination to the shyness of the child who will not try to make new friends. While in this respect they may behave similarly to *Lycopodium*, the root cause is different. A *Lycopodium* child fears a loss of social status, whereas in *Natrum muriaticum* the pressure to succeed comes from within. The **self-recrimination**, the emotional self-punishment for being a bad person, would be too much to bear.

Teenagers may be able to articulate these self-flagellating thoughts very clearly, and perhaps during the interview the whole scenario will be re-enacted. If the child makes a mistake in speech or answers a question improperly, even if it is because the question was not properly understood, the child may readily blush, especially if the youngster is a boy.

Because the *Natrum muriaticum* child is so very self-conscious, intensely aware of himself in every interaction, he is aware of every little faux pas he makes. Tension and self-condemnation quickly fill the room; be sensitive to this, as the remedy becomes clear at this point. One can almost hear him say, "I am an idiot, this is proof that I am an idiot, I am worthless. Never again will I make such a mistake." All this happens with a mature attitude, unlike responses by the more childish *Lycopodium* or *Pulsatilla* personalities. Or, for that matter, *Sulphur*, who will shrug or laugh at the mistake along with everyone else.

It is this tendency toward self-blame that pushes these children to perfect any endeavors they take on. Theirs is an inner drive to achieve, the likes of which few other remedy types possess. They may choose poetry, music, the visual arts, or sports—it does not really matter what the vehicle of creative expression is. What is consistent is that they **excel at whatever they choose.**

This drive to succeed is born out of the child's **dissatisfaction with her own performance or creation.** The dissatisfaction leads her to push her abilities ever further toward perfection, always criticizing any finished piece or performance, never hearing the compliments or applause. In athletics the child may not care for team sports and instead will favor individual pursuits such as track or gymnastics.

Because of their perfectionism and dedication, they often finish first in competitions—but the praise can go unheard. They may be **embarrassed by the attention** it brings or they may focus only on their mistakes. It is not so much for these accolades, then, that they choose individual pursuits, but because they feel as if they stand out too much in group activities, that they never really quite fit in. But here it is again! All the applause and the spotlight—and once more they are "sticking out."

The overly conscientious nature of *Natrum muriaticum* may cause **anxiety attacks** in the youth. One adolescent patient, Peter, had severe stomachaches and headaches whenever he became anxious about his mathematics class. He had panic attacks before exams from fear that he would not receive good grades. His fears were not based on reality, as he was an excellent student and his parents had never pushed him to perform. Again, this instance is not one of a performance fear, as can be found with *Lycopodium* or *Silicea*, but rather of a self-generated need to do well, which goes along with other apparently inborn needs and signs of perfectionism: **cleanliness, order, and organization.** It is not that the parents force them into it; this is a natural state for them. However, as a symptom, this perfectionism points readily to *Natrum muriaticum* as a remedy because, though it is a natural state for them, it is not a natural state for a child to be so fastidious.

Profound Emotions

Natrum muriaticum children experience emotions very profoundly, and are especially predisposed to **sadness.** A death in the family, separation or divorce, or siblings and friends moving away can all trigger this predisposition. Grief alone is not enough to warrant the prescription of this remedy; they need to respond to the grief with symptomatology that fits the *Natrum muriaticum* picture.

Whenever a child develops **disease after a severe depression or when depression accompanies an illness**, *Natrum muriaticum* should be considered. One child developed a depression with his eczema, another developed arthritis after a bout with depression. One child had dysmenorrhea after a death in the family, another had headaches after the parents divorced, while yet another had chronic upper respiratory tract infections after her best friend moved away. One should always ask about what has been occurring in the child's life as it will often provide a window into the internal emotional state. Grief and sadness are etiologies for *Natrum muriaticum* illnesses as much as suppressed eruptions are for *Sulphur*.

With such profound emotions, they become very **sensitive to the slightest criticism**, from which they shut down and become defensive. After they have been corrected they may act very hurt and withdraw to sulk for some time. The offender may not even realize what he or she has done and ask, "What happened?" to which the reply is, "Nothing." "Did I say something wrong?" "No." Yet the child or teenager may glare at the parent, slam the door, and wear a disgusted look. The slightest offense can rock their fragile self-concept to the core and throw them into the pattern of self-denigration for which they are so well known.

Introversion

Above all else, *Natrum muriaticum* at any age is a **loner**. When relating to others, they like to interact on a one-to-one basis, hating and fearing larger groups. The young *Natrum muriaticum* may never like going to parties because of shyness and introversion and a feeling of being out of place. Often they do not have many close friends and feel that no one understands them. They typically have only one or two good friends at most.

They are budding artists, poets, or musicians who **take their creativity very seriously**. Because they push others away in fear and hypersensitivity, others begin to think of them as aloof and seemingly too serious for such young people. They may act as though they carried the burden of the world's cares upon their slender shoulders—though resentfully!

This emotionally sensitive and reactive nature combined with great shyness makes the youngster seem closed and emotionless; this could not be further from the truth. **Intense and deeply felt emotions** pour out onto the pages of diaries, the canvases of paintings, and the ethers in the singing of woeful songs as they release their pent-up emotions through artistic expression. Children of this type are shy with people and often have a natural love for and become very close to animals.

They seek any activity that allows them a **refuge** from ridicule and an opportunity to vent their emotions. The fantasy world waiting for them in books is one reason why they are often voracious readers. They like to inhabit the world inside their heads, a world where they can be emotionally open and share feelings easily with others. The books they choose, therefore, often have a great deal of active dialogue between children, such as is found in the currently popular Baby-Sitter's Club series.

Children universally go through periods of introversion. In *Natrum muriaticum* individuals, however, this phase is **protracted and seemingly addictive**; reading stories and going to movies or watching television allows them to feel a wide range of emotions without the risk of getting emotionally hurt or anyone else being involved. This pattern becomes commonplace for *Natrum muriaticum* people as they grow up.

Family Affairs

At school functions one may find a *Natrum muriaticum* sitting next to her parents and avoiding the gaze of everyone else; or on the contrary, embarrassed by her parents and refusing to acknowledge or speak to them throughout the entire affair. As the parents describe this episode, the child will be seen either slumping in her chair with a sad, faraway look in her eyes or glaring at her parents with a look that could kill and a mind that could be read as thinking: "God, you are awful! Why are you saying this? Are you trying to embarrass me to death?"

"It is my fault that this terrible thing is happening, I caused this divorce." "My brother died because of me." These are the kinds of thoughts that plague such children about their families. In the alcoholic family, they often cast themselves as the heroic savior: "There is only one thing to be done: I must take care of them. It is my responsibility, my fault alone." It is incredible and sometimes tragic that one finds such **guilt and remorse** in a child of perhaps seven years.

Grudges against and **hatred of certain family members** can often be seen in an adult who claims to have forgiven offending kin but even forty or fifty years later cannot forget early indignities and injustices. When one finds the resentment against family members or hatred and guilt in the peacekeeping child, *Natrum muriaticum* should come to mind.

Weeping

If they are scolded or if the parents are harsh with them, it may bring on torrents of tears. They are so **sensitive to reprimand** that they may weep if merely **looked at the** "wrong way." If they are punished, it reinforces their feelings of resentment, self-condemnation, and worthlessness. This and the desire for anonymity in order to escape ridicule is why *Natrum muriaticum* is found under the rubric: Mind; Looked at; aversion. In the interview the child will most likely not look at the doctor but more often gaze out the window or at the floor, especially when speaking. For the most part, it is enough for a mother just to look at her child to keep him in line.

They weep not only when chastised but also when they are mad or frustrated with their own perceived lack of ability. When they weep from anger like this, they may also storm off to the bedroom or bathroom to be alone and cry.

The hyperactive *Natrum muriaticum* is enraged at being contradicted and weeps from that rage. This should be added to Kent's *Repertory* under the rubric: Mind; Weeping, anger, from. It is this type of *Natrum muriaticum* child who insults his parents during the interview.

The child weeps easily and exhibits an **aversion to being held**, having a desire to be alone rather than consoled. Crying may alternate with laughing. Sometimes, when hearing something sad and moreover when having to tell someone else disheartening news, a **smile inappropriately** and helplessly comes to the lips. This is very characteristic of this remedy type and explains why *Natrum muriaticum* is found under the rubrics: Mind; Laughs; immoderately, and Mind; Laughs; involuntarily. The child may also smile involuntarily with every question asked of him during the interview. Laughter at these times is not the robust mirth seen in *Sulphur* children, but a tense and nervous titter.

Aggravation from Consolation

They often resent being handled or interfered with as toddlers. Later in life, this turns into a negative reaction to consolation. They may actually desire consolation from their parents, but they never ask for it. They stand apart from others or run to their rooms if upset. "I am the rock of the family. No one must know that I am needy, that I feel insecure." Attempts to console them precipitate an even greater sadness, making a bad situation worse. Since they feel that no one *really* understands them, consolation is not accepted as valid. Some actually have tantrums or violently push the consoling person away.

They may also be averse to consolation for merely a short length of time until they resolve their internal conflicts: "After an argument, I want to be alone for two hours, and then I want to talk to my parents about it." With acute disease this **close-mouthedness** may be absolutely maddening to the attending adults. The child may moan, cry, and groan but not say what is disturbing him. The parents justly become frustrated when they cannot figure out what is ailing their dear child.

The picture is **sulky**: with the description that "she can't bring herself to be happy" in the *Materia Medica*, Kent goes right to the heart of the matter. *Natrum muriaticum* children tend to cling to a certain belief about themselves, such as that they are so bad, every negative event or consequence must be their fault. Much of their psychology revolves around dealing with this issue; they are very serious children with adult-sized conflicts.

Anger

Angry grudges may develop, especially after being ridiculed or experiencing sadness. When hurt, they reexperience the humiliation over and over again, burning with each fresh revelation and fuming as every nuance of the conflict slaps them in the face. It may take years for them to forgive and forget this insult.

Anger may provoke yelling, but of a less violent variety than that typical of *Nux vomica* or *Tuberculinum*. If, however, the parent yells back, sensitivity takes over again and the child shuts down quickly, as if coming back to reality. He or she might disappear into a private corner to mope and sulk, taking hours to come out of it. Insolent *Natrum muriaticum* children are irritable not only when consoled or scolded, but also occasionally upon awakening.

Anxiety

A **fear of evil** or that something awful will happen is common. There is a feeling with these children that something will inevitably prove that the world is cruel and harsh, thereby confirming their basically harsh world view.

"Where are you going?" "When will you be back?" "When do we get there?" "How should I act?" "I don't want to go to a new school." These are examples of the anxiety of *Natrum muriaticum* concerning **family members** and **the unknown**. Anxiety about parents who do not arrive home on time is symptomatic of this type, as is the sometimes voiced desire that a parent drive more slowly and watch the road carefully. It is as if they cannot bear the thought of losing a loved one and so try to prevent what they nonetheless fear is unavoidable. This symptom is found in the Kent's *Repertory* under Mind; Fear; happen, something will.

Typically, there is partial compensation for this fear in the form of an **attempt to control events**. They must know what is going to happen next, what schedule is to be followed. This knowledge gives them the opportunity to plan a change of activities without becoming upset. These are children who, like *Calcarea carbonica*, need to finish all tasks once they are begun.

They are **irritated by excitement**, by strong emotions, and by loud noises such as thunder. Their nervous systems are so tense that strong stimuli wreak havoc with them. This is why *Natrum muriaticum* children may need *Ignatia amara* acutely; their nerves are strung so taut that with too much strain they develop *Ignatia amara* symptomatology.

Fears

Fears similar to those of *Phosphorus* may haunt them: **fear of the dark, of being alone, of thunderstorms, of snakes, spiders, killer bees, and insects with large mandibles; fear that the cat will die; or fear that there is something scary around the corner.** They have a great fear of **robbers**, imagining that within each evening shadow there hides a thief. Such a child may come home and breathlessly inform her parents that she matches perfectly the description of a child who is likely to be **kidnaped.**

They may be anxious about having to **speak in public.** Anxiety about health may be apparent, though this is found more commonly in adults. One of their strongest fears, if present, is a fear of **heights**, as strongly presented as one would find with *Sulphur* or *Calcarea carbonica.* Eight-year-old Cyrus became terrified when having to cross a bridge. He would scream, cry, and beg to hold his father's hand as he walked, trembling, over the bridge with his eyes closed. This same boy also had nightmares about bridges coming apart and he himself falling into the abyss. While this may seem to be an extreme example, similar experiences of equal vividness can be found in many *Natrum muriaticum* children.

The child may also have **claustrophobia** or a fear of being pinned down. This is experienced most often during wrestling, tackle football, and other sports that present an opportunity for such contact and constraint.

Slowness

Occasionally the *Natrum muriaticum* child is slow to develop mentally or physically. He may walk and talk later than most children and may exhibit dyslexia. It can be a real struggle for this child to become a good student, especially in mathematics and other subjects that require much abstract thinking. Rochelle, an adolescent student with this dysfunction, miscalculated all the ingredient amounts while attempting to make bread from a recipe. The bread was, of course, a complete failure—and Rochelle, overcome with frustration, cried bitterly.

The main problem, as bluntly explained by another teenager, is that she herself felt that she was just too dense and slow at school. She could not concentrate well and responded slowly to questions. To the *Natrum muriaticum* child these **mistakes are unbearable** and make her weep with frustration and humiliation, as did the youth who would be a baker. The slowness may have an etiology of brain injury during a difficult birth or in early childhood. This trauma to the brain may help us understand the relationship between *Natrum muriaticum* and *Natrum sulphuricum*, a remedy well known for helping to heal the aftereffects of head injuries.

Sleep

The sleep of *Natrum muriaticum* children is **often troubled**. Many find it hard to fall asleep in the first place and sometimes lie awake in their beds for several hours before succumbing. There are several common obstacles to sleep. Some **stay awake to recapitulate** the social and emotional encounters of the day. It is as if the emotions that were repressed during the actual exchanges can finally be experienced in their full magnitude. They go over the details of every conversation as if from phonographic memory, finally letting themselves feel the emotions they could not allow earlier. Besides rehashing the events of the day, they may do the same thing by thinking over the next day's plans and activities. They sometimes talk to themselves during this time, being thoroughly engrossed in this fantasy life. During this time of aloneness, a child may pore over novels about teenagers, experiencing adventures vicariously through such books.

Some children, like some *Natrum muriaticum* adults, **force themselves to stay awake** at night rather than relinquish a wakeful mind busy constructing social scenarios to unconsciousness. Sometimes the forced wakefulness is the result of great anger, which makes the child act out; to spite the parent, he forces himself to stay awake, sitting up in bed and making enough noise so that the parents have no doubt that he is not asleep. Often after the remedy has acted, this type of child reports that he is able to fall asleep at an earlier hour. This can be taken as a confirmation that the child is spending less time in the world of make-believe and more in the present. *Natrum muriaticum* children may also complain of waking up in the middle of the night and thinking about things that need to be done.

They usually sleep on the **left side** or on the **back**. Some stay covered because of chills that develop in bed or just to feel secure being buried in their blankets, while others may uncover. They can **talk** (sometimes revealing secrets) **and walk** in their sleep. *Natrum muriaticum* and *Phosphorus* are the two most common remedies for sleepwalking found under the rubric: Mind; Somnambulism in Kent's *Repertory*. In *Natrum muriaticum*, sleep-walking typically involves children getting up from bed and going into the living room to converse with parents for several minutes with the eyes open—but the conversation does not make sense completely. They then go back to sleep for the rest of the night and in the morning do not recall the incident at all.

Occasionally, *Natrum muriaticum* children **perspire** heavily on the head or all over while asleep.

Enuresis in little **boys** who are shy and fine skinned and who dislike being looked at will often respond to the remedy *Natrum muriaticum*. This is a common syndrome, something that I have observed many times, yet it is not described in homeopathic reference books. These are the soft-spoken boys who turn their feet in out of coyness in the interview and are picky eaters. It is interesting that the enuresis of this remedy type is marked by the fact that the child, though ostensibly asleep, finds some kind of receptacle in which to urinate. Some children walk up to a plant in the room and urinate into the pot, while others find a sink or a wastebasket.

Many *Natrum muriaticum* children experience **anxiety-fraught dreams**. They dream of being chased, of being behind enemy lines during a war, or of a ghoul such as Dracula breaking in and seizing them. They dream of robbers, as do the adults, or of fires after fire drills or other possible, if implausible, disasters. They may dream that the school has moved and they cannot find it, that they are late for class, that the teacher ridicules them, or that an important exam is given when they are unprepared. Others may dream that they have been kidnaped, or that their parents cannot see them or just do not notice them, or that they have been abandoned. While these last symptoms resemble those of *Pulsatilla*, the *Natrum muriaticum* aversion to consolation and a strong thirst helps to easily differentiate it from *Pulsatilla*, who craves consolation and is thirstless.

Their sleep, even when thus disturbed, is mostly **refreshing**, although some will awaken in the morning unrested. In these cases, they may wake up irritable, though not as grumpy as *Lycopodium* or *Nux vomica*. They may likewise not wish to speak much until later in the morning.

Vertigo

The child may experience vertigo with his headaches and from becoming overheated in the sun. This may be aggravated by reading, walking, and looking up.

Physical Symptomatology

Head

Skin **eruptions** often develop around the margins of the hairline and behind the ears, which ooze a thin, watery fluid that coagulates to a slightly yellow-tinged scab. The rash may be eczema or psoriasis and may flake or itch terribly, especially when the child becomes overheated.

The **hair** may be very dry and brittle and easily split on the ends or may be fine and oily, but will most always be well groomed.

Often *Natrum muriaticum* children will **not wear hats**, not needing them for warmth as well as not wishing the hat to ruin their fine hairstyles. The only time they do desire hats is when they are out in the full sun. Without a hat in this case, the child is destined for a headache, heat prostration, or sunstroke.

Headaches

Headaches are a **frequent complaint** of the *Natrum muriaticum* child. They may accompany any acute illness or occur periodically every week or two or every month. The headaches may begin, as do migraines, with visual loss on the contralateral side. The rubric in Kent's *Repertory*: Vision; loss of vision; headache at beginning of, is too limited and lacks the remedies *Natrum muriaticum*,

Phosphorus, Sulphur, and *Tuberculinum,* all of which should be listed in bold type.

The actual headache may start just as vision returns. The sufferer is often not able to focus the eyes and may become unable to read as letters become fuzzy and scattered on the page. The eyes may hurt. Wherever the pains may be located in the head, they are intense. The head throbs violently with the sensation of pressure, as if it were held in a vise.

Headaches that occur from **reading too much,** such as during school, are frequently seen. These are often worse at ten o'clock in the morning or at three o'clock in the afternoon: just as school lets out. The headaches can also begin due to a weakness in the eye muscles when aggravated by strain during intense concentration, as is also found with *Calcarea carbonica* and *Tuberculinum.*

Natrum muriaticum children, like the adults of this type, may have headaches from exposure to the **sun** and **before the menses.**

A physician typically finds frontal headaches that are worse on the right side or localized in the right temple area. They may be vague, migratory, stitching pains that seem to move about the skull, now manifesting here, now there. Another common location for headaches begins at the vertex and extends down the back of the skull to the neck, or just as likely from the right forehead area extending to the vertex.

The *Natrum muriaticum* headache is **aggravated by exertion,** sports, jarring motion, **sharp noise,** and **bright light,** as it is in *Bryonia alba* and *Phosphorus.* Also as in *Phosphorus* and *Bryonia alba,* they are often accompanied by a thirst for cold drinks and a **desire for cold** compresses to be applied to the head. *Bryonia alba,* being a common acute remedy for *Natrum muriaticum* individuals, will often cure these acute headaches—but will stop working when they become pure *Natrum muriaticum* headaches. The differentiating point with regard to *Phosphorus* is seen in the response to food. In *Phosphorus,* the desire for food precedes or accompanies the headache and subsequently develops into a ravenous appetite; in *Natrum muriaticum,* the child becomes **nauseated and loses any appetite for food.**

The face becomes **pale** and the afflicted person desires to be **alone** and to **lie down flat with cold and pressure against the** head, and occasionally to have the neck rubbed. During the headache the child is **irritable** and may weep, which may either ameliorate the headache or bring on a worse one. The headache may also be brought on or aggravated by strong odors such as perfume and diesel exhaust.

Eyes

One can see **great sensitivity** in the eyes of *Natrum muriaticum* children. There is a definite sparkle there, yet it is intermixed with sadness and anxiety. The child may develop dark circles under the eyes, as well as Denny's lines: the **creases under the lower eyelids** that typify allergies.

They can be quite **photophobic** and need to wear sunglasses. The photophobia is of graded severity; some have extreme sensitivity to light, while others develop headaches when in the sun. Others just prefer the shade. But all squint in bright light. In the doctor's office, many will move their chairs to get out of the path of the sun's rays if direct sunlight is streaming in through the window.

The *Natrum muriaticum* type tends to develop **myopia** at an early age. Ruby was brought in for migraine headaches and myopia. Both problems arose after an event that caused great grief. It was as though she no longer wanted to see as far and wished to close off her sensorium to the detriment of her eyesight. As is common in these cases of myopia, the vision may be corrected with a homeopathic remedy, especially if the child is still very young.

Ears and Nose

While the **ears are rarely affected**—perhaps the commonest symptom is an **increased wax production**—the **nose is frequently troubled**. *Natrum muriaticum* children often have many **allergies** to the environment, developing hay fever-like symptoms from dust, molds, and pollen. Paroxysmal attacks of sneezing may recur every spring or fall.

There may also be **allergic reactions to foods**. Some children are allergic to bananas, to legumes such as peanuts, and to milk. Such foods make the palate itch and cause a postnasal catarrh. A frequent complaint is of a postnasal catarrh that is watery and clear, albuminous, or white. The throat becomes sore and the nostrils alternate between being clogged and discharging mucus.

The allergies may lead to **sinus infections** and sinus headaches, especially during a change in weather. Symptoms are generally worse in the morning, when children may hawk up white mucus that often tastes bad or salty. The throat, nose, and all their upper mucous membranes feel dry, explaining the intense thirst that such children often experience.

Face

Adolescent girls can develop a distinctive **rash along the jaw line,** something I have come to call the "estrogen rash," a symptom that becomes worse before the menses. This rash is made up of either red pimples or hard, white papules that come and go periodically, coinciding with the menses and aggravated by eating sweets.

Acne and rashes on the face tend to be centered on the **forehead.** The skin is often very greasy with a greenish tinge, or else the child, especially a boy, is quite fair.

Natrum muriaticum should be added to the rubric: Face; **Freckles.**

Urticaria may also be a chief complaint. Hives may develop from each and every exposure to the sun or may occur only during the first three or four weeks of summer sunshine. The hives itch and then disappear. The discomfort of these hives is eased when the skin is cooled.

The **lips** are often **dry,** cracked, or sore, and frequently develop a fissure in the center of either the bottom or the top lip. With colds, influenzas, and fevers, blisters or herpetic **sores** develop that recur around the lips.

Mouth

The mouth may feel **dry and sore** and the **tongue may be geographically mapped** with red and white areas that constantly change boundaries and positions. With the dry mouth there is a periodic or constant thirst for ice-cold water or soft drinks, which are consumed by the glassful. In active girls there may be a thirst for cold milk as well as for other cold drinks. Children may also complain of canker sores and aphthae aggravated by acidic foods.

Lower Respiratory System

Asthma

The asthma of *Natrum muriaticum* is not discussed in the old books, nor is it found in the *Repertory*, but it is commonly found in practice today. Asthma may be related to allergies or found after exertion. It begins with a dry, hollow cough that is described as sounding like a dog's bark. This is accompanied by shortness of breath that is aggravated by exertion; dust; evening time; open or dry, cold air; and summer and fall weather in general. The chest tightens with any of the above instigators and a cough quickly ensues. Allergies to cats is a common complaint as well. Shortness of breath, worse when lying on the left side and better when leaning forward or bending double, like that found with *Arsenicum album*, may respond well to *Natrum muriaticum* if the general symptoms agree with a *Natrum muriaticum* picture.

As might be expected, asthma in this remedy type is often triggered by **emotional causes**. Annamarie, a teenager, would develop asthma whenever she came to tears. As the nasal mucosa began to moisten from the tears and the nose began to run, asthma would follow as a matter of course. For this reason she suppressed her tears, not crying for many years no matter what happened.

It is uncanny how often a *Natrum muriaticum* picture develops in cases where the child must suppress sadness, and in so many ways. Another girl would have an asthma attack whenever her divorced mother would come to pick her up for the weekend. The asthma first began when the parents first filed for divorce. The parent may describe, and the doctor may notice in the interview, that the child seems to control her breath as much as she controls her emotions.

The child may develop **allergic coughs** that do not progress all the way to asthma. Eight-year-old Frank coughed daily for two years. No reason could be found for the cough by his pediatrician. It was a little cough caused by a tickle in the throat, according to Frank. The cough was aggravated by each preceding cough, by eating, and by heat. It was found upon questioning that the cough had started soon after the boy's best friend had moved away. This was a terrible blow to him, although he told no one how he felt. Nor did he tell anyone how his feelings were being hurt even more by his siblings every day by their callous disregard—he just closed himself off emotionally. The remedy *Natrum muriaticum* stopped the cough for good.

Alimentary System

Food Cravings and Aversions

Natrum muriaticum children have strong **desires for salt and sweets** as well as weaker desires for **bread, chips, fruit, chocolate, yogurt, and ice cream.** Some like sour foods such as lemons.

They may intensely **dislike milk, fat, and slimy foods, as well as meat, cheese, some fruit, seafood (especially anchovies), and bitter foods.** They dislike dishes that are prepared from many food elements, such as casseroles. One patient called them with disgust, **"mixed-up foods."** They like their foods separated and neatly arranged on the plate. They are found to be neat eaters and not prone to making a mess on the bib, high chair, or floor as a baby or toddler.

Many *Natrum muriaticum* children are **lactose intolerant,** evidenced by indigestion or a respiratory allergy to milk. Nausea, abdominal cramps, and diarrhea after drinking milk are common indications of this.

They may have a great **appetite** but not gain any weight. In fact, they may lose weight, especially around the neck area. They may also have little appetite and snack throughout the day rather than sitting down to a meal, becoming the picky eater in the family. This child is typically the thin and lanky type in the *Natrum muriaticum* group.

They may get hungry at about **eleven o'clock in the morning,** as do *Iodum* and *Sulphur* children. They have a strong **thirst for cold** to ice-cold drinks and may often be found drinking copious amounts with meals.

Stomach

A large number complain of **recurrent stomachaches or abdominal cramps.** Some children complain of an "acid stomach" with heartburn after eating certain foods or spices, such as pumpkin, seafood, and cinnamon; or after a very salty meal. In these cases the stomach symptoms may be accompanied by a postnasal catarrh or a full sinus infection. The stomach feels better after drinking ice-cold drinks.

Nausea before or with the menses is fairly common. A frequent complaint is **motion sickness**, especially during any long drive. The nausea becomes worse if the child is cinched in with a seat belt and the sun is shining into the car. These are the children who cannot be spun around in games due to nausea and who find no pleasure in riding fast or whirling rides at carnivals.

Abdomen

Clinically, one finds that the abdominal area **cramps easily** in the *Natrum muriaticum* child. The symptoms fit an **irritable bowel syndrome** very well, often leading to a full-blown case of it in older teenagers and adults. The abdomen becomes hard to the touch, cramps up, and is accompanied by severe pain as if the colon were being grasped and squeezed by a tight fist. The pain is occasionally localized to the splenic flexure. Those afflicted are compelled to double up with this acute attack, which is followed by the passage of flatus and eventually stool. The pains are often precipitated by the abdomen becoming full of gas (often due to a malabsorptive condition) and sometimes by constipation.

Rectum

Occasionally one encounters a baby with severe colic. Milk or wheat cereal bring on the symptoms. This baby does not want to be fussed with or held. *Natrum muriaticum* as a remedy in these cases may be effective.

There is a tendency toward **constipation**. The stools are dry and the child strains and may cramp before passing a hard stool. The bowel movement is painful because of the dryness and impaction of the stool, causing the anal sphincter to tighten involuntarily, making it even more painful. This makes the child not want to go to the bathroom, and so habitual constipation develops. With such a history, these children develop many tiny **anal fissures** as well.

The old materia medicas describe **chronic diarrhea** in young *Natrum muriaticum* children. Due to the scant information about the diarrhea, it took several years for these children to receive the remedy *Natrum muriaticum* from me, having missed the correct prescription many times. To expand upon this complaint, in my practice, I find that the diarrhea acts very much like a celiac sprue: it occurs first thing in the morning, is odorless, and may be projectile. The diarrhea is aggravated by the ingestion of milk or wheat and is accompanied by much flatus and cutting pains in the lower abdomen.

Urogenital System

Boys
Urination irregularities are not often marked in this remedy type except in two instances. The **shy** child, especially the **adolescent boy, will**, as the old books describe, **find it difficult to urinate in a public rest room**. It is as if the sphincters involuntarily spasm due to the embarrassment the child feels. The other irregularity is **bed-wetting**, described in the section on **Sleep**.

Girls
Nondescript vaginitis in a young girl is not uncommon, and sometimes comes up as a complaint of the mother during the initial interview.

The **premenstrual syndrome** plays a big role for *Natrum muriaticum* adolescents. Before the menses, sadness and irritability prevail. They may experience abdominal cramps, "spotting" before the flow, nausea, or diarrhea. Teens may also develop an oily face replete with acne before the flow commences.

The actual **menses may be painful**, with backaches that get better while lying flat on the back on a hard surface. Abdominal pains that come with the menses extend down the thighs to the knees. Localized uterine pain is aggravated by the slightest jarring motion and is lessened with heat, as with the application of a heating pad or hot water bottle directly to the lower abdomen. *Natrum muriaticum* dysmenorrhea may sometimes be ameliorated by the remedy *Belladonna*, as the symptoms are so similar for both remedy types in this regard.

The menstrual blood may be bright red with no or few clots, as in *Lycopodium*, or be dark with dark clots as is often the case with *Pulsatilla* and *Ignatia amara*.

Occasionally, the **flow is affected by shock or grief**. Fourteen-year-old Barbara, brought in for primary dysmenorrhea, was found to have had her menarche at nine years of age, three months after her grandfather's death. This was a major episode of grief that only became resolved after the remedy *Natrum muriaticum* was given, which put an end to not only her depression but her menstrual pains as well. One may assume that the grief brought on the flow prematurely as well as the pain associated with it.

Musculoskeletal System

Extremities

The toddler may be small or emaciated and may be slow to learn to walk and talk, occasionally as slow as a typical *Calcarea carbonica* youngster, learning to walk at seventeen months or later. When they finally do walk, they may turn an ankle frequently, a symptom that may be noticed in adults as well as children. Such weakness may follow a strain or sprain to the ankle. A patient developed eczema after he turned his ankle very badly. The ankle remained weak and susceptible to being turned easily until *Natrum muriaticum* was given. It was interesting that no other helpful symptoms were elicited aside from a few keynotes: photophobia, a desire for sweets, and, of course, a concomitant rash. The remedy was given and ended the chronic ankle-turning episodes as well as the rash.

Clinically, a syndrome that should often bring the remedy *Natrum muriaticum* to mind is frequent or easily induced **tendinitis**. The most commonly affected tendons are those of the left shoulder, the knees, the ankles (especially the Achilles tendon, from the heel to the calf), and the fingers. When the wrists are involved, the adolescent may also develop ganglions in the affected tendon. The pains that accompany these inflammations are often sharp and will be ameliorated by cold and pressure, reminiscent of *Bryonia alba*.

Rheumatoid arthritis has also been successfully ameliorated by the administration of *Natrum muriaticum*. Any of the extremities may be affected by this condition as well as the neck.

The onset may follow grief and may progress through all the joints very quickly.

In typical *Natrum muriaticum* fashion, ten-year-old Craig, noticing the swelling of the joints of his fingers, became frightened of what this could mean, but did not tell anyone about it for several weeks. He feared the attention, the scrutiny, the effect on his parents, and the prodding and probing of the doctor. Craig wrote in his private journal about what he thought was going to be a quick end to him so that his parents could read it after his demise. He documented what he thought was a fait accompli that, when discovered, would answer his parents' questions as to how much he loved them and about his pains, yet spare him possible humiliation and public notice.

Besides the frighteningly rapid spread of the arthritis, there is usually an abundance of sharp, stitching pains in all the affected joints. Whereas most *Natrum muriaticum* complaints are ameliorated by cold, in the case of this disease, cold is contraindicated because it stiffens up the joints even more.

Many *Natrum muriaticum* children develop very **stiff neck muscles**. Whereas in *Ignatia amara* this is found mostly in girls, in *Natrum muriaticum* this is found mainly in perfectionistic teenaged boys. The boys often cannot resist the desire to "pop" their neck muscles to relieve the tension felt there.

They **bite their nails** frequently, and as adults can develop recurrent hangnails, ingrown toenails, or dryness and cracking of the skin around the nails.

Skin

The skin is often **dry, cracked, and predisposed to the development of eczematous rashes**, as previously described. People who have eczema on their hands, elbows, ankles, hairline, or behind the ears; and which is red, raw, cracked and weepy, frequently benefit from a dose of *Natrum muriaticum*. The eczema itches intensely, especially when the child eats a food that she is allergic to or when she becomes hot. The rash also tends to be aggravated in the wintertime, mostly due to dry indoor air.

There may often be a problem with **hair loss**, such as **alopecia or morphea**, or **shrinking of tissues** such as lichen sclerosus et atrophicus. In alopecia cases, the scalp around the hairless patch is dry and flaky and itches a great deal.

Alopecia areata following an emotionally stressful situation may be aided by this remedy. Seven-year-old Harry developed morphea with alopecia after the divorce of his parents. He and his father were very close and, as a result, the divorce absolutely crushed the spirit of this youth. He became very sad and would cry endlessly over his missing father. The remedy not only stopped his hair loss, but also allowed the child to face his father's absence quite well, as if he had successfully resolved the conflict within himself.

Natrum muriaticum children often complain of **warts**, plantar and otherwise.

Urticaria aggravated by exposure to the sun is another complaint found within this remedy type. The hives are often aggravated by exertion and by becoming overheated and are soothed by cooling down.

Except during sleep, when sweating can be profuse, the *Natrum muriaticum* child tends to show **scanty or uneven perspiration**. It is common for the child to become quite hot while running and playing, yet perspire only lightly, even in the summertime.

Psoriasis

Psoriasis develops readily on the *Natrum muriaticum* body. Often there is a specific **emotional etiology** such as grief that brings on the lesions. Scenarios commonly observed by the doctor include examples such as a girl of ten developing psoriasis after her parents sought a divorce, and a boy of the same age developing this condition after moving away from his friends to a new city.

The psoriasis may be unusual in several respects. It may be extremely **painful**, burning with each new outbreak, or it may be the rarer form of pustular psoriasis. In general, exacerbation from new grief or emotional trauma is the rule. **Pustular psoriasis** may have a very rapid spread accompanied by strong chills and headaches. Lastly, the lesion, while it remains curable, may behave paradoxically to all other types of psoriasis lesions. It is pathognomonic for this disease that the ultraviolet light of the sun ameliorates the rash. In *Natrum muriaticum*, however, the opposite may be found: the rash becomes **aggravated by the sun's rays** and the lesions grow on skin surfaces that have been exposed to the sun.

After the child has had the disease for several years, especially if strong medications have been used, this last modality is lost and the rash then becomes ameliorated by exposure to sunlight. This should make the prescriber view the case more cautiously, as the lesion is now less likely to be cured completely. With this change, one understands that the homeostatic mechanism of the individual is no longer concerned with the rash. In a few words, the body is in the process of giving up on the rash and learning to live with it rather than to fight and attempt to vanquish it.

Physical Generals

Warm-blooded for the most part, *Natrum muriaticum* children dislike heat and stuffy rooms, although their allergic or respiratory symptoms may be activated by the cold. When very young, they can be so warm-blooded that they, like *Sulphur*, *Medorrhinum*, and *Pulsatilla*, walk about barefoot whenever possible.

Some may like a warm bath but many prefer cool ones. A minority become extremely chilly when coming out of a bath, before the onset of acute illness, and during sleep.

Natrum muriaticum children prefer the shade and dislike **and are aggravated by direct sunshine.**

Many children are thin, pale, weak, and anemic.

There is a general aggravation time from three to six o'clock in the afternoon.

Notes on *Natrum muriaticum* Infants

These infants are by far the rarest of the eight common childhood remedies. I have the least information about these infants of the types here presented.

I notice that children seem to be about four to six years of age before *Natrum muriaticum* pathology begins. What may be found as clues in infancy are few.

Infants and toddlers with *Natrum muriaticum* tendencies are reserved at home as well as in the doctor's office. They cry little, talk little, or try to keep communication to a minimum. They may like to be alone and not wish to be interfered with. They dislike being handled and fondled.

Their desire for cleanliness may begin early; toddlers of seventeen months may toilet train themselves. They may like to wear bibs and are the cleanest eaters of all the eight types.

Canker sores and aphthae of the mouth are common.

They dislike milk; it causes nausea, vomiting, colic, and diarrhea. Diarrhea may also be caused by eating wheat products, resembling celiac disease. The diarrhea may be chronic. It is characteristically odorless and projectile, and usually occurs in the morning. A great deal of flatus may accompany diarrhea. This syndrome is noted especially in small babies who eat well but do not gain weight normally.

Infants can be overly thin and late learning to walk and talk.

They dislike heat and perhaps sunlight, and appear pale and anemic.

Natrum muriaticum Outline

I. Mental/Emotional Characteristics
  A. Perfectionism
    1. Well groomed
      a) Clothes
      b) Hair
    2. Well behaved and reserved
      a) During the office interview
        (1) Answer appropriately
        (2) Often very polite
        (3) Quiet and adultlike in the waiting room
      b) In general
    3. Neat and tidy
      a) Toilet train early
      b) Like rooms to be neat
      c) Like possessions in order
    4. Become very good at whatever they do
      a) Perfect homework; they make sure it is correct
      b) Excel at solitary pursuits
        (1) Sports
          (a) Track
          (b) Gymnastics
        (2) Arts
        (3) Literature
  B. Extreme Introversion
    1. Nervous about answering questions
      a) Almost whisper their answers
      b) Become more tense when asked about emotional issues
    2. Few friends
    3. Difficulty connecting with others
  C. Self-consciousness
    1. Fear of ridicule
      a) Doubt causes intense self-reproach
      b) Cannot play in groups because of this; end up alone
      c) Fear of making mistakes

      (1) Fear that others will laugh at them
      (2) Fear of criticism
      (3) Great emotional pain from oversensitivity
      (4) Feel as if they are "bad people" for making mistakes
  2. Cannot urinate in public rest rooms
D. Emotions intensely experienced
  1. Sadness
    a) May have difficulty with expression
    b) May have difficulty weeping
    c) May become severely depressed and wish to be alone
    d) Martyr themselves; think everything is their fault
    e) Aggravation from consolation
  2. Grief
    a) Kept private
    b) May cause illness
  3. All emotional pains are aggravated by consolation
E. Loners
  1. Due to self-consciousness
  2. Choose activities that can be mastered alone
  3. Like to read in their rooms
  4. Befriend animals
    a) Often
    b) Rather than people
F. Anger
  1. Weep if angry, especially if scolded
  2. May hold angry grudges for a long time
    a) Replay events in their minds
    b) Become upset with parents
      (1) Glare at them in the office interview
      (2) Ostracize them at public events
        (a) Due to anger
        (b) Due to embarrassment
G. Fears
  1. General
    a) Something "bad" will happen
    b) A grief will arise

2. Specific
   a) The dark
   b) Thunderstorms
   c) Spiders
   d) Snakes
   e) Bees
   f) Insects with big mandibles
   g) Thieves
   h) Kidnapers
   i) Heights
   j) Closed-in places
   k) Public speaking
H. Sleep
   1. Fall asleep with difficulty
      a) Due to overactive minds and imaginations
         (1) Mentally replay past events
         (2) Plan conversations and events to come
      b) Force themselves to stay awake out of spite
   2. Sleep positions
      a) On the left side
      b) Occasionally on the back
   3. Commonly walk or talk in their sleep
   4. Shy boys may wet the bed
   5. Anxious dreams
      a) Being chased
      b) Being behind enemy lines
II. Physical Symptomatology
   A. Head Area
      1. Head
         a) Headaches
            (1) Common
            (2) Frequent migraines
            (3) Can be periodic
            (4) More frequently found in the right temple area
            (5) Causes
               (a) Overuse of the eyes, as during school
               (b) Being in the direct sunlight

(c) Strong odors such as diesel exhaust
(6) Accompanying symptoms
    (a) Visual loss or blurring
        i) Before a headache
        ii) During a headache
    (b) Thirst for ice-cold drinks
    (c) Loss of appetite
    (d) Irritability
b) Warm-blooded
    (1) Do not like to wear hats
        (a) Because of heat
        (b) Because of hair grooming
    (2) Cannot be in the sun without a hat for shade

2. Eyes
a) Sensitivity evident in the eyes
b) Denny's lines
    (1) Under the eyes
    (2) Point to allergies
c) Photophobic; must squint
d) Myopic
    (1) From an early age
    (2) Must wear glasses or develop headaches

3. Ears develop cracks behind them due to eczema

4. Nose often affected by hay fever
a) Itchy palate
b) Postnasal catarrh with a discharge
    (1) Clear
    (2) White

5. Face
a) Premenstrual rash along the jawline
b) Acne develops mostly on the forehead along the hairline
c) Face may shine with excess oil production
d) Hives
    (1) From being in the sun
    (2) During the first exposure to sun in spring
e) Fever blisters

(1) With dry, cracked lips

(2) Very common

6. Mouth

    a) Geographic tongue

    b) Frequent canker sores

    c) Dry mouth: thirst

        (1) Frequent

        (2) For ice-cold water

B. Torso

    1. Lower Respiratory System

        a) Asthma

            (1) After exertion

            (2) Allergic

            (3) Emotional causes: allergic cough following grief

                (a) Chronic

                (b) Due to a tickle in the throat

                (c) Aggravated by grief and crying

            (4) Presents as a cough like a dog's bark

            (5) Aggravated in the evenings

    2. Alimentary System

        a) Food cravings and aversions

            (1) Cravings

                (a) Salt greatly craved

                (b) Sweets

            (2) Aversions

                (a) Fat

                (b) Slimy foods

                (c) Mixed foods such as casseroles

                (d) Milk intolerance

                    (i) Stomachaches

                    (ii) Allergies

            (3) Thirst for ice-cold drinks

        b) Stomach

            (1) Babies with failure to thrive

                (a) Large appetite with little or no weight gain

                (b) Diarrhea

      (c) Talk little

      (d) Walk late

    (2) Stomachaches and heartburn

      (a) Recurrent

      (b) From eating aggravating foods

    (3) Motion sickness and car sickness

  c) Abdomen

    (1) Irritable bowel disease with cramping

    (2) Pains from drinking milk

  d) Rectum

    (1) Stools

      (a) Regular

      (b) Hard with constipation

    (2) History of anal fissures

    (3) Diarrhea in infants with malabsorption syndromes

3. Urogenital System

  a) Do not like to urinate in public rest rooms due to shyness

  b) Boys: bed-wetting if shy

  c) Girls

    (1) Premenstrual syndrome

      (a) Sadness

      (b) Irritability

      (c) Acne

      (d) Oily face

      (e) Cramps

    (2) Menses

      (a) Backache

      (b) Severe uterine cramps

      (c) Bright red menstrual blood

C. Musculoskeletal System: extremities

  1. May learn to walk late

  2. Readily turn their ankles

  3. Frequent tendinitis

  4. Arthritis

    a) May follow grief

    b) Joints affected

        1) Very swollen

        2) Deformed

    c) Stiff neck

  5. Problems with the nails

    a) Bite the nails

    b) Develop hangnails easily

D. Skin

  1. Texture

    a) Dry

    b) Cracked

    c) Predisposed to eczema

  2. Psoriasis

    a) Painful

    b) Aggravated by exposure to sunlight

  3. Hives

    a) From exposure to sunlight

    b) Amelioration from cool applications

  4. Alopecia

  5. Morphea

  6. Premenstrual rash on the jaw

  7. Occasional oily face

  8. Acne on the forehead

III. Physical Generals

A. Illnesses with emotional etiologies such as grief

B. May be weak and anemic

C. Warm-blooded

D. May like cool baths

E. Aggravation from exposure to sunlight

Natrum muriaticum Confirmatory Picture

These are perfectionistic, introverted children who are well groomed, self-conscious, and fearful of ridicule. They feel sadness deeply, become depressed, and blame themselves for any disaster that befalls the family. They refuse consolation. They fear insects, robbers, and emotional hurt.

Confirmatory Checklist

- Sleep on the left side
- Headaches with visual distortions from eyestrain or from being in the sun
- Photophobia
- Dry mouth with a thirst for cold water
- Crave salt and sweets
- Avoid fat, slimy foods, and milk
- Lactose intolerance
- Bed-wetting in shy boys
- Tendinitis
- Skin eruptions aggravated by the sun
- Warm-blooded
- Illnesses with an emotional etiology such as grief
- May like cool baths
- Aggravation from exposure to direct sunlight

Phosphorus

Mental/Emotional Characteristics

As a group, *Phosphorus* children are the most enjoyable to treat. They tend to be very **communicative, excitable, and expressive.** They are emotional, like *Pulsatilla*, but also mischievous. One can readily see that the *Phosphorus* child, bright eyed, follows with curiosity everything that occurs in her environment and reacts with quick, easily read facial and bodily expressions.

Phosphorus children are generally **good-natured** and happy from birth. They are **warmhearted** and like to be picked up and hugged. Love is a four-way street for them; they like to give as well as receive affection, and those around them like to give and receive love from them.

The children have **good manners**, so their parents do not hesitate to bring them to public places. I remember treating two brothers who both responded well to the remedy *Phosphorus*. When the boys were alone in the waiting room they wrestled around, but as soon as an adult entered the room they quickly scurried off to their respective chairs and "behaved." In this, the natural playfulness of children of the remedy type combined with the self-control they are able to muster when necessary can be discerned.

This little point may make the difference as to whether one prescribes *Phosphorus* or *Tuberculinum*. *Tuberculinum* is a remedy type with a physique and symptomatology similar to that of *Phosphorus*, yet one that lacks such self-control.

Extroversion

It is the nature of the *Phosphorus* child to be extroverted. In our waiting room one day, a new patient by the name of Rose walked up to the receptionist and spontaneously proceeded to tell her, "My father does not work for the flower shop anymore. He has hay fever and cannot work around flowers and now we do not have enough money for me to be able to go to the amusement park like we used to." The receptionist, taken aback for a moment by the child's forthrightness, rallied an appropriate response in reaction to the child's charm and asked what she did now instead of going to the amusement park. The child, given the okay for further communication, responded with the first thing that came to mind although it was unrelated to the previous statement: that she had many friends. When the secretary jokingly asked, "Many?" Rose's mother backed her up with, "Yes! She *does* have a lot of friends."

The child is very impressionable as well as warm, outgoing, and affectionate; qualities that **attract others** like iron filings to a magnet. The mother states that the child never hurts anyone and gives love easily and freely to all. She is expressive and affectionate both physically and verbally. She hugs others easily and is hugged readily in return. It seems that this child's natural charm is so potent that even *Natrum muriaticum* adults cannot defend their interpersonal barriers against its penetrating power.

The *Phosphorus* child appears bright, answering questions quickly and asking many questions of her own. She **extemporizes** on anything, often straying from the topic at hand. It is common for the child to simultaneously answer a question and begin a new sentence on a separate, though perhaps related, topic.

A question was once put to the mother of an eight-year-old *Phosphorus* girl as to whether the child tended toward diarrhea or constipation. "Neither," was the mother's response. The child, however, interjected, "But Mom, don't you remember when we were in Mexico and I was swimming across the pool and I was sick and I pooped in the water and it was all runny and mushy and not hard. . . ." This soliloquy continued for about two minutes until I interrupted. The answer had such energy and the delivery such life that one could easily imagine being there in the pool with the child (whether this was an appealing idea or not).

Another mother was asked if she had any problem getting her *Phosphorus* child to take a bath. Before the mother could respond, the child chimed in, "It's fun to wash! I *love* to take a bath!"

Openness

As a doctor, one can experience the child's openness and observe the ease with which she floats through the world, able to **establish rapport** easily with just about anyone. The child is very accepting and does not hold grudges; if accidentally hurt, she is able to quickly let go of any offense or grief experienced. Even though the child has brief moments of anger, sadness, or shyness, extroversion will remain the overriding character trait.

When ill, if not seriously so, the child tends to **remain outgoing** physically as well as verbally. Most *Phosphorus* children will tell their parents or the doctor when and how they do not feel well. They may yell in the middle of the night, "Mommy, my stomach hurts!" With those big, wet, doe eyes they gaze up at a parent and say, "My legs hurt. The only thing that will help is if you rub them and help me fall back to sleep."

Expressiveness

It is remarkable how specifically the child will express a desire to be rubbed, tucked in, or sung to. Young Sam, pointing to his forehead, approached me and said, "Paul it hurts here" in a most pathetic tone, reminiscent of high drama. Such appealing pathos often causes the doctor to put down the pen, pick up the child, and give a heartfelt hug.

To better visualize this quality, *Phosphorus* behavior during sickness should be juxtaposed with that of an ill *Natrum muriaticum* child. Parents of the *Natrum muriaticum* have to pry the symptoms out of the child. Whether it is a severe headache, asthma, or gastroenteritis, the child will not easily volunteer information. The parents are occasionally shocked to find that the child has had an asthma attack the week before and did not tell them about it. The *Natrum muriaticum* in severe pain may also scream or cry, but to find out exactly what is wrong will be nearly impossible. Consequently, the parents feel irritable and irked with the *Natrum muriaticum* because of this resistance to communication. On the other hand, with *Phosphorus*, **health prob-**

lems are clearly expressed, and thus the parents can greatly empathize with their child.

The only time such openness is not the case is during severe illness, especially during high fever states. The *Phosphorus* child may effectively "shut down" emotionally in such a situation and wish only for loved ones to remain in the room. This is still considered a *Phosphorus* state, though. The illness is so great that the patient becomes very fearful, and it is then impossible for the child to remain open to others.

Leadership

These bright children are often **group leaders** when playing games. While in *Sulphur* this leadership trait is due to sheer mental strength, in *Phosphorus* it comes from a love of others as well as a love of the game. The affection that the child emits toward others unconsciously draws them closer. The child loves company and so naturally attracts a crowd.

When a child previously needing *Calcarea carbonica* or some other remedy evolves into a *Phosphorus* state, personality changes will often be dramatic. Parents may recount that a child who was previously always shy, timid, or headstrong has become very outgoing and is all of a sudden picking up more friends, talking to strangers, and being unusually affectionate. This change of personality toward openness is so characteristic of *Phosphorus* that it is a key confirmation of the remedy.

Center of Attention

The child is often found to be the center of attention, whether at school, with friends, or at home. Talking too long or too loudly in the office (though not obnoxiously) or doing cartwheels in the waiting room all place her in the limelight. The parents say that the child is always in the middle of the action and never left out. If someone tries to exclude her from the game, the child cries loudly until included. Even if the *Phosphorus* child is too young for a particular task, she perseveres until she can master it.

In one example, all the other children were riding bicycles and having fun. The *Phosphorus* child, Leon, was too young to know how to ride but began to cry foul play, protesting that he was not getting his fair share of the riding. He mounted a bicycle and began to ride and fall, ride and fall, over and over again until he could indeed ride the bicycle!

This particular event illustrates two aspects of the *Phosphorus* personality. First, they **love being the center of attention**. They desire to have all those older children watch them and then cheer when they prevail. And second, they **strongly prefer to not be considered "just average."** Concerning Leon, it was this distaste for being relegated to the sidelines and being thought unexceptional that drove him on to accomplish something that, because of his developmental age, he should not have been able to perform.

When praise is earned in situations such as these, the recipient **relishes** the **achievements** and the glory. Whereas the *Natrum muriaticum* child melts away with embarrassment at such accolades, refuting or minimizing praise, the *Phosphorus* will enjoy it for all it is worth.

There are negative aspects to this **self-centeredness** as well. For instance, the child may occasionally show signs of being too proud of herself, of selfishness and a lack of desire to share appropriately, as in *Pulsatilla*. Or the child may become very demanding and want things her own way, weeping if she does not get it, as in *Calcarea carbonica*. What is distinctive about *Phosphorus*, however, is that it is easy to stop her from crying by diverting her attention to something else and hugging and kissing her and letting her know that she is loved.

Excitability

Phosphorus children are **very enthusiastic about new environments**, people, or activities. If the mother tells them it is time to go shopping, time to go to the park, or time to go just about anywhere, they become extremely excited. The stimulation of a new environment fills their aesthetic sensibilities and they lose themselves in the excitement of the experience. They love going to shopping malls, game arcades, and playgrounds. At times the excitement makes them almost uncontrollable. They love to play with all the toys, video machines, and games.

Phosphorus children may be quite **restless** from sheer excitement. They fidget around all the time, constantly moving about in the chair during the interview. Parents tell the doctor that their child "can't keep still for one minute" and cannot focus on a task long enough to finish it. These youngsters can become easily excited and unable to maintain the composure normal for children of that age, especially when captivated by a new object, person, or task. Teachers may tell parents that, although the child is delightful, he or she should be taking Ritalin. This is in sharp contrast to the restlessness that one finds in *Tuberculinum* or *Lycopodium*, in which cases the child becomes nasty and unruly.

The more energetic children try to **bargain with their parents** to get money to spend on games and toys. They do extra chores around the house for an allowance and try to bribe a parent. Statements such as, "I ate all my food, give me a toy," or "I did good in school, let's go to the arcade," if offered in a pleasant manner, are typical pleas of the *Phosphorus* child. The *Lycopodium* child will also ask for such things, but not nearly so sweetly; rather, with an edge of irritability and a domineering tone.

The child may **get up many times during the night** to ask for water or to go to the bathroom, or anything else that gains an audience with the parents. While this is the same sort of behavior that one might find in *Pulsatilla*, in *Phosphorus* it arises from excitement, whereas in *Pulsatilla* it arises from an anxiety or fear of being alone even while asleep.

The child usually **spends all of his allowance** as soon as he gets it. The parents tell the doctor that the child buys as if there is a fire in his pants pocket; he must spend every penny. If he uses his money on a toy and has a quarter left over, he will buy candy with the remainder. If the doctor looks at the child as the parent is giving this description, he may find the child grinning self-consciously. If the doctor should ask how many toys the child has, the parent may reply that he has a great number and yet is constantly adding to his collection.

The parents of a *Phosphorus* child may tell hilarious anecdotes of the child's excitable tendencies. Before going out on a special occasion, Sabrina brought down all of her clothes from her upstairs bedroom and had her mother watch and critique how she looked as she dressed in one outfit after another, exhausting her wardrobe with the dress rehearsal.

Sabrina's example illustrates the difference between *Phosphorus* and *Pulsatilla*. While neither child may be sure of what to wear, the *Phosphorus* will be extremely active and substantially more energetic than the *Pulsatilla*, and in her excitement will actually empty her closet in an all-out search for the perfect outfit. The *Pulsatilla*, in contrast, may whine or cry and beg the mother to come upstairs and help her decide. Likewise, the *Pulsatilla* child may try on just one outfit, and if the mother is not crazy about it, be crushed. The mother will then have to spend time trying to piece the child back together again. The *Phosphorus* will be much less daunted, and although perhaps momentarily upset, just as quickly appeased before hurrying to try on something else.

The excitability is easily **noted in the interview. The child speaks openly and demonstratively** with hand, eye, and whole body gestures. The child may wander off the topic and, if very excitable (as are those labeled with attention deficit disorders), will begin to blink often, flare the nostrils, and confuse the proper order of words in speech; for instance, by starting in the middle of a sentence and finishing with the beginning. The patient may become flustered when this happens.

If already excited when they come into the office, *Phosphorus* children **may not be able to restrain themselves** during the interview. One day when I was wearing a colorful pair of socks, one such patient exemplified this trait. As I was asking the father about the child's food cravings, the child blurted out, "Oh, I like your socks, Paul!" The timing of this statement was utterly surprising and illustrated well how her excitability had gotten the better of her.

I remember another example that was even more telling of this extroverted, excitable trait. A child was sitting in the waiting room as I came in to use the telephone. Before the receiver could be picked up, the child quickly started a conversation. "Hi, Paul! Are you going to be finished with my father soon? When is it going to be my turn? James wants to play with me today and I do not like him but my mother says that I should be nice to him because he is nice to me and he has an extra bicycle that I can ride and. . . ." The girl's soliloquy was astounding. It was both endless and captivating, and the excitement in her eyes and bub-bliness in her voice were extremely hypnotizing.

Anticipation

Excitability is also heightened by upcoming events. The antici-pation *Phosphorus* children experience can be great. Before a team game, public singing event, ballet recital, or other event, the *Phosphorus* child becomes anxious. He may even become **physi-cally ill from anticipation**. He may develop headaches, nausea and vomiting, or irritable bowel disease.

Twelve-year-old Kim had continuous hiccoughs for weeks. The hiccoughs were more intense when she was anxious, aggra-vated by emotions or excitement such as the anticipation she felt before a piano recital. The remedy *Phosphorus* not only stopped the anxiety attacks, but also put an end to the hiccoughs as well.

Many of these children will not be able to relax due to think-ing of the upcoming event, sometimes to the extent that they are kept up at night. The difficulty falling asleep may also become chronic after a sudden, intense, exciting incident. If relocating, many times the knowledge that the family will be moving is enough to keep the child awake for weeks before the departure date. Long after the move it may be found that the child is still too excited in the evening to get to sleep.

This typical *Phosphorus* excitement is further illustrated when parents have guests over for the evening. The child senses the energy in the household and refuses to go to bed, falling asleep instead on the couch in the living room among the guests.

The child may also develop illnesses or fears after being in emotionally charged situations. In particular, strong frights or strong emotions in the environment such as a fight between the parents can bring on an acute illness.

Generosity

The children may, in excitement and or in sympathy, give away favorite toys and other possessions. They are often carried away with good will during these moments and later regret such actions. They may then weep with remorse and feel that the benefit they received from such a gesture was too little. Even though they experience regret, it will not stop them from repeating it again and again throughout their lives.

This **generous giving away of personal possessions** is a reflection of the sensitive and giving nature of *Phosphorus* and a precursor to the famous rubric in Kent's *Repertory*: Mind; Sympathetic. The child is deeply caring, taking responsibility for siblings or animals that are in need, as does the *Phosphorus* adult. The doctor is told that the child has been sensitive and thoughtful of others from a very early age. As an example, the mother of one patient stated that her four-year-old son Alex climbs into bed with her to comfort her when she feels under the weather. This behavior shows the result of a sympathetic nature combined with anxiety about the welfare of family members, which these children feel keenly.

Curiosity

Curiosity is another **expression of combined natural excitability and extroversion** in *Phosphorus* children. In the office they play all over the floor with their siblings or friends, touching everything and exploring one toy or game after another. This is done in a far neater fashion than *Sulphur* children exhibit. It also lacks the destructiveness found in *Tuberculinum*, although they may tear apart toys and machines to find out how they work with a straightforward curiosity. If they wish to know something, they will ask the doctor point blank, as shyness will not prevent inquisitiveness from manifesting for very long. The questioning will seem appropriate and not irritating as might be found in *Medorrhinum*.

Distractibility

Some *Phosphorus* children develop the **lack of mental focus** for which this remedy type is well known. This may be observed in the short attention span and easy distractibility of the child. In the classroom the teacher complains that if a pencil is dropped or if someone taps on a desk the *Phosphorus* student is automatically distracted.

Occasionally the confusion is deeper, verging on that associated with **petit mal seizures**. One child stood poised over the bathroom sink with a moistened toothbrush in hand, not recalling

183

what she was supposed to do, and just remained there in that pose for several minutes until her father found her immobilized in that trance-like state.

If this state of confusion becomes worse or frequent, it can be associated in adolescents with a feeling that they are not really here, that everything is happening without their real participation, as if it is all a movie that they are merely watching. If this **extremely detached state** is attained by a teenager, it shows a deeply ingrained pathology for which the cure may be a long time coming.

More commonly, one finds the less intense problem of a child who cannot concentrate at all times on the environment. This child becomes startled again and again even by identical stimuli, especially noises.

Extroversion/Introversion

Another major aspect of the *Phosphorus* child is **shyness**. This may be particularly noted in the initial interview. When the doctor first meets the child, it is likely that if he or she catches a glimpse of the *Phosphorus* patient out of the corner of an eye, the youngster will be found inquisitively watching every move the doctor makes while walking around the office finishing paperwork or doing other tasks.

When doctor and patient are finally introduced and proceed with the interview, the doctor will note that this child is very shy and blushes easily. Mild-mannered boys look down at the floor and do not say anything, in a manner similar to *Natrum muriaticum*. The shiest children look at the mother or father at all times and with every question, as if they need the support of an adult to be able to answer. They answer with a whisper in a sweet, timid voice, just as one may expect with *Pulsatilla*. The remedy type *Lycopodium* also answers shyly, but in a manner that is somewhat irritating to the prescriber. While one has the underlying feeling that the *Lycopodium* is being childish and pestering, with *Phosphorus* children one only feels their preciousness.

The answers *Phosphorus* gives come more easily as one-to-one rapport is quickly established and the child cooperates with the whole process. As the interview continues, one notes that the shyness quickly fades and excitement builds within the child. While at first he was able to sit still with his hands neatly folded in his lap, containing his inquisitiveness, now he becomes restless and fidgety. By the midpoint of the interview, if not before, the child may stand up and move closer to the doctor. After some more time the child may be on the doctor's lap having the doctor stroke the hair or rub the back of the patient. The mother chuckles as she tells the doctor that this always happens, even with strangers. It is amazing how the unique *Phosphorus* magnetism attracts others regardless of their reservations.

Another example shows this feature more amusingly. Once I was treating a family over lunch. One of the three children of the group was nine-year-old Liz. At the beginning of the interview she was very shy, whispering and looking to her father for answers and not ever looking at her questioner. By the second half of the interview she was answering questions herself and beginning to pick at my food. As I watched this girl unfold and finally win my affection as well as my french fries, all I or anyone else present wished to do was hug her. This **instantaneous feeling of affection** quite often helps me identify and prescribe *Phosphorus*.

Weepiness

Phosphorus children **change moods and cry easily**. Common causes of crying arise when they are tired, spanked, fearful, or left out of the fun, and also when the anger of others is directed toward them. They need affection and consolation and can cry easily and openly in front of others. They need to share their sadness as they share their happiness. The parents, from their side, need to hug and reassure their *Phosphorus* offspring and build them up; this is similar to what is required by *Pulsatilla* children.

The *Phosphorus* child **recovers more quickly** than the *Pulsatilla*, and plays openly throughout the time of sadness. The child also tends not to turn the grief inward and blame himself, as does the *Pulsatilla*. The *Phosphorus* child, unlike the *Natrum muriaticum* who harbors resentments privately, expresses hurt openly, as did a girl of eight who walked up to the offending person and said bluntly, "You hurt my feelings."

Aesthetics

It will be obvious that these children have a strongly developed aesthetic sense both from the way they appear and in the interests they pursue. The body structure alone gives one this impression. The child is usually tall and thin, with finely textured skin and hair and refined features evident even in infancy, giving the impression of being a natural actor or dancer. They dress nicely from the start, choosing coordinated colors and patterns like *Pulsatilla* and grooming themselves neatly like *Natrum muriaticum*, though usually donning more eye-catching, colorful garb than a *Natrum muriaticum* would dare to wear. They are attracted to artistic endeavors such as painting, music, and (sometimes to the detriment of the larynx) singing.

Fears

The *Phosphorus* child becomes **terribly fearful with the slightest provocation**. The parent and even the child may say that he is a worrier. As the child describes his fears, he often looks at the parent to assess the appropriateness of his response. Such a child will seem tense and anxious at these times, as tense as a *Natrum muriaticum* child can become. When interviewing a child who seems to need the remedy *Natrum muriaticum* due to unfounded fears but who craves consolation, one should consider that he may be a fearful *Phosphorus* instead. I once interviewed an anxious *Phosphorus* boy who, in the middle of narrating his fearfulness, said, "I always worry. Oh, by the way, Mother, the parking meter is about to run out."

As a parent gives an account of the child's fears, one often sees the actual terror consume the child. The eyes open wide while the mother sketches the child's reaction to a thunderstorm, as if the hapless child is reliving the experience. Some children become hysterical when describing their fears, as did thirteen-year-old Alison who started wailing, "But wwwhatt iiff I gggetttt kidnappppped?" The child was so terrified that she completely fell apart from dwelling upon her own projection.

The strongest and most common fears are of **the dark, being alone, ghosts, and thunderstorms**. "In a thunderstorm," tells the parent, "Donald screams loud enough to wake the dead with his bloodcurdling cry." The child may jump into the parents' bed or cover his head with a bedspread when thunder is heard. Even *Phosphorus* infants fear the loud noise of a thunderclap.

The fear of **ghosts** may be as strong as that found in *Calcarea carbonica*, and accentuated by watching horror movies or listening to ghost stories. As do *Calcarea carbonica* viewers, they may develop nightmares from such movies. The child will go to the parents and cry, "I'm scared," and then tell them exactly what is needed to remedy this: "Take me and hug me and tell me you love me."

The fear of **the dark** and of **being alone** in the dark can be understood as an outgrowth of this fear of ghosts. When children are alone in the dark, every shadow or noise stirs up the imagination, and they begin to actually see the ghost, goblin, witch, or monster lurking in the shadows. At night they sleep with the lights on and often creep into their parents' or sibling's bed. The sibling does not need to be older than the *Phosphorus* child to make him feel secure, as may be the case with a remedy picture like *Lycopodium*, for any company is enough to help.

The child may be frightened of the **doctor the first time** he goes in for an office visit, as implied by the initial shyness discussed earlier.

The child also commonly fears **insects, especially bees and spiders.**

If the child **falls**, he gets such a fright that he begins to cry and runs to his parents. This fear is much stronger if the child is about to undergo a procedure in which the parents are not allowed into the room, such as an operation. Crying and wanting hugs, kisses, and consolation are observed even in older children who should have outgrown such behavior.

They fear **being alone in the house** and compulsively check the doors to make sure that the house is locked and that there are no robbers, again behaving similarly to *Natrum muriaticum* in this regard. The major difference regarding the shared fears (robbers, insects, thunderstorms) between these two remedy types is that the *Phosphorus* cannot help but talk about the fears with dramatic expressions that pull the listener right into the experience, whereas the *Natrum muriaticum* child will largely keep his fears to himself, being closed in this way as well as others. The *Natrum muriaticum* may merely mention to the parent, "Perhaps you should lock the door." Such a comment does not betray the deep and intense fear felt inside.

Many of the *Phosphorus* fears can be distilled down to the single fear that **something "bad" will happen**. This is experienced as a general foreboding that encompasses many facets of the child's daily life. The poor *Phosphorus* child is often left with an overactive imagination with which to fantasize what this threat might be.

If pushed further, this **wild imagination** makes the child fear the **future**, especially possible illnesses. When asked what he was afraid of, twelve-year-old Paul said he feared AIDS. Having heard that it killed people and not knowing how one developed the disease, he became anxious over the prospect of dying from it. Besides the irrationality of assuming he would contract such a disease, the fear of death in one so young is quite unusual and peculiar to this remedy type.

During an illness the child may become especially anxious, fearing the sickness itself and the severity of it. He may try to be brave, but if he is pushed very far, the fear of the disease becomes evident, and he begins to openly display his terror by crying.

As a corollary, a parent may tell the doctor that the child **loves going to doctors** and loves taking pills, even if the child is six years old or younger. When a sibling is ill, the *Phosphorus* child sometimes begs to go to the doctor's office with the brother or sister. As the parent describes this, one may note once again that the child acknowledges this trait with a grin.

Phosphorus youngsters crave company and physical contact when suffering from illnesses. One may find them in the office holding onto a parent, usually the father, for dear life. This is not the fear of abandonment found in *Pulsatilla*, but the desire for reassurance and love that lets them know that they will be alright. During this state of fear the child will make eye contact with the doctor or the parent, as if that visual and intimate contact is required by the child to be assured that she will be well cared for.

The child may likewise develop great anxiety and fear if a family member is ill, due to a strongly sympathetic nature. And if the sibling or parent is late or missing, the child may begin to panic. Such a fear was described earlier in the case of four-year-old Alex, who would get into bed with his mother in order to comfort the ill parent. This type of behavior, showing anxiety and **concern about a parent**, has often led me to the correct prescription of *Phosphorus*. While behavior such as this is pleasant and perhaps even desirable, when taken to the extreme that *Phosphorus* children sometimes take it, that is, by actually becoming ill themselves, it becomes pathological—and therefore treatable as well.

This child may develop a **fear of an event that has caused trauma** in the past. A child may remain in fear of dogs or, more commonly, insects after being bitten or stung. A child of my acquaintance feared threaded needles because they reminded him of a fall when he was four years old in which he cut himself and subsequently had to be stitched up. A child may fear "that terrible stove" upon which he burned his hand when he was younger.

A very common fear among *Phosphorus* girls is that of **being raped** after hearing of a rape in the area; this is found even in a seven-year-old. After a program at school on abductions a child may cling to the parents or not be able to sleep alone at night for months after the event. One child feared male strangers, believing that all men would abduct her.

A fear of rival drug gangs had sweet Stuart, a boy of nine, terrified because he thought he would be forced to take drugs and kill other students in his class. Hearing of an escaped convict, one child was sure the fugitive lurked behind a neighbor's house. These fears can be summarized by a feeling that something awful will happen to them, some horror will beset them.

Fears may affect the stomach, as they do in the remedy types *Pulsatilla*, *Lycopodium*, *Kali carbonicum*, and *Mezereum*. Nausea, stomachaches, vomiting, ulcers, or diarrhea may develop with these fears as they become **somaticized**.

Others will develop an autonomic nervous system response (fight or flight reaction), including heart palpitations and severe perspiration of the hands and feet. Yet others begin to obsessively flare their nostrils and blink repeatedly. Many will bite their nails and become restless or seem anxious in the office when fear sets in.

Sleep

Sleep and behaviors related to it offer many strong symptoms that point to the remedy *Phosphorus*.

The children **do not like to go to sleep alone**. Even infants and toddlers may fuss until a parent lies down with them, ostensibly to go to sleep as well. In the dark they fear that the room, the bed, or the closet is filled with monsters or ghosts, and every changing light and shadow pattern gives them a start. This again illustrates the strong imagination observed in these children. For this reason they often report that they **sleep with a light on.**

Phosphorus is one of the most common remedies given to the child who, even though eight or ten years old, still sneaks into bed with his or her parents due to nighttime fears. Such a child may also have a difficult time falling asleep if emotionally troubled or excited about an upcoming event. The child may need to talk to the parent and to be rubbed to sleep if anticipating an important event the next day. It is not uncommon to have a thirteen-year-old *Phosphorus* girl still wanting to be tucked in at night.

The **sleep position** is normally characteristic in *Phosphorus* people. While it is common to find *Phosphorus* adults sleeping only on their right sides, in the pediatric population the position is evenly split between the right side and the abdomen, one or the other being favored by a particular child about ninety percent of the time. Only occasionally will they be found lying on their backs, and even more rarely lying on the left side.

They tend to talk in their sleep, and many will **sleepwalk.** *Phosphorus* and *Natrum muriaticum* will be found to be the two most common remedies for somnambulism, and both remedy types will walk into walls and into the parents' bedroom or down to the living room during their midnight rambles. Both remedies are found in Kent's *Repertory* in bold type in the rubric: Mind; Somnambulism.

Sleep may be **restless**, as they have many **nightmares** centered around monsters, ghosts, and animals. The dreams may also include ominous episodes with chase scenes, murders, or other frightening, macabre happenings. Many of the dreams take root from a movie or event that the child has just experienced.

The child, even if fifteen years old, may go to the parents' bed when awakened by these dreams. She may wake up frequently, asking of the parent ten or twenty favors a night: "I need a drink of water, I need this . . . and that . . . " In short, anything to keep an adult around until she finally falls asleep. While this is similar to the behavior of *Pulsatilla* children, in that remedy type it stems from childishness and a fear of abandonment, whereas in *Phosphorus* it is rooted in a craving for comfort in the face of the evils produced by their own active imaginations.

If *Phosphorus* children have an acute respiratory or digestive complaint, they may moan in their sleep; perhaps it is the phosphoric element in *Calcarea phosphorica* that gives that remedy type the keynote of moaning in the sleep as well.

Phosphorus infants and children usually **wake up refreshed**, though perhaps **hungry**.

Vertigo

Tall, thin children frequently complain of **orthostatic hypotension**—low blood pressure upon arising—that causes vertigo. When they rise quickly from a reclining position, especially when they are hot, they feel light-headed and dizzy, as if their feet do not touch the ground.

Older girls may also feel this way when they menstruate heavily.

Physical Symptomatology
Head

The **heads** of *Phosphorus* children **share three similarities with** those of *Calcarea carbonica*: the head of *Phosphorus* may often be covered with fine, silky, shiny hair; baldness occurs in certain areas when the child is experiencing tremendous illness such as pneumonia or bronchitis; and finally, the child may perspire profusely from the scalp.

Headaches

These children tend to develop headaches, even to the point of **migraines**. There are quite a few keynotes of *Phosphorus* to be

elicited in connection with these headaches. They may be heralded or joined by many **visual changes** such as photophobia,
flickers, lightning flashes, or black and white floating spots, as
found in *Natrum muriaticum, Sulphur,* and *Tuberculinum.*

The headaches are commonly preceded or accompanied by
hunger; the child describes an empty feeling in the chest or stomach area. If the child, especially a teenager, misses a meal, he will
probably develop a headache just as *Lycopodium* and
Tuberculinum teens do. The parents tell the doctor that if the child
eats too much sugar at any one time, he gets a headache an hour
or two later. The rapid increase of insulin in the blood causes a
quickly lowered blood sugar level (hypoglycemia) and a subsequent headache. Due to this low blood sugar level, a common
concomitant of these headaches is, ironically, a craving for sweets.

The other common type of *Phosphorus* headache occurs due to
a **sensitivity to the environment.** This headache may be set off by
strong odors such as perfumes, car exhausts, and tobacco smoke.

Very thin, anemic children may also complain of headaches
after exertion, even from simply reading for too long.

With all types of headaches, the *Phosphorus* will crave ice-
cold compresses applied to the head, as do those needing the remedy *Bryonia alba, Natrum muriaticum,* or *Pulsatilla.* This is the
case even if the headache is caused by severe sinusitis or encephalitis. **Amelioration** of a headache by **cold** is a big clue to this remedy, as most people with sinusitis crave heat applied to the head.

During severe headaches of all kinds there may characteristically be **nausea and vomiting.**

Congestive headaches due to vascular or sinus causes are
aggravated by motion and by being in a warm room, and are ameliorated by pressure and by sleep. And, while the faces of most
Phosphorus children flush with the headache, others become pale
as a sheet with dark blue circles around the eyes.

Eyes

The eyes of infants and children are **bright and wide open,** shining with a glimmer and brilliance all their own.

As is found with all remedies used to treat the tubercular
miasm, *Phosphorus* types have **long eyelashes,** even from birth.

Another feature that may be observed is **blue-tinged rings** of discoloration around the eyes of a pale-faced child. These rings may be slightly puffy, growing puffier yet when the child is ill and receding during recovery.

While *Arnica* should be the first remedy considered for **subconjunctival hemorrhages** in infants and children, *Phosphorus* should be especially considered if the bleeding recurs often, whenever the children strain during coughing or blowing the nose or with slight trauma.

Paralysis of the optic nerve causing gradual blindness is also a complaint that should make one think of *Phosphorus*. The paralysis may be due to an unexplained degeneration of the nerve or may occur after a brain tumor causes papilledema with loss of visual fields. As mentioned in relation to headaches, the child may have in this case many **visual distortions** such as "floaters" of any shape, color, or size.

Finally, the child may complain of eczema or seborrheic dermatitis on **the eyebrows**, both of which are exfoliative.

Ears

The ears are not often affected in these children. Occasionally a child will be seen for fluid in the ears, which can cause the echoing of sounds or even deafness. The parent often notices that this muffling occurs every time the child has a cold. The response to questions directed at such a child will often be "what?" This is the only syndrome commonly found in children exhibiting a famous old *Phosphorus* keynote; namely, that they cannot hear the human voice.

In the taking of the health history, the parent of a *Phosphorus* child may state that the child at one time had an ear infection that caused the eardrum to rupture and give forth a **bloody discharge**. Thus, *Phosphorus* should come to mind for both infants and children who presently have or once had a very bloody ear infection.

Nose

In contrast to the ears, the nose is **frequently problematic** in *Phosphorus* children and adolescents. Many of these children have a history of **nosebleeds**. The blood is bright red and profuse to the point of actively gushing. The left nostril is slightly more susceptible to bleeding than the right. Most youngsters tend to experience them more commonly during sleep and in the wintertime, summertime, and evenings.

Adolescent girls may have nosebleeds along with their menstrual flow. Nosebleeds can also occur from the slightest trauma to the nose and from any straining, such as that which accompanies coughing or sneezing. Even though the effluence is bright red, in the morning when the blood has coagulated, the pillowcase may be stained a dark red.

It is common to elicit the fact that the child develops **many colds** each winter that begin in the nose. The infection may progress to full-blown sinusitis, either acute or chronic. The mucus from the nose may be blood-tinged, thick, greenish-yellow, and burning to the point of excoriating the mucous membranes of the nose.

For some, the cold quickly drops into the larynx and chest, and not uncommonly develops into full bronchitis.

Hay Fever

Phosphorus children may have hay fever caused by different pollens and grasses, especially from May to July. The nose becomes very dry and stuffed up, resulting in congested sinuses until the body begins to release histamine and profuse mucus begins to run, accompanied by paroxysms of sneezing; this is exactly the opposite of what is found with *Sticta pulmonaria*, where the mucous membranes become painfully dry as quickly as possible.

Phosphorus hay fever continues with the eyes itching even more intensely; both the eyes and nose redden and the throat becomes scratchy. The discharge is the same as it is with colds: a bloody, green mucus—though it may be more watery than is usually found with a cold. *Phosphorus* children commonly have nosebleeds along with the fits of sneezing. When they are older, nasal polyps can also be associated with the periods of hay fever.

Olfactory Acuity

During times when the nasal area is not congested, the child may have a very acute sense of smell and may develop headaches from strong odors.

A keynote symptom belonging to the nose is that, during acute infections, fevers, and weakened states, as well as when the child is healthy but nervous while speaking, the nostrils flare, as is found with *Lycopodium* children. This should not be considered a *common* confirmatory symptom, however, as only a small percentage of *Phosphorus* children exhibit this trait.

Face

The *Phosphorus* face of both infants and older children is often particularly **beautiful, with fine features and fine skin.** The skin may be almost transparent and pallid at rest, but will flush full of color with embarrassment, shyness, or excitement. This pinking of the cheeks also occurs with fevers and acute infections anywhere in the body.

Children with allergies to food and airborne particles develop allergic "**shiners**": dark, often puffy, circles under the eyes.

The face perspires, just as it does with *Ignatia amara* and *Tuberculinum*, especially if the child is nervous or participating in athletic activities.

The **lips tend to become red, dry, and cracked** (especially the lower middle lip), just like they do in *Natrum muriaticum*. This is especially true in the wintertime. Because of this dryness of the lips and mouth the child can become very thirsty.

Mouth

The mouth favors the development of frequent **canker sores** throughout, brought on by lip-biting and from eating acid foods.

The **tongue** is **long and thin** and may be thickly coated in acute diseases. Such a coat will discolor the tongue to a white with a dirty-looking yellow or brown color at the back of the tongue.

The shape of the **teeth** is similar to the shape of the typical *Phosphorus* body: **long and thin.**

The **gums** may show a tendency to **bleed easily**, especially if an adolescent does not floss.

The child may drool during sleep and wake up with bad breath in the morning, as does *Pulsatilla*.

Throat and Neck

When *Phosphorus* children develop **sore throats** (which they do often), they are inevitably accompanied by **hoarseness**. Pain is aggravated by talking too long and by coughing. Children tend to develop **laryngitis** with these infections, reporting frequent episodes of losing their voices. The sinus infections cause a post-nasal catarrh that irritates the larynx. This irritation causes a child to clear the throat often during the interview. The throat feels raw, dry, and burning. With this parched feeling, the child must drink often for relief and will especially favor cold drinks.

Lower Respiratory System

The chest is one of the most affected parts of the body in this remedy type. It is noted that, from an early age, **any cold quickly drops into the chest** to cause a cough, bronchitis, or pneumonia, even in infants. The coughs are aggravated by cold air, by lying on the left side, and by any excitement, such as when the doctor enters the room to auscultate the lungs. The cough is also aggravated by eating, drinking, or talking. The paroxysms of coughing will be worse in the morning and will decrease during the day, only to worsen again at night from sundown until about midnight.

Since the **cough can be quite painful**, one may observe the child trying to hold her breath because every time she inhales, she coughs. An interesting rubric that illustrates this is found in Kent's *Repertory*: Cough; Fears to, and seems to avoid it as long as possible, children with bronchial catarrh. Sufferers often hold their chests when they cough, just as *Bryonia alba* children with a cough do, again because coughing causes pain to the rib cage due to motion. If the motion is limited by holding the chest, the pain is minimized.

Pneumonia

Phosphorus is one of the main remedies to be considered for pneumonia in **infants**, especially malnourished, emaciated babies who lose weight and become very thin. With pneumonia, the nostrils flare during labored breathing. Pneumonia in older children pro-

196

duces the harsh cough mentioned above. In addition, they develop a feeling of "heaviness" in the chest, as if a weight were resting there that prevented easy breathing. Some will experience the sensation of a tightening band around the chest as well.

During the crisis stages of pneumonia, infants and children often have bright red faces, act very anxious, and are not able to lie down or sleep comfortably. Upon closer observation, one can see that they are using all the accessory breathing muscles in the chest and neck, the chest wall is straining, and the nostrils are flaring as they struggle to breathe.

An X-ray often confirms that the pneumonia is mostly in the **lower lungs**. While the right lung is more vulnerable to attack, the remedy *Phosphorus* can cure irrespective of the location of the infection. The old materia medicas were so adamant that the site of the infection be in the lower right lobe of the lung that many a homeopathic physician prescribed (and still prescribes) incorrectly, misled by this inflexibility.

During these attacks there is also a **burning sensation** located anywhere in the chest, felt especially during inspiration. A strong concomitant feature that will help find the correct remedy is the great **craving for ice-cold drinks** during these attacks predominant among *Phosphorus* individuals, young and old alike. The remedy types *Sulphur*, *Bryonia alba*, and *Tuberculinum* all share this symptom.

Asthma

The remedy *Phosphorus* has also been used successfully for asthma, though it is less well known for this than for other conditions. *Phosphorus* is often the remedy for the classic narrow, stoop-shouldered, hollow-chested asthmatic youth. In *Phosphorus*, asthma is often related to **allergies** (such as to pollens and molds) that are prone to be worse in the spring and fall. Other asthma attacks are set off by **upper respiratory tract infections** that drop into the chest, leading to the spasms.

The asthma is often worse on humid days, especially during exertion and inspiration. The chest tightens, feeling as if a weight were placed on the sternum. Curiously, with allergic asthmas the sternum may itch as well as feel tight.

When the child lies down at night he begins to wheeze, becomes congested, and develops a wet, unproductive cough due to a tickle in the throat which causes the feeling that he needs to clear it often. He may sometimes develop heart palpitations with the attack that make him nervous, jittery, and weepy.

Alimentary System

Food Cravings and Aversions

Phosphorus children **crave ice-cold foods** such as ice cream, frozen yogurt, cold milk, and often just plain ice cubes. They desire **chocolate**, and refreshing **snacks** such as cucumbers, sweets, salty things, and various delicacies. They also love **spicy foods** such as pickles and pickle juice, and **sour foods** such as lemons.

Many of these children also love **bubble gum**. They will stay clean, clean their rooms, potty train, or carry out other parental requests all for the reward of a stick of gum. Some of the more mischievous boys even steal it from hiding places such as their mothers' purses.

They **dislike eggs** and bread.

About half the children have an inordinate taste for fat while the other half have an aversion to it. Kent in his *Materia Medica* indicates that *Phosphorus* will be averse to sweets and to meat; in practice, the opposite is most often elicited. And some dislike fish just as much as others find it delectable.

This is one of the most **thirst-prone** remedy types in the entire materia medica, drinking many glasses of liquid a day and even waking up at night to drink. Most of the drinks will be cold to ice-cold. Many of the children will drink more than a gallon of water a day. While one may try to justify this thirst by assuming that children are thirstier than adults because they are more active, if one compared a *Phosphorus* child to other children, one would still find a great difference in the amount imbibed.

Stomach

In general, the child has a **good appetite**. Being acutely sensitive to the blood sugar level, any time the child abstains from eating he or she will develop **hypoglycemic symptoms**. When a meal is skipped, dizziness may ensue, a headache may develop, or mild irritability may be noted. The *Phosphorus* child will be among the first to arrive at the breakfast table, and somewhat anxious until getting some food to eat. He or she may also want to eat before going to sleep or may wake up in the middle of the night longing for a snack and a drink.

The stomach is **one of the weakest areas** of the *Phosphorus* constitution. With any acute infection such as influenza the child develops **nausea and/or vomiting**, retching at the slightest provocation.

I once saw a patient, ten years of age, who had developed an acute respiratory tract infection that seemed to fit the symptoms of several remedy pictures. Along with the infection he had also developed heart palpitations and easy bruising. These symptoms pointed the way to the remedy *Phosphorus*. The symptom that finally cinched the case was that by the time he reached my office he had developed abdominal cramps followed by vomiting and diarrhea. He did well on the remedy *Phosphorus* in all respects.

While such digestive tract problems can occur during a viral or bacterial infection, they may also occur from anxiety or stress. The keynote *Phosphorus* symptom of **vomiting** is further verified if it is aggravated by anything warm and **ameliorated by anything cold**; in fact, the colder the better. The afflicted youngster will drink ice-cold drinks or eat ice cream for relief, but as soon as the drink warms up in the stomach (in about fifteen minutes), the nausea returns. This keynote may be found in Kent's *Repertory* under the rubric: Stomach; Vomiting, drinking, after, soon as water becomes warm in stomach.

Hypoglycemia

Children who miss meals or fast for holidays or for other reasons may become not only nauseous but also weak, trembly, and susceptible to headaches. Because of a **rapid metabolism**, the *Phosphorus* child seems hypoglycemic and needs to eat often.

If extenuating circumstances intervene with their meals, there may be a noticeable lack of ability to concentrate in addition to the physical symptomatology. It seems that, as in *Tuberculinum* and

Iodum, the metabolism is quickened, rapidly burning up especially the sugars ingested. The need for food may be understood in light of how quickly these children gain height, becoming very tall though lean for their age.

Many of these children will not be able to fall asleep because of hunger, while others will wake up in the middle of the night for want of food. What they crave at these times are sweet and cold foods. Other symptoms of hypoglycemia that often crop up are snacking throughout the day or remaining hungry even after a substantial meal.

Resembling the remedy type *Sulphur*, the teenagers may become faint and dizzy at around eleven o'clock in the morning from lack of food, "starving" for their lunch. The point of differentiation will be seen at the breakfast table; most *Sulphur* children and adolescents do not relish breakfast and pass it up because they just do not see the point of it. This is in sharp contrast to *Phosphorus*, who will be the first one to the breakfast table and will relish the morning meal after having "starved" the night through. A *Phosphorus* will become **voracious** almost to the point of anxiety, eagerly eating almost anything on the table. While other remedy types may have blood sugar problems, it is unique to a few remedies such as *Phosphorus* that this may be found in youngsters five years of age or younger.

Abdomen

Many **pains** are experienced **in the lower abdominal area**, anywhere from the umbilicus to the hypogastrium. Emotional upheaval in general exacerbates these discomforts, and so these pains often coincide with stress, fear, anxiety, or even just excitement. As with nausea, such problems will be **ameliorated by any ice-cold drink**. These pains may herald the onset of peptic ulcers in the adolescent, being the physical manifestations of deep and painful emotions, such as the grief of a broken heart.

With these repeated attacks of pains and nausea may come black, tarry stools that indicate a bleeding **ulcer**. It is noteworthy that historically, homeopaths of the last century believed *Phosphorus* individuals crave ice-cold drinks not only because the ice numbs the stomach, but also because it constricts the blood vessels in the stomach, thus slowing down any tendency for bleeding there.

The pains may awaken the child at night and drive him to the parents' bed, crying that he has a stomachache. Amusingly, the same story may be told by a *Phosphorus* child who does not really have any pain at all. Since the child craves affection and attention and has fears of being alone in the dark, he can effortlessly fabricate a fictitious stomachache that wins the much-desired attention.

Abdominal pains may be associated with hepatitis in young children.

The children may develop **stomachaches from** drinking **hot milk**. Finally, one point that may confuse the prescriber is that *Phosphorus*, like *Pulsatilla*, may develop stomachaches from eating **pork**; the thirst of the former and the thirstlessness of the the latter should differentiate these two remedy types with regard to the stomach.

Rectum

The rectum gives a few keynotes to the remedy as well. The *Phosphorus* child tends to develop **diarrhea** quite easily. The diarrhea tends to be painless, watery, and somewhat offensive smelling. It gushes, shooting out of the rectum as it does in a *Podophyllum*. As found in *Sulphur*, this condition tends to be aggravated in the mornings. The diarrhea may be a symptom of an acute bacterial infection or other organic cause, but may also be caused solely by strong emotions.

In *Phosphorus* **infants**, watch for **recurring diarrhea**. It may accompany any illness and may last for a long time after the illness is resolved. Sometimes a toddler who used to be robust loses weight dramatically after an illness such as chronic diarrhea and becomes gaunt.

Less well known is the *Phosphorus* **constipation**. In this case, the stools tend to either be small pellets or long, thin stools that the child must strain to expel. This constipation occurs most often in fevered states when the child is dehydrated or in children who are born with a redundant colon.

There may also be some **aberrant behavior** regarding the

stool, using the passage of it to get rewards or just staying in the bathroom for an hour at a time, even though the child is not actually constipated. And, as mentioned in the next paragraph, the child may soil his pants during exciting play, forgetting that he has control of his sphincter.

Urogenital System

Enuresis

There are two types of problems with bed-wetting. The rarer state is found in the child who has or is vulnerable to kidney or bladder disease, bed-wetting in this case being only one symptom of the disease. The more common state is found in the child who loses bladder control **when excited** while awake during the day as well as when asleep at night in bed. This type of youngster may even lose stool during exciting play.

Boys

While the male genitalia does not offer many distinctive symptoms, the female genitalia does.

Girls

Quite often in teenaged girls the **menstrual flow** will be affected. The flow tends to be very heavy and consists of a bright red flow throughout the entire period. The flow may be so **heavy** that the adolescent becomes anemic, pale, and, quite commonly, dizzy while menstruating. This is especially noted in tall, thin girls.

The cycle may also be shortened by quite a few days. It is a common story to hear that the girl, from the first menses onward, has had a cycle of twenty to twenty-three days. Or the periodicity may be abnormally short: a girl may have a one-week flow, followed by one week without a flow, and again a flow, **fluctuating** like this for months at a time. The teenager may also bleed between menses, typically having breakthrough bleeding at ovulation time. Conventional hormonal treatment for any of these conditions will either be wholly unsuccessful or will regulate the cycle temporarily; as soon as the hormones are stopped, the flow becomes excessive or irregular again.

Phosphorus teenagers may also develop nosebleeds, increased appetite, diarrhea, or hot, feverish feelings before the menses. The remedy should also be considered for severe right-sided ovaritis with sharp, stabbing pains that cause a girl to cramp and double up, along with the other symptoms mentioned here.

Musculoskeletal System

Extremities

The **feet may sway** in the interview, gently flowing back and forth. This is partly out of nervousness, partly to get the doctor's attention, and partly from the fact that the knee joints tend to feel as though they "tighten up" if the child sits too long.

The remedy *Phosphorus* has cured types of **arthritis** that share similar modalities with *Rhus toxicodendron* and *Tuberculinum*. Arthritis symptoms are aggravated by first motion and by cold, and are ameliorated by continued motion. While this is still observed in youngsters, it is much less common than the older materia medicas indicate. This discrepancy may be attributed to the fact that there are far fewer cases of tuberculosis in our society these days. Many children with joint pains will have a positive family history of tuberculosis. *Phosphorus* is found to be one of the main remedies able to remove the inherited miasmatic condition for these progeny. Since the decline in frequency of tuberculosis in the Western world, there has been a proportional decrease in the use of *Phosphorus* in these joint afflictions, though by all means it is still used. It is of interest that homeopathic physicians in countries that are still plagued by tuberculosis such as India use the remedy *Phosphorus* for joint afflictions much more frequently than do their counterparts in Europe and the Americas.

In children who **grow too rapidly** there may be **pains in the shins**, just as are found in the remedy type *Phosphoricum acidum*. Infants may be thin to begin with; or they may, though seemingly healthy, lag behind in weight as they grow in height, creating a tall, thin, string bean-style body.

The child tends to acquire **plantar warts** on either foot. The **hands and feet perspire profusely** any time the child is anxious or excited.

Skin

While the skin is not often affected, the keynote is sometimes observed that this remedy is known to both create and cure: *Phosphorus* types will produce the **driest skin and flakiest eruptions of all the polychrests**. This can range from simple dandruff to extensive ichthyosis, in which the whole skin flakes off constantly and resembles fish scales. In the old materia medicas and repertories, this type of skin condition was termed "furfuraceous," meaning covered with scales.

The child tends to develop warts on the hands, face, and soles of the feet.

As mentioned before, the child will **perspire profusely**, especially on the head and chest and, if nervous, on the palms and soles.

Physical Generals

Phosphorus children are generally tall, thin, and beautiful. One often feels as though they are etheric, even translucent. One can almost see right through them, as if they are not totally present. They usually have fine-textured skin and refined features and look a bit elfin, though perhaps anemic elves.

The *Phosphorus* remedy type is vulnerable to **bleeding problems** and hemorrhages of any sort.

Phosphorus is a remedy to be considered, along with *Tuberculinum* and *Natrum muriaticum*, for children who lose a lot of weight when they develop acute problems.

Likewise, *Phosphorus* should be considered for the child who appears quite robust as an infant only to suddenly sprout upward to rate in the ninety-fifth percentile in height for that age while remaining in the tenth or twentieth percentile in weight.

Another typical history would be that of a fat child who becomes malnourished or starved. Once thin, the youngster begins to project many *Phosphorus* symptoms. Yet another history may be of a fat child who developed diarrhea from having parasites for more than a year and needed to be orally rehydrated for that span of time, but became thin and *Phosphorus*-like in the process.

Phosphorus children tend to be chilly and crave open air and sunshine.

The conditions of *Phosphorus* children tend to be aggravated by lying on the **left side**, and at **dusk** and **twilight**. This applies to both mental and physical syndromes. *Phosphorus* conditions are ameliorated in general by lying on the right side, and by **drinking cold water** or eating cold food, which are ameliorating in action in both the mouth and the stomach. *Phosphorus* children are helped mentally and physically by **consolation**, being rubbed, and sleep.

Notes on *Phosphorus* Infants

Phosphorus infants are good-natured and happy from birth. Affection runs both ways easily; they like to give love as well as receive it. They are expressive, and they like to be picked up and hugged.

They fear sudden loud noises, such as thunderclaps.

Infants and toddlers often hate to sleep alone and may fuss until a parent lies down with them. They wake up refreshed, though perhaps hungry. Toddlers may awaken at night thirsting for a drink.

Babies are born with long eyelashes and brilliant eyes. They may develop subconjunctival hemorrhages easily.

Toddlers contract ear infections accompanied by a very bloody discharge.

Coughs, bronchitis, and pneumonia are all common ailments. More serious infections happen with greater frequency to malnourished or very thin *Phosphorus* children. Pneumonia causes the nostrils to flare with labored breathing and is accompanied by a red face.

Acute infections anywhere in the body often lead to vomiting and diarrhea. Diarrhea often recurs. It may accompany any illness and may last for a long time after the illness is resolved.

Infants are typically fine skinned, fine featured, and thin. Robust toddlers may suddenly develop chronic diarrhea or another problem that causes them to lose weight dramatically and become gaunt. Also, infants can seem healthy yet fail to gain the amount of weight appropriate for their height; therefore they often appear too thin.

Phosphorus Outline

I. Mental/Emotional Characteristics
  A. Enjoyable children during the interview
    1. Well mannered
    2. Good-natured
    3. Expressive
  B. Extroverted
    1. In the office
      a) Able to talk to everyone easily
      b) Answer questions merrily
      c) May talk a great deal during the interview
    2. In general
      a) Lead groups and perform
        (1) From excitement and anticipation
        (2) Seeking praise
      b) Center of attention
      c) Many friends
      d) When ill
        (1) Remain open
        (2) Communicative
  C. Excitable
    1. Enthusiastic
      (1) About everybody
      (2) About every task
    2. Severe anticipation; ailments stem from excitement
    3. May generously give away favorite toys in excitement
    4. Spend entire allowance
    5. In the doctor's office
      a) Excited, extroverted curiosity
      b) Go from one object to another
  D. Shyness during the initial interview
    1. For the first few minutes
    2. Behavior observed
      a) Whispered answers
      b) Blushing
      c) Glance toward parents for support

206

3. Quickly passes
E. "Spacey"
  1. Short attention spans
  2. Easily distracted
F. Emotionally resilient
  1. Recover quickly after an emotional hurt
  2. Do not harbor hate
  3. Weep easily
G. Fears
  1. Many
  2. Sudden noises; startled easily
  3. Thunderstorms
  4. Ghosts
  5. Monsters
  6. Being alone in the dark
  7. Products of an overactive imagination, such as being kidnaped
  8. Insects
  9. Robbers
  10. Worry about the well-being of their families
  11. During illness they may worry about their own health
  12. All fears are easily dispelled by parental attention
    a) Hugs
    b) Reassurance
  13. Fears often somaticize to the stomach
    a) Nausea
    b) Abdominal pain
H. Sleep
  1. Fear of the dark
    a) Want the light on
    b) Sneak into the parents' bed
  2. Sleep positions
    a) On the right side
    b) On the abdomen
  3. Walk and talk in their sleep readily
  4. Nightmares of monsters
    a) From reading

b) From watching television
c) From an overactive imagination
5. Moan during sleep
6. Wake up refreshed
I. Vertigo: orthostatic hypotension
  1. In tall, thin children
  2. Upon rising
  3. With the menses
II. Physical Symptomatology
  A. Head Area
    1. Head
      a) Headaches
        (1) Accompanied by visual changes
        (2) Due to hypoglycemia
        (3) Due to stimuli
          (a) Smells
          (b) Noises
        (4) Amelioration
          (a) From cold applications to the head
          (b) From eating
      b) Similar to *Calcarea carbonica*
        (1) Fine hair
        (2) Baldness
        (3) Perspiration
    2. Eyes
      a) Tubercular
        (1) Brilliant appearance
        (2) Long eyelashes
      b) Discoloration
        (1) Blue
        (2) Around the eyes
      c) Hemorrhages
        (1) Anywhere in the eye
        (2) From slight trauma
      d) Paralysis of the optic nerve
      e) Flaky eruptions of the eyebrows
    3. Ears
      a) Rarely affected

b) Ear infections
    (1) With a bloody discharge
    (2) Occasional
4. Nose
    a) Frequently recurring epistaxis
    b) Colds that progress
        (1) To sinus infections
        (2) To chest infections
        (3) Blood-tinged discharge
    c) Hay fever
        (1) Begins with a very dry nose
        (2) Progressive
            (a) To copious mucus and sneezing
            (b) Discharge
                i) Blood-tinged
                ii) Greenish
            (c) Nosebleed
    d) Acute sense of smell
    e) Flaring of the nostrils
        (1) During respiratory infections
        (2) With nervousness
5. Face
    a) Fine featured
    b) Transparent skin
    c) Flush easily with excitement
    d) Lips dry and crack
6. Mouth
    a) Dry mouth
    b) Thirst
        (1) Great
        (2) For very cold drinks
    c) Canker sores
    d) Tongue coating
        (1) Dark yellow
        (2) Brown
        (3) During infectious illnesses
    e) Bleeding gums
7. Throat and Neck

a) Sore throats
(1) Accompanied by hoarseness
(2) Painful with speech
b) Laryngitis
(1) Frequent
(2) With respiratory infections
c) Postnasal catarrh
(1) Irritates the throat
(2) Causes the child to clear the throat often
B. Torso
1. Lower Respiratory System
a) Colds drop into the chest, causing chest infections
b) Coughs
(1) Aggravations
(a) Cold air
(b) Lying on the left side
(c) Excitement
(d) Eating and drinking
(2) Painful, causing children to hold their chests
c) Pneumonia
(1) With the above symptoms
(2) Additional symptoms
(a) Heavy feeling in the chest
(b) Red cheeks
(c) A strong thirst for ice-cold water
d) Asthma
(1) Allergic or infectious in nature
(2) Feels as if there were a weight on the chest
(3) Sternum may itch
(4) Possible palpitations during the attack
(5) Anxiety
(6) Aggravated by humid days
2. Alimentary System
a) Food cravings and aversions
(1) Cravings
(a) Cold foods

i) Ice cream

ii) Cold milk

(b) Cucumbers

(c) Salt

(d) Sweets

(e) Spicy foods

(f) Delicacies

(g) Fish

(h) Bubble gum

(2) Aversions

(a) Eggs

(b) Fish

(c) Bread

(3) Thirsty for a great deal of cold water

b) Stomach

(1) Good appetite; eat every meal

(2) Hypoglycemic symptoms if a meal is missed

(a) Headaches

(b) Nausea

(c) Weakness

(3) Easy vomiting

(a) With any illness

(b) With anxiety

(4) Aggravation from warm drinks

(5) Amelioration from cold drinks

c) Abdomen: pains near the umbilicus

(1) With emotional stress

(2) With excitement

d) Rectum

(1) Diarrhea

(a) Develops easily

(b) Accompanies any illness

(2) Constipation

(a) Rare

(b) May consist of long, thin stools due to a
    redundant colon

(3) Issues around bowel habits: wishing bribes
    for good habits

3. Urogenital System
   a) Bed-wetting
      (1) Excitement causes the child to lose urine even if awake
      (2) Kidney disease may show this symptom
   b) Girls
      (1) Heavy menses
         (a) Frequent flow, occurring every three weeks or less
         (b) Bright red blood
         (c) Anemia due to heavy menstruation
      (2) Ovaritis
         (a) Right-sided
         (b) Severe, sharp pains
C. Musculoskeletal System: extremities
   1. Gentle motion of the legs during the interview
   ⁻2. Arthritis
      a) Aggravated by first motion
      b) Ameliorated by continuous motion
   3. Plantar warts
   4. Perspiration of all extremities
      a) If anxious
      b) If excited
D. Skin
   1. Driest of skin and flakiest of eruptions all over the body
   2. Perspiration of the extremities
   3. Warts
      a) On the extremities
      b) On the face
III. Physical Generals
   1. Tall, thin children who may become emaciated, especially during illness
   2. Easy bleeding from anywhere on the body
   3. Slightly chilly
   4. Aggravation from lying on the left side
   5. Amelioration from consolation

Phosphorus Confirmatory Picture

These are friendly, good-natured, extroverted, excitable children. They complain of many fears, especially of the dark, thunderstorms, insects, their family's well-being, and an ominous, unknown something that will "get" them. All complaints are ameliorated by consolation.

Confirmatory Checklist

- Sleep on the right side
- Fear of the dark; sneak into the parents' bed, sleepwalk, and have nightmares
- Nosebleeds
- Colds that cause bronchitis and pneumonia
- Sore throats and laryngitis
- Crave ice cream, cold foods, sweet and salty foods, delicacies, cucumbers, and fish
- Avoid eggs and sometimes fish
- Very thirsty for ice-cold drinks, which ameliorate digestive complaints
- Complaints from missing meals
- Prone to vomiting and diarrhea
- Heavy menstrual flow
- Tall and thin
- General problems with bleeding and respiratory infections
- Aggravation from lying on the left side
- Amelioration from consolation

Pulsatilla

Mental/Emotional Characteristics

Insecurity

At a glance, one can easily see the *Pulsatilla* youngster's **gentle, clingy, fearful** nature. The first characteristic noticed about these children is how close they sit to their parents in the doctor's office. In a waiting room full of toys and other distractions, the *Pulsatilla* child chooses the chair closest to the parent and then leans toward the mother or father. The sicker the child is, the closer she leans—until she finally sits on or lies across her parent's lap.

As the doctor approaches the family, the fearful child may lunge toward the mother and burrow into her bosom. Another scene could just as easily find a group of children playing together with only the *Pulsatilla* child sitting and being held by her mother. Immediately, even the casual observer sees that the **child must remain close to the parent** as the little one does not feel secure alone. There is a core weakness that makes the *Pulsatilla* child **sensitive to perceived possible abandonment** by a parent. This sensitivity plays a major role in the child's psychological makeup.

If a *Pulsatilla* toddler is on the floor at the parent's feet and the parent stands up to get a glass of water, the child begins to cry. The doctor comes out to greet the new patient and finds the child crying and the mother caressing and rocking him in an attempt to reassure the youngster. Parental cuddling almost always manages to staunch the flow of tears, which begins again as soon as the mother tries to put the child down. The mother's story is that she goes through this sort of thing all day long; she cannot put the child down or leave his eyesight lest the tears begin to flow. She is

215

unable to shop, cook, or do housework because **she has to hold the child in order to prevent continuous crying.**

Bashfulness

From infancy through the teen years, the child is **oversensitive and cries easily.** As a parent so informs the doctor, the child may look down at the floor or at his shoes and **blush.** When asked if this is true, the child blushes again, looks at the floor, and tells the doctor that it is, in a voice so soft it can scarcely be heard.

The *Pulsatilla* patient appears very **anxious before every answer.** When asked a question in the interview, a boy of nine turned to his mother and said, "You tell him, Mom," and promptly crawled into her lap. When asked a question, timid six-year-old Harriet looked at her mother and moved in order to sit on her lap, but would not answer. Throughout the interview I had to ask the mother the questions, and she in turn had to ask the child, who whispered the answer back to her mother, who then relayed it to me. **Timidity** as pronounced as this is one of the bridges between *Pulsatilla* and its complement, *Silicea*—the child strains to attempt an answer.

One clue to this weakness of character is that all will **look at the mother or father** to see if they answered correctly or in order to ascertain the "right" answer. They may have one foot planted on top of the other in a nervous, coy sort of way, or they may sit with the toes curled under the rest of the foot. From the cumulative picture that emerges from such observations, one begins to feel that these children are **immature** for their age, similar in this way to *Lycopodium*.

When asked if the child is always so shy, the parent either answers yes or says that the child is only this way in unfamiliar surroundings. *Pulsatilla* children may be quite reserved around others in a new classroom or playground situation. They want to be liked but often **lack the initiative** to begin a dialogue or interaction themselves. They must bashfully wait until a *Phosphorus* or *Sulphur* comes along and scoops them up into the fun. From that point on, the barrier of shyness is broken in that circle of friends, as they play well with the other children and enjoy themselves.

Because he seems to be so quiet in the office, it may surprise the doctor that, according to the parents, at home where the child is relaxed, he "yaks away" and communicates well with family members all day long.

The only time *Pulsatilla* children are not talkative at home is when they have taken offense at something and are upset. At that time they may refuse to talk to anyone and mope about pouting instead. Such a tendency is characteristic of a **follower, not a leader.** This quality, if strong, will shift the case automatically from a remedy type with a strong personality, such as *Sulphur*, toward *Pulsatilla*. For example, if a coach is unfair to a *Pulsatilla* child and will not let her play, she often **mopes and cries.** *Sulphur* and other remedy types try to find a creative solution to the problem or even confront the coach directly. This natural ability to challenge unfair practices does not belong to the *Pulsatilla* child.

Eager to Please

These children are very friendly within an intimate, familiar group such as the family, **showing and needing lots of affection.** They like to sit with the parents and have stories read to them or songs sung—anything, really, as long as a parent rubs them and hugs them during the activity. Often, as a book is read, the *Pulsatilla* child will rub an arm against the parent ever so slightly so that unconsciously the parent begins to rub the child in return—this makes for the perfect evening.

The *Pulsatilla* child finds out early how to get what she or he wants by being **affectionate, yielding, and submissive**—essentially, by producing **whatever behavior it takes to win the attention and security so craved.** Even in the interview, if the child is relaxed the doctor may be the lucky recipient of a neck rub!

The child likes to be **neat and tidy** and often wears coordinated outfits. The shoes are clean and the socks neatly pulled up, as on a doll, including the boys. The hair is combed perfectly, as it is in *Natrum muriaticum*. To differentiate the two remedies: in *Pulsatilla*, cuteness of style prevails; there is a **childishness to the dress** that lacks the seriousness of the *Natrum muriaticum*. *Pulsatilla* children may be messy in their other habits, but personally they are usually neat. Neatness is mostly another tool used in order to be liked and, for the most part, is not imposed by the parents.

The mother proudly proclaims that her child is **easy to handle, mild, and quickly persuaded to complete his chores.** He helps around the house, makes his bed, and cleans his room. Always such help is accompanied by questions such as "Is this how you want it?" and "Am I doing it right?"

In contrast, the *Natrum muriaticum* child cannot help but clean his room; the drive comes from within. In *Pulsatilla* children, it is strictly an action for which they seek an emotional reward. They want parents to praise them again and again the whole day through. "How do you like the triangle I drew?" "Watch me dance!" "See my new dress?" They **need constant attention and affection, without which they wilt into feelings of worthlessness,** demonstrated by tearstained faces and endless crying jags. The *Phosphorus* child also seeks constant attention, but more so that she can be the star and shine out the way *Phosphorus* does so well. *Pulsatilla* children seek an audience in order to reap the **emotional rewards** of hugs, kisses, love, and affection, which, if won effectively, allay an underlying fear of abandonment.

Fear of Abandonment

The fear of abandonment can become very strong as the children grow up. This pathology can take **several forms,** such as **feigning illness** to get attention. What I find amazing is the fact that if they feel that no one is paying attention to them, they may actually produce a fever. A child will ask the parents over and over again, "Do you really love me?" "Do you love my brother more than you love me?" "Who is your favorite?" Parents must reaffirm on a daily basis the fundamental premise, "Yes, I do love you. Yes, you are very precious to me."

As will be mentioned under **Sleep,** a very common manifestation of this insecurity is the **refusal to go to bed alone.** The children want a parent to sleep with them until they are quite old. They may wake up at night and either go to the parents' bed or get into bed with a sibling.

Occasionally one finds a *Pulsatilla* child of very strict, harsh parents sitting during the interview with hands folded, perfectly dressed and not moving in the slightest. This unnatural behavior in a child is indicative of the **intense desire for acceptance by the parents** and the equally intense fear of alienating them.

Shock of a New Sibling

All these different ploys are aimed at one thing: to put to rest the supreme fear that they will be left to their own limited devices in the great, unknown world. One major shock that frequently pushes this fear into an acute state is the birth of a sibling. There are **five main expressions of this shock: jealousy, irritability, obstinacy, somaticized symptoms, and regression.** With the natural diversion of affection and care to the newborn member of the family, the *Pulsatilla* feels that she is losing her connection with her parents, since they "obviously" love the new baby more.

Jealousy and Selfishness

The child may become extremely jealous of the newborn. Every time the parent wants to change the baby's diapers, the *Pulsatilla* **asks for something from the parent:** "Can you draw me a cat?" "Let's play now." "I want a drink." I want this and I want that. When the parent does not comply, the *Pulsatilla* youngster is devastated by the clear confirmation that the other child is loved more than she is. She hates her sibling. She sobs pitifully to the parents "You don't love me anymore" and cannot be convinced otherwise.

Pulsatilla children become obstinate with this jealousy, demanding the mother's attention. They become **selfish** and, at times, **possessive** to the point of kleptomania, claiming wrongly that a toy is theirs rather than their sibling's; telling siblings that the parents do not love them or that they are adopted; or just not letting siblings play with their toys. They may even scream in their sleep, "That's mine! Do *not* touch it!"

They become very attached to material possessions. They carry around a favorite stuffed animal or blanket that they will not let anyone else touch, even to let the mother wash it. Jealousy is usually aimed only at children born after the *Pulsatilla* child and not at the siblings born before, as the latter do not disturb the established flow of love from the parents—the bond they worked so hard to secure.

The selfishness of the remedy is found in the **constant desire for attention**. She becomes possessive of the parents' time and love. The child becomes manipulative, learning early that "to be `Daddy's girl' all she has to do is turn on the tears," as one mother tells it.

Irritability

Due to this jealousy, irritability and anger develop, which naturally promote **aggression against the younger sibling**. Five-year-old Samantha had recurrent upper respiratory tract infections and earaches. The mother reported that the child was very irritable and bossy, hitting others with no apparent provocation. Although specific symptoms of the earaches fit a *Pulsatilla* picture, the behavior did not. During one office visit, Samantha opened a door while her sister played behind it, making sure as she did that her younger sibling would be knocked down. To a direct question, the mother replied that the child only behaved like this with her younger sister; with everyone else she was extremely sweet, desiring the hugs and kisses so typical of *Pulsatilla*. The remedy *Pulsatilla* helped the girl immensely. Until I realized how deep the jealousy ran, it seemed strange to see this aggressive acting-out behavior in an otherwise very sweet, passive girl.

Obstinacy

While some *Pulsatilla* children become jealous, others may become **obstinate in order to secure the desired attention.** This is particularly true of **hyperactive boys**, a phenomenon that only **angers most parents** further. The boy demands attention so strongly and for so long that the parent finally becomes annoyed and pushes him away, and may even hit the "pestering" child. Such a negative interaction harms the relationship and causes the child to feel even more abandoned and misunderstood.

This obstinate behavior may also begin a trend that is occasionally found in adults: they become "**hardened**" **and opinionated**, even to the point of strongly fixed ideas. In his *Materia Medica*, Kent describes adults who will not marry or who develop a strong repulsion to the opposite sex or an unreasonable aversion to certain foods.

Though in children one will not find this intensely fixed, rigid behavior on a grand scale, one may find minor aberrations such as that exhibited by a *Pulsatilla* child who refused to write with a pen. No matter what resistance she had to exert in order to do so, she only allowed herself to write with a pencil. This was singularly peculiar in the case. The mother said that ever since the child was left with in-laws while the parents were on vacation, she would not use a pen and had become clingy, weepy, and irresolute. The rest of the case confirmed the appropriate remedy. It was then understood that this aversion for pens was the well-known *Pulsatilla* aversion or **disgust for certain objects**, here found in a child of eight years.

Somaticized Symptoms

Another peculiarity often noticed within the first two months of a sibling being born is that the child will develop "real" physical illnesses, usually of the **respiratory** variety. Such illnesses typically begin with an earache, bronchitis, or fever, all of which have typical *Pulsatilla* modalities and characteristics. An older child or an adult *Pulsatilla* may present with a health history revealing that the **asthma** from which they have suffered for so many years began soon after the birth of a sibling.

Regression

Regression is particularly acute in *Pulsatilla* children when they experience a **major stress**, such as the birth of a sibling. Other common stresses for all children but to which the *Pulsatilla* child is particularaly sensitive and that can cause regression include changing the sleeping place (such as from a crib to a bed, or from the parents' bedroom into a private room), weaning from the breast or bottle, toilet training, beginning school, and going through puberty.

Different forms of regression are manifestations of the **acute fears** that the *Pulsatilla* child feels **at developmental milestones**. There is a **resistance to growth** and the attainment of maturity: a *Pulsatilla* child will wet the bed after being "dry" for years. Another child will begin to suck a thumb again while rubbing the nose with a forefinger or a small piece of soft rag. Another may roll his fingers around in his hair while rocking. By far the most common syndrome is that the child exhibits basic babylike behavior. These children may begin to babble like babies, want to breast-feed or sleep in the parents' bed again, or whine and cry in the ways that used to work so well to get what they want—attention and affection. Perhaps it is due to this general regressive tendency that the remedy *Pulsatilla* has a reputation for stopping **thumb sucking** in children too old for this behavior.

Grief

The reaction to intense grief in the *Pulsatilla* adolescent may, as in the adult, render them **inarticulate**. They feel left alone in the universe, forsaken by the positive forces of life. They just sit in their rooms or mope around the house. "Is there anything wrong?" the parents ask. "No." "What happened?" "Nothing." They respond monosyllabically as self-pity engulfs them. They become blind to the people who care about them and are trying to help, much as *Natrum muriaticum* children do. The difference is that the *Natrum muriaticum* child resents the interference that consolation implies to him, while the *Pulsatilla* may not notice it at all. For *Natrum muriaticum*, one refers to the rubric: Mind; Consolation; aggravates. For *Pulsatilla*, one consults the rubric: Mind, Inconsolable.

This very **deep, morose state** can be **especially dangerous for a *Pulsatilla* teenager.** One must be careful here that the child does not entertain thoughts of **suicide**; it is precisely while in this inconsolable state of shock that *Pulsatilla* adults are most likely to kill themselves.

Some of the children who seem inconsolable have a **grief they have not shared with others.** Nine-year-old John began to have headaches after moving to a new neighborhood. He confided during an office visit that when he moved, he left behind his best friends and that he missed them very much. He would cry every day and was unable to shake this dark mood. He would wish to be alone and grieve. After prescribing *Natrum muriaticum*, a remedy that seemed to fit the other symptoms but did not help at all, it became apparent that this was a *Pulsatilla* child manifesting the behaviors previously mentioned. After eliciting other confirmatory symptoms, the remedy *Pulsatilla* ended not only his headaches but his grief as well.

School

School is a big cause of stress for *Pulsatilla* children. They become **sad and forlorn if an older sibling goes away to school**, leaving them at home by themselves. It disturbs the harmony they have known as they become alone more of the time. They act as if they have lost one of their possessions: their older sibling-playmate. They are also a bit jealous, as they too want to come home and share all the exciting news of the day with the parents.

Even so, when it comes time for them to go to school, they develop a strong **fear** of it. When left off at school in the morning by a parent, the *Pulsatilla* child cries nonstop for the first few days. This is followed by a **period of shyness** until she becomes comfortable in the new setting, after which time she becomes a pleasure in the classroom both to her teacher and to other students. The report from school will be very positive as the **teacher receives near-complete compliance** from the *Pulsatilla* child with regard to schoolwork and behavior. A possible exception here may be that the child talks to her neighbors too much.

One last problem can arise after school is over for the day: if a parent is even five minutes late to pick her up, the child **fears that she has been forgotten** and begins to wail hysterically.

Although she may not be the most popular child in the class, the *Pulsatilla's* **friends will be close to her**. If **favorites change**, as they frequently do, the child feels **emotionally destroyed**. If for some reason she believes a friend has ignored or slighted her, or if perhaps she is not invited to a friend's birthday party, she will surely arrive home with a tearstained face and near hysterics. The tears flow so freely and with such deep emotion that the mere recounting of such an incident in the doctor's office may bring those tears back for the *Pulsatilla* child, who sheepishly pulls one tissue after another from the box on the desk.

One little boy cried several times during the initial interview while trying to explain his actual chief complaint: the other boys at school caused him to cry too much! Six-year-old Bill began to whimper when he revealed that he was concerned about what

223

other people thought of him, especially one girl in his class who did not seem to like him at all.

The child may often **dream or talk in his sleep about** school, parties, and all sorts of **situations** that involve his sometimes problematic relationships.

Weepiness

Emotions flow freely in the *Pulsatilla* child, especially in the form of sadness and tears. Whereas *Natrum muriaticum* sadness can be exquisitely controlled and private, the *Pulsatilla* child expresses sadness openly and with ease. It is surprising to see how old these children can be and still cry like babes. Equally striking is the ease with which these children, **boys and girls alike**, talk about their weeping. "I cry because my feelings are hurt," said Alan*, without hesitation or inhibition, as though weeping were a natural language with which he communicated.

It is interesting to find **weeping in older boys**, given that our society has such strong mores prohibiting it. For instance, one sensitive boy wept in the office while describing how he was not allowed to wrestle along with the other boys in his class. The dichotomy of personal sensitivity with the aggressive wrestling play he sought pointed to *Pulsatilla*.

The tears that so easily flow help the child both physically and emotionally. The **consolation** that he receives from **displaying sadness** re-establishes the bonds of love so critical to his emotional survival. Any time the child is angry, sad, irritable, frustrated, or perhaps just teased by siblings or parents, he breaks down and sobs; this is an act that renders him great psychological relief. This twofold amelioration comes from both the actual physical relief crying affords and the acts of consolation it elicits from others.

The *Pulsatilla* youngster is **easily offended**; and when she is, she begins to weep, sulk, or pout. The parents ask, "What's wrong?" The child answers, "Nothing." "Are you sure?" "Yes." If the parent probes further and asks, "Why are you behaving this way?" more often than not, the peevish sulkiness breaks down and the child begins to weep involuntarily, throwing herself on her mother's bosom and soaking up all the love she can. **Receiving sympathy** and consolation puts her, just as it would a tiny infant, at the center of the universe again.

These children easily become discouraged in their work and give up projects they have begun with genuine enthusiasm. Disappointment in themselves and feelings of failure feed into fears of not being a "good person," not being worthy of love, and that people they love and depend on will inevitably abandon them. How upset they become, moping about until they begin to cry, causing the parents to console them—at which point they confess their minor "crime" of real or imagined disability. In a moment they are fine and happy, joyful and bouncy, while their parents feel as if they were living with a schizophrenic.

Weeping is also seen as a reaction to pain. As a rule, these children are very sensitive to pain, just as is the *Lycopodium* youngster, and cry continuously and hysterically when hurt until an adult picks them up. This is especially true regarding earaches. Eight-year-old Betty was seen for recurrent earaches and sinus infections. With every hint of illness she would cry dramatically, running to her father to be picked up. While the otitis media symptoms did not give any special clues to the remedy, the intense sensitivity to pain—expressed in the form of needing consolation—put the rest of the case in order and pointed to *Pulsatilla*. After the remedy was given, Betty's next earache was her last.

With every instance of otitis, three-year-old Donna would hold her head just behind the ears and cry, "Mommy help me! Mommy help me!" over and over again. She would not be put down to nap and had to be carried around the house, even though the motion hurt her head even more.

Six-year-old Tommy had gastroenteritis accompanied by vomiting, stomach cramps, and diarrhea. The symptoms of the case weighed equally between *Sulphur* and *Pulsatilla*. The symptom that sent the verdict to *Pulsatilla* was that Tommy was ultrasensitive to the pain. He had to be held and rocked to ameliorate the hurt. If his mother left the room while his stomach was hurting, he would yell for her until she returned.

As an aside, after practicing for a time I found that God has been merciful to the homeopath; in acute cases one usually finds that the physical symptoms and modalities are so strong that they unequivocally give the remedy away. In the cases where this is not true, especially those involving children in a great deal of pain (as in the case of little Betty just described), the mental and emotional symptoms accompanying the physical symptoms point to the correct remedy. It is wonderful to discover that the **necessary information to find the remedy needed is always there** to be found.

Irresoluteness

It seems that the **emotions rule** this child to the extent that the mental faculties suffer. **When upset**, she becomes irresolute and **unable to make any decision**, trivial or important. When she goes to a restaurant, she cannot decide what she wants to eat, and the parents must make the choice for her. When she has to decide what game to play, she is unable to do so—and therefore her playmates will decide. When she needs to dress herself, she cannot make up her mind what to wear.

Pulsatilla children may change their clothing several times a day or ask the mother to pick something out for them. While this changing of clothes may be observed with *Natrum muriaticum* as well, the reasons are completely different. *Natrum muriaticum* children do not wish to be laughed at or be conspicuous, so they try on outfit after outfit, looking for the "appropriate" one. In *Pulsatilla*, however, the **decision-making process is faulty**; they cannot decide which one looks better. Someone else will have to choose, or they will finally pick one out only from time pressure. Then, when they are out in public and someone merely looks at them, the first thing they think is, "Oh no! I picked the wrong one!" *Pulsatilla* not only has difficulty making decisions, but doubts the decision finally made at even a stranger's passing glance.

"Soft" Boys

It is interesting to note the quandary in which *Pulsatilla* children find themselves in because of their irresoluteness. Because they are not able to make a true decision on their own, they **can never stand up for a particular belief** either verbally or physically. When this quality is pronounced in a boy, the child may **seem effeminate** and softer than his peers. The other boys at school may pick on him because he seems incapable of defending not only his opinions but himself.

Eleven-year-old Tony was seen for bowel incontinence and handling of the genitals, both of which had begun after the birth of his sister five years earlier. Besides the two problems mentioned, Tony's father complained that the child was a "sissy" and too effeminate. "The child likes to play with his mother, not me," he confided. "The other boys at school pick on him." The father was agitated because the child cried hysterically when upset, "his voice screeching like a girl's," and he began to talk like a baby and act childish. Every time the child was teased at school he burst into tears, which only egged on the taunting children more.

In another case, ten-year-old Nathan was seen for recurrent diarrhea. When probed about his feelings, his mother volunteered that he wept easily. Asked if this was true, Nathan burst into tears, becoming totally uncontrollable with loud, racking sobs. It was easy to see that he had been told he was too old for this type of behavior, because he tried to cover his mouth so that no one would see him crying hysterically. "It is because my sister hurts my feelings on purpose, calling me a sissy," he finally managed to say. What a dilemma in which the *Pulsatilla* boy finds himself, placed in our society and having to **stifle these natural inclinations in order to conform to a sex role.**

The way some of these tenderhearted boys respond to taunting is by developing a temper as they grow, finally fighting anyone who picks on them. The closest that they come, however, to regular fighting matches may be with a younger sibling who, in their eyes, took a parent's love away from them. This shows up as shouting matches, tussles, and not letting the sibling use his toys or wear his clothes.

When reading materia medicas of the past, one often finds many descriptions of what has just been described for *Pulsatilla*; easily led or persuaded, mild, gentle, submissive, timid, yielding, and sweet are all common adjectives. The child gives in on most issues if there are differing or louder opinions. This yielding nature combined with clinginess, if taken to the extreme, may drive a parent to distraction. Parents and materia medicas all describe the same basic psychology using different terminology. The children all act as they do from an insecure nature, the fear of abandonment, indecisiveness, and easy, strong emotionality.

Consolation

With these core weaknesses ruling the child, one can see why there is such a strong amelioration from consolation. All actions and ideas are held together by a common theme: if a *Pulsatilla* child is connected to the ones he or she loves, the world is secure and everything is fine. Likewise, one observes that when they feel their attachment to loved ones threatened, these children become suspicious, envious, and jealous of anything that might undermine their **sense of security**.

Hyperactivity

A small number of *Pulsatilla* boys may also be hyperactive, running around all over the house, unable to sit down in a chair, but always hanging around the parent. "Watch this, Mom!" is a favorite gambit. In one respect, *Pulsatilla* is very different from other hyperactive remedy types in that *Pulsatilla* children exhibit their **sweet qualities** even if they are hyperactive. Some of these children seem to be "set off" by eating foods that have dyes, especially red ones, added to them. One should pay special attention to any comments about foods and **food allergies** when querying the children or their parents.

Fears

The fears that rule *Pulsatilla* are mainly of **abandonment and all its derivatives**, such as being **left alone** in a room or house or in the dark, and should be added to the rubric: Mind; Fear, alone, dark, children. The fear may arise acutely in certain situations. If the **parents go away** on vacation, the *Pulsatilla* child does not understand that they will return, only that they have left him— leading to many hours of sorrow and crying. One boy refused to go to sleep in his bedroom from that point on, sleeping only on the living room couch where he could keep an eye out for thieves. Another child had a complete **relapse** of migraines and enuresis when her mother had to go to the hospital for several days. Besides all the other *Pulsatilla* symptoms that she exhibited even upon her mother's return, she acted like a fearful baby, not at all happy to be taken to school or to the baby-sitter. She now had to sleep with her parents again.

The *Pulsatilla* child not only develops illnesses from these traumas, but also the **shock of** the temporary or permanent **loss** of a family member **may act as an antidote to a dose of** *Pulsatilla* previously given with curative effect, and thus will need to be repeated. Death of a loved one may be experienced as a deep grief, but can have an aspect of selfishness as well, exhibited in an attitude as if to say to the world, "Now, what do I do?"

They may fear robbers and **being kidnaped**, and even dream of this theme. Naturally, they will be **afraid to go to bed alone**, frightened to be in the dark alone, and may need someone to scout out the house for intruders. They may wake up crying with these bad dreams, calling for a parent to come get into bed with them. Others cry, get out of bed, and work their way into the parents' bed, all the while sucking a thumb, twirling bits of hair, and carrying a favorite stuffed animal. This problem may become so great that they are unable to sleep over at a friend's house for fear of abandonment and end up calling home at bedtime to be picked up.

Pulsatilla should also be added to the rubrics: Mind; Fear, dogs; Mind; Fear, **insects**; and Mind; Fear, **snakes**. They also experience fear in the **evening** of **monsters, ghosts**, and **large animals**. These last fears are very similar to those of *Phosphorus*, *Causticum*, and *Lycopodium*.

Several materia medicas describe the fear of **looking up**. In practice this is very rarely seen in *Pulsatilla*, being more commonly found in *Calcarea carbonica* and *Silicea*.

Two Types

Two main sets of *Pulsatilla* children are observed in practice: **those who will need the remedy** *Calcarea carbonica* **after** *Pulsatilla*, **and those who** will require *Sulphur*. Each behave somewhat differently as the underlying second remedy interplays with the prevailing *Pulsatilla* layer, altering it slightly.

The ones having *Sulphur* underneath develop very **red lips** and/or a rash around the mouth. They may also tend toward **pos-**

sessiveness and hyperactivity. Those who will eventually have a need for *Calcarea carbonica* have a definite fear of snakes and insects and may dream of them. This subset also has more of a natural desire for cleanliness. They might keep their shoes and socks neat and clean and all their toys picked up. This stems from a basic sense of order rather than the compulsive fastidiousness of *Natrum muriaticum*.

Sleep

Sleep offers many keynotes to the remedy. One finds that *Pulsatilla* babies need to be rocked and nursed in order to fall asleep. Every time the infant awakens, it cries for the mother who must rock, bounce, caress, or nurse the child back to sleep. Finally the baby falls asleep, but as the mother puts the child down again, the crying begins anew. The mother often has to sleep with the baby even when the "baby" is now a child of seven, eight, or nine years old.

Older children may have difficulty falling asleep for several reasons. Fourteen-year-old Anna started to weep as she described her nights: she worried for hours if she had studied enough for the next day's test; would she do well, and would her parents think less of her if she did not? Another child described staying awake night after night to review her old, secret griefs, as one would find in *Natrum muriaticum*. The thoughts keeping these children up are rooted in the fear of losing the love of their parents. When they finally do fall asleep, their dreams may be full of the same topics that kept them awake.

Likewise, when a parent announces bedtime and time to be tucked in, the child often resists because sleep separates him or her from the parent. Such children pretend that they need a glass of water, need to urinate, need yet another bedtime story, or that they are scared. After an hour of these sincere pleas, when the parents are finally relaxing on the living room couch, they hear the voice of their little *Pulsatilla* wafting through with some final comments: "What are you doing?" "Can you come here?" "Can I come out?" Anything as long as it brings a parent into the room. Eventually they fall asleep out of exhaustion.

When the child becomes old enough to walk, waking up and **finding the way to the parents' bed** will be common. As mentioned before, many of these children have a fear of the dark and a fear of being alone, so the easy migration into the parents' bed is natural. *Pulsatilla* children may need to **sleep with the lights on** because they are **afraid** of the dark, of monsters, and of the moving shadows of trees on the walls and the like.

They generally fall asleep on their backs, possibly with their **hands above their heads**; or on the **abdomen** with their hands tucked under their abdomens. They **dislike covering up** and will kick off the covers, especially from their warm feet. Babies who are covered up and become too warm will cry until the parent understands and pulls the blanket back a bit to let them cool off. They may not tolerate those currently popular footed pajamas from the first year on, and may eventually struggle their way out of them.

These children may **weep, talk, or drool in their sleep**; the latter trait also belongs to *Sulphur*. They usually **wake up happy and refreshed**; generally conditions are ameliorated in the mornings.

They may have **nightmares** if there is **stress in the family** such as a possible divorce or anything else that threatens their sense of security. The fear of separation often makes its way into the sleep state with dreams such as the mother getting into an accident and dying. They wake up terrified by these dreams and run to their parents' room for consolation.

The sleep of *Pulsatilla* children is affected during **fevers**. The children may become slightly **delirious**. They may dream and talk of **black cats or other animals** or just of ominous, amorphous dark shapes.

Vertigo

The closest these children approach vertigo is **orthostatic hypotension**, which commonly occurs in closed rooms where the air is still. When they bend over and reach down for a book on a low shelf in the library, for instance, dizziness can occur.

Physical Symptomatology

Head

The head remains **relatively free of problems** in *Pulsatilla* children with only a few exceptions. Girls may develop **schooltime headaches** accompanied by digestive upsets, aggravated by eating too much ice cream, meats, or fats, as described in the old materia medicas. These headaches, like those of *Natrum muriaticum*, will also be caused or aggravated by watching television, reading, or becoming overheated, and especially by lingering too long in the sun. A child may complain that headaches only develop in one particular class. If the doctor asks a little more specifically, it will usually be revealed that the child finds this particular **classroom too warm**.

Teenaged girls may complain of **headaches associated with the menses**, occurring either just before, during, or immediately after the flow. The pains will be felt on one side or temple and be congestive in nature; the adolescent feels a constant throbbing. The hot head is relieved by cold packs, pressure, and sitting up. The amelioration from cold is a point that aids in differentiating *Pulsatilla* from its complementary remedy *Silicea*, who craves heat on the painful head. This congestive type of headache may often be confused with that of *Belladonna*, as the two remedies share the modalities of aggravation from quick motion and stooping. Also, as is found in *Belladonna*, the face becomes red during the congestive headache and the eyes feel engorged, as if there is pressure pushing them outward.

Lastly, *Pulsatilla* children sometimes have headaches that are associated with **upper respiratory tract infections** such as sinusitis, similar to those of *Calcarea carbonica*.

The headache may be **aggravated by lying down and ameliorated by outdoor activity**, by getting the mind off the pain and moving about in the open air—both of which help enormously. A key point to ask about or observe if one knows the child goes outside in the wintertime is whether or not the child keeps a hat on. Parents of a *Pulsatilla* state that the child always **takes the hat off, even in the coldest weather**. This may be an important differentiating point when treating a child in an acute respiratory crisis, as the other common remedy types such as *Lycopodium* and *Silicea* keep their hats securely on.

Eyes

The eyes are **frequently affected** by various problems in the *Pulsatilla* child. **During any disease**, especially of the upper respiratory tract, the child may develop either **conjunctivitis, dacryocystitis, or marginal blepharitis.** The symptoms of these diseases match perfectly the symptoms of *Pulsatilla*. The eyes become **inflamed, even in the newborn.** Children rub their eyes continuously, which they say **burn and itch, especially at night.** They may feel and describe the sensation that there is sand in the eyes, similar to what children needing *Sulphur* report with eye problems.

Colds can settle in the eyes and produce a thick, purulent, yellow-green, bland **discharge.** Agglutination of the eyelids during the night is common. When the child awakens in the morning, the lids must be moistened with warm water to loosen the dried, crusty mucus away. Profuse lacrimation is associated with any eye complaints, noticeable especially in the open or cold air. *Pulsatilla* children may also become photophobic with eye complaints.

Some children develop **styes that recur** over and over again. Although materia medicas only describe styes of the upper lid, they may be found as frequently on the lower lid. As the stye progresses, it discharges thick, yellow pus. Aside from lacrimation, all *Pulsatilla* eye symptoms are **aggravated** in a warm room or **by warm** bathing, and are tremendously ameliorated **by cold** air, bathing the eye in cold water, or applying cold compresses. Even small babies will push away a warm cloth if it approaches the troubled eye.

While there are many remedies that affect the eye, it will be found that if the symptoms are ameliorated by cold applications, the great majority of these children will do well with the remedy *Pulsatilla*. The temperature modality is the most important factor to ask about because the answer will help to differentiate *Pulsatilla* from other common homeopathic medicines that alleviate eye problems.

Ears

Pulsatilla cures many ear symptoms as well. It may be considered the prime remedy for otitis media along with *Belladonna* and *Chamomilla*. The inflammation may begin with a cold or an exanthem such as measles. Other children develop earaches after being out in a cold, dry wind or playing in the rain. The external ear may be red, hot, and swollen; and the tragus may develop red sores. Severe throbbing pains in the ears become worse at night and with the warmth of the bed, and feel better outdoors and with cool applications. Some cry with the pain and can be soothed by being held, rocked, or carried around.

Older children who can describe the feeling may report a sensation of something crawling out of the ear or pressure pushing outward from inside the ear. If the inflammation is allowed to progress, the ear will produce a copious, thick, bland, yellowgreen discharge that sometimes gives off an offensive odor. This is similar to *Kali sulphuricum*, except that the *Kali sulphuricum* discharge is more of an orange-yellow color and usually more watery.

The pus and mucus may cause deafness along with the feeling of the ears being stopped up, the child only hearing a distant roaring noise synchronous with the pulse. With very young children it is obviously difficult to elicit such detailed symptomatology, so the remedy will be prescribed on the basis of what one observes in the office, what a parent can describe about the etiology, the child's behavior, and the patterns of sleep, thirst, and temperature.

Lastly, *Pulsatilla*, *Silicea*, and *Hepar sulphuris* are the common remedies that help the outer ear, curing otitis externa or "swimmer's ear."

Nose

The nose is involved in almost every upper respiratory tract infection. *Pulsatilla* children develop repeated colds accompanied by much sneezing. Six-year-old Sally was typical in her infection, which began with repeated sneezing, followed by a clear mucus discharge from the nose. Her conjunctiva became red and her eyes began to itch. Her lips dried out quickly and began to crack and bleed over the next few days. She then started to have sharp, pressing pains in the ears accompanied by a high fever. During the inflammation she also developed vaginitis and became lethargic, wanting to be held much of the time by her mother. *Pulsatilla* prevented this girl from developing any further infections and stopped her cycle of upper respiratory tract breakdowns.

Aggravation of cold symptoms is found **at night**. When the child lies down to sleep the nose plugs up, forcing him to breathe through his continually open and drying mouth. This is a very common symptom for both children and adults in acute or chronic *Pulsatilla* states. In the morning the nasal passages are completely obstructed, even if the nose is blown frequently.

During acute states, the mucus is dislodged easily: a thick, yellow-green, bland discharge that may form greenish, bloody crusts. In chronic states, however, sufferers blow and blow to no effect. The main amelioration of nasal and sinus symptoms is found in open air. The only exception to this is found during hay fever season when conditions grow worse outdoors.

Due to a perpetually **clogged nose**, the sense of smell is often diminished. Curiously, older children and adults may comment that although they cannot smell, they do sense a terrible, sour, putrid odor originating from within their own noses. They may have **nosebleeds** at night or bleeding from the hard nasal crusts that develop. The blood in this case tends to be dark and clotted.

Hay Fever

Pulsatilla is one of the most useful remedies for curing hay fever. Hay fever in *Pulsatilla* types is aggravated in the open air and at night. It begins with **itching of the upper palate**, especially noted at night. This itching causes those afflicted to make clucking sounds with their tongues while trying to scratch the upper palate. The eyes then begin to itch and lacrimate greatly. At first the tears are acrid, but after a few days a dacryocystitis develops with a thicker, more bland discharge. They also develop a postnasal drip, which causes a dry, tickling cough at night.

The nose itches, as well as the eyes and palate, and it discharges clear, bland mucus, especially in the morning and when the child is outside. At night the nasal passages become obstructed and may only be cleared if the child wakes up in the middle

235

of the night sneezing, clucking, and blowing the now watery mucus out of the nose. In the morning the dryness is gone and the child is able to hawk up the mucus with ease.

All hay fever symptoms are aggravated out of doors by being around grasses, by the change of seasons, by hot days, and by direct sunshine in the eyes. The attacks are ameliorated by cool days and by splashing cold water on the face.

Face

The face can be either pale and anemic or red and plethoric. In anemic children one observes dark circles under the eyes. With every cold these circles grow darker and larger. **Plethoric girls** have periodic edematous swellings of the face and the lips. They may also have **flushing of the face**, with swollen lips, just before the menses that subsides as soon as the flow begins.

A subset of *Pulsatilla* children have very **red, dry, and cracked lips** with or without an accompanying red rash around the mouth. This dryness (noted especially in **boys**) makes them lick their lips frequently, which further exacerbates the dry lip syndrome. After prescribing the simillimum *Pulsatilla* to these children, the dryness disappears only to later reappear along with a constellation of symptoms that now point to *Sulphur* as the new simillimum. This rash, then, forms one of the **bridges** between the two remedies.

With **fevers** the face becomes **flushed**. Occasionally only **one cheek** becomes flushed while the other becomes pale, a peculiar symptom that *Pulsatilla* shares with *Aconitum*, *Chamomilla*, and *Ipecacuanha*.

While quite rare in these times of antibiotic use, one may find a patient with **mumps** in which the face is **very flushed** and the inflammation has **metastasized to the breasts or testes** and is accompanied by much swelling and pain. *Pulsatilla* will be one of the main remedies considered along with *Rhododendron* and *Abrotanum*.

Mouth

The mouth provides a few keynotes for *Pulsatilla*. **A dry mouth yet lack of thirst is classic**. Children who have obstructed noses and so have become obligatory mouth-breathers will awaken with totally dry palates unless they wake up at night and drink a few sips of water to wet the mucous membranes. Even in this situation, however, they still will not drink much. The *Natrum muriaticum* child in comparison will drink the whole glass and even ask for more.

The **breath** can be quite **foul** when these children get up in the **morning**, even in the very young. While examining *Pulsatilla* children, one can often see a thin, white or lacy coating on the tongue just as they open their mouths. A thick, ropy strand of saliva stretching from one lip to the other may also be present.

Pulsatilla children occasionally develop **blisters on the tip of the tongue.**

Lower Respiratory System

The **chest is the site of many problems** for the *Pulsatilla* child, both acute and chronic. There may be a history of **bronchitis or pneumonia**. The remedy *Pulsatilla* also cures a type of croup, although this is not usually discussed in the old literature, being more often assigned to *Aconitum* and *Spongia tosta*.

The croup typically begins with a dry cough that is aggravated at night and accompanied by the sensation as if the throat were closing off at the larynx. It is aggravated during sleep while the child is lying down, forcing her to sit up during the attack. The cough may also cause retching and vomiting.

Bronchitis may begin similarly to the croup with a dry, raw throat and irritation of the trachea. This may develop after or along with a childhood exanthem or rash that is suppressed by ointments and does not fully develop. The cough is caused by a dry tickle in the trachea, which is worse when the child lies down at night or becomes warm or overheated, as from exertion. The cough usually subsides when the child walks in the cool, open air; sits up; or becomes active (though not to the point of overheating). The cough eventually becomes productive, offering up a thick, purulent, yellow, bland expectoration that is easily dislodged with every spasm.

A **keynote** of *Pulsatilla*, as well as of *Calcarea carbonica*, is the common complaint of a **dry cough** throughout the entire day and night and a loose, **wet cough only upon awakening**, accompanied by much expectoration at that time. Such children also develop a bad taste in the mouth during these morning bronchitis attacks.

The *Pulsatilla* child is often very **allergic to the environment**, developing **asthma** from any bark dust or pollen in the air. At first the child only manifests **hay fever**, as described previously. Eventually, the hay fever stops and the child progresses to asthma. The asthma may also be a sequela to influenza, pharyngitis, or bronchitis. Many of the symptoms of the asthma will be the same as those described for bronchitis, especially the wet cough with its attendant modalities.

Asthma is aggravated at night and by lying on the left side, by cold and wet or humid weather, and by overheating. An aggravation time of one o'clock in the morning may also be reported.

Alimentary System

Food Cravings and Aversions

It is interesting to note that **many of the foods *Pulsatilla* children crave aggravate problems of their digestive tracts.** They **desire cheese, ice cream, eggs, butter** (even more commonly than is found in *Mercurius vivus*), **pastry and cakes, peanut butter, and sweets.** They are **aggravated by pastry, ice cream, lemons and very sour foods, fats, and meat (especially pork).** Many of these foods cause vomiting, diarrhea, and headaches. They are **averse to eating fruits, milk, bread, fats, warm foods, and meat (especially fatty meats such as pork).**

A commonly confirmed keynote is that the child is quite **thirstless**, even though he may have a fever or a very dry mouth.

Stomach

The stomach is troubled as often as is the respiratory tract in the *Pulsatilla* child. **Gastroenteritis** is accompanied by severe abdominal cramps that are ameliorated by rocking, consolation, and in some cases, cold drinks. During the attack most children will not wish to eat or drink and will become droopy and clingy. Some may also develop a coryza that accompanies the enteritis.

The stomach of *Pulsatilla* **digests both food and emotional interactions slowly.** Any time there is a strong emotional stress, the child develops stomachaches, nausea, and/or vomiting, similar in this regard to *Phosphorus*. The child may also develop ulcers in the stomach from strong emotions that remain unresolved.

Ten-year-old Roy developed **ulcers** after his older brother left for college. This secret grief made him cry often, though he never told anyone why he was sad or why he was crying. The ulcers would pain him at night, and he felt better if he opened the window and took a breath of fresh air. Although the boy had been grieving and struggling with the ulcers for two years, he became symptom-free within one month of taking the remedy *Pulsatilla*. While Roy remained a sensitive young man, his grief and subsequent weeping were finally resolved.

The stomach is easily **upset by eating rich foods** such as meat, fat, oil, and butter; and unfortunately, by foods *Pulsatilla* children enjoy immensely, such as ice cream, cake, and cheese. These foods may be eructated for hours after being eaten and may cause vomiting or diarrhea. These are foods that sit in the stomach for a long time and feel to the child as if there were a lump there.

Frequently a doctor will treat a child who complains of early morning nausea, vomiting, and diarrhea. The history often shows that the previous evening the child went to a party and had ice cream and pastries or other rich foods. One parent described her daughter's sensitive stomach as "Post-Halloween-Birthday-Easter-Christmas Syndrome." After coming home from such a celebration, the child becomes very sick from the foods eaten. The youngster may cry, complain, and come to the parents' bed whimpering during the night. At first the parents may think that the child has appendicitis, but eventually they perceive the pattern that follows every binge of eating rich foods.

One last distinctive digestive symptom, often observed in *Pulsatilla* **infants**, is that most will **hiccough after they eat**. I have created a new rubric for this symptom: Stomach; Hiccough; eating, after, in infants; and have listed *Pulsatilla* in bold type, with *Calcarea carbonica* and *Lycopodium* in italics and *Nux vomica* in plain type.

The remedy *Pulsatilla* should be considered for **motion sickness** as well.

Abdomen

Infants with colic often respond well to the remedy *Pulsatilla* when other symptoms match. The abdomen distends and there is audible rumbling and gurgling. Gas bubbles can be seen rippling across the abdomen. Older children often complain of full, swollen bellies after eating rich, fatty foods.

Adolescent girls may complain of abdominal bloating that accompanies the facial bloating typically found before the onset of the menses.

Rectum

The **infant** may develop **diarrhea** easily or have the chief complaint of infantile colic. Before the diarrhea, the abdomen distends painfully. The stools are watery and full of mucus. They vary in color between green and yellow, but their basically slimy character remains. The colic may be worse at night. Infantile diarrhea may **alternate with constipation**, conforming to the adage **"No two stools alike."** While this is a bit of an exaggeration, what one does find is that there is **no predictability** as to what type of stool will emerge next. **Older girls** may also have **diarrhea along with the menses.**

The children may develop constipation with large, hard stools. Very often a homeopath will observe these symptoms of constipation and prescribe *Pulsatilla* only to find that it does not work—but that *Calcarea carbonica* will. Likewise, many times *Calcarea carbonica* will not work and *Pulsatilla* will; as usual, the general symptoms lead and must prevail in the selection of the remedy, as the local symptoms often overlap between remedies.

Urogenital System

Pulsatilla cures, in the *Pulsatilla* child, **nocturnal enuresis** that is aggravated by the child lying on her back. As the topic is discussed with the doctor, the parent will state that this problem makes the child cry from shame. Stresses that affect the child emotionally may precipitate enuresis. Two common causes of such stress are school beginning again after a vacation and sleeping over at a friend's house.

240

Pulsatilla is a key remedy to consider for children who develop **recurrent cystitis** and for those who may have a history of **kidney infections**. The trilogy of weakness of the bladder muscles, a small bladder, and infrequent drinking leads to recurrent problems. Frequency of urination that is aggravated at night by lying down accompanies this cystitis. As an aside, scanty urine that burns when the child finally does urinate would burn less if the child drank more.

Little Mary developed a bladder infection two weeks after her sister Susan was born. When it started, she became very droopy and weak and began to cry more than usual. She then developed a fever along with more regressive behavior. The next day she had urinary frequency accompanied by blood in the urine. The case was clearly *Pulsatilla*, as illustrated by the regression, the sibling rivalry, and the clinginess. Her mother reported that even when the child urinated more frequently and thus should have experienced dehydration, her thirst decreased instead of increased. This modality, contrary to what would seem to make sense physiologically, pointed especially to *Pulsatilla* as an effective remedy, which it proved to be.

Boys

Boys may be born with **hydroceles** or may develop **mumps that metastasize to the testes**, although the latter is quite rare now.

Girls

Even at an early age, girls may develop a thick, creamy, offensive-smelling, bland or excoriating **leukorrhea**. This is often associated with an upper respiratory tract infection. Every time they catch a cold or develop bronchitis, they contend with this leukorrhea as well.

Many girls have a case of **chronic vaginitis** a year or two before their menarche. At other times the parents may complain of the girl's strong vaginal odor, even though there is no discernible discharge. The leukorrhea and concomitant odor often cause the doctor to mistakenly prescribe *Calcarea carbonica*, a remedy type that also shares these symptoms.

The *Pulsatilla* picture tends to develop more fully during

puberty or at the menarche. Along with the emotional and mental changes that first emerge during this time are some specific menstrual problems that are commonly seen.

The menses may **begin late**, some not experiencing menarche until sixteen or seventeen years of age. The first year's menses can be irregular for girls of all types, with cycles commencing from every twenty-odd days to every six months as the hormonal system "gets into gear." For *Pulsatilla*, however, this **irregularity** is particularly pronounced and may last for several years.

Before the menses, girls become **weepy and morose** for no apparent reason. Everything seems to be fine when suddenly the thought arises in them that there is no purpose in living. At this time they pout and need to talk to their mothers or fathers and establish the contact of love and purpose so central to their lives.

Adolescents may also have facial, abdominal, and breast swelling; chilliness; excessive yawning; and diarrhea right before the menses. Older girls sometimes say that this **premenstrual feeling** stays around all month long, including the swelling of the abdomen and breasts, and the melancholy mood.

The **flow** may consist of only a little dark, watery blood with clots, or a flow that stops and starts erratically. The catamenia (when the menstrual blood flows freely) may become lengthy and profuse as well.

The menses are accompanied by much **pain**, causing the girls to double over, toss and turn in bed, or pace the floor. A special keynote is that the pain may be aggravated by hot applications and ameliorated by cold ones; an unusual finding, as most girls report amelioration of menstrual pain by heat.

Menstrual pains will not reduce during the flow, which is also peculiar, for most menstrual pains decrease or stop after the catamenia is established. The girls may cry with pain, walk the floor, and become very gloomy with a "woe is me" attitude reflected in both their tone of voice and facial expressions. Restlessness may be quite marked during the pain.

The old materia medicas describe the occasional flow of milk in nonpregnant girls. **Lactation** of this sort has become rare due to the routine hormonal treatment of pituitary gland dysfunctions. A seven-year-old girl who came to see me suddenly developed this type of breast discharge. The breasts oozed clear liquid that crusted up to a slightly off-white color. At the same time the nipples became itchy, raised, and very tender to the touch. The rest of the case fit *Pulsatilla*, which restored the breasts to normal in short order.

Musculoskeletal System

Extremities

The most common *Pulsatilla* symptom in the extremities is the **warmth** found there. The children want to walk around barefoot even in the wintertime. They often stick their feet out of the covers at night. In the summertime, the feet aim for the air conditioner or touch the walls for coolness.

Pulsatilla infants often have feet that are purplish and cold to the touch—but the sensation of the children is that the feet feel warm; they resist putting them under the covers.

The hands may show that the child bites the nails.

Frequently, the *Pulsatilla* child manifests all the foot symptoms of *Silicea*, including **foul perspiration of the feet** that corrodes the skin. A bridge to *Silicea*, the complementary remedy of *Pulsatilla*, is thus formed by this symptom. The differentiating point leading to *Pulsatilla* is found in the nails of those sweaty feet: in *Pulsatilla*, the perspiration will not affect the integrity of the nails; in *Silicea*, however, when profuse foot perspiration is found, the nails are also often affected by cracks or other disfigurement.

Pulsatilla may be used to treat juvenile **rheumatoid arthritis** with migratory joint pains that are aggravated in the morning, by warmth, and by lying in bed at night. The pains are ameliorated by motion and by cool air. The joints are swollen, red, and hot. Nodules develop during the early stages of the disease. Of course, the mental picture must also be consistent with *Pulsatilla* before it is assumed to be the correct remedy.

Skin

Pulsatilla **babies** have a characteristic feature of the skin: it takes on a purplish, marbled, **mottled appearance** most of the time. While this condition may become less pronounced when they are warm, in a cool office one will see the mottling very easily. This remedy type also develops large hives, especially from strong emotional stresses, but also from aggravating foods, as do *Lycopodium* and *Urtica urens*.

Pulsatilla is quite valuable as a remedy in many childhood **exanthems** such as measles, chickenpox, fifth disease, and roseola. The rash will commonly be accompanied by otitis media, conjunctivitis, or bronchitis. All the skin problems are aggravated by warmth (especially at night in bed) and by contact with wool. These problems are ameliorated in the open air.

The parents state that the child itches terribly in bed at night when she becomes warm and may scratch until she begins to bleed, as is found with *Sulphur*. These rashes, like hives and other *Pulsatilla* complaints, may come and go, reappearing even after it seems that they have left for good.

The child may also be afflicted with a terrible odor that can emanate from virtually any portion of the body. The parents are likely to be astonished at how bad their child smells, even when regularly bathed.

Fevers

High fevers may accompany any acute disease. A delirium may occur during fevers in which the child imagines, for example, big things falling on him, or large, dark animals nearby. The child may try to run away, to escape from the bed in his sleep. With a typically flushed face, he may resemble *Belladonna* very much in this circumstance.

Girls sometimes "spike" a fever at will. Parents may rightly suspect that any time the child wishes attention or feels insecure, or any time there is turmoil in the house, she develops a fever.

Physical Generals

Pulsatilla weaknesses are aggravated by the following: becoming **overheated**, remaining in stuffy rooms, taking hot baths, performing fast exercises, getting wet and chilled, and from **suppressed skin eruptions**; and during a change of weather from hot to cold, evening and nighttime, summer, **puberty**, and the premenstrual syndrome (due chiefly to chronic anemia).

Pulsatilla youngsters are **warm-blooded** children who wear few clothes, love to run around naked even in the wintertime, and hate to wear hats! They may say they are chilly with their acute illnesses, even though these conditions will often be ameliorated by cool air.

Symptoms in general may be experienced only on one side of the body or may migrate or change modality from time to time. Occasionally when one reads over the case of a patient who has not been helped by various remedies, it is observed that there is no consistency to the symptoms given; in fact, the patient gave contradictory information over time. This inconsistency is a very important clue to the adult *Pulsatilla*; it is much less frequently found in children. I mention it here simply as a point to keep in mind.

Pulsatilla presents a picture of a child whose nature is ameliorated by sleep, walking slowly, **cool applications**, and **being carried or gently rocked**; as well as in the morning and in the **open air. Weeping ameliorates** many *Pulsatilla* pains and illnesses, or at least will usually be present in these instances.

Notes on *Pulsatilla* Infants

Pulsatilla infants, though pleasant, cry a great deal. Infants need to be held all the time: they cry whenever they are put down, even for short periods, and are content only when picked up again. The crying, though it may become wearing on the nerves after a while, does not have an annoying quality to it. It makes parents pay more attention to their babies and lavish love upon them, which is exactly what these babies want all the time.

Toddlers, craving the company of parents, hate to be transferred to bedrooms of their own and will cry until a parent comes in to lie down with them. Babies may also cry and fuss when weaned from the breast. Young children of this type fear the separation from parents that such changes appear to bring. Toddlers also fear being alone in the dark and will cry until a parent comes in to comfort them with hugs.

Babies and infants may be very sensitive to pain, screaming in agony with every minor earache or injury. Again, they feel better if picked up, rocked, or carried about by a parent.

Babies need to be rocked and nursed in order to fall asleep. Every time infants wake up they cry for their mothers, who must rock, bounce, caress, or nurse them back to sleep; yet nonetheless they wake up again when put down. Mothers may have to sleep with their *Pulsatilla* babies. *Pulsatilla* children like to sleep on their backs with their hands above their heads, or on their stomachs with their hands either above their heads or tucked under their abdomens. They awake refreshed and in a good mood. During fevers they may fear dogs; one thirteen-month-old patient fearfully whimpered the word "dog" often during a fevered sleep.

Infections of the eyes recur. The eye area becomes readily inflamed, producing a great deal of thick, yellow to green discharge that agglutinates the eyelids. Toddlers will cry if a warm application is used to remove the discharge; heat aggravates any pain felt in the eye area. The discharge should be removed with cool, soothing water in these cases.

Recurrent otitis media may result from a cold. The pains are much worse at night when the child is warm in bed, and cause the child to cry.

This is ameliorated by parental comforting, gentle bouncing of the child, and cool applications. Ruptured eardrums exude a great deal of thick, bland, yellow to green discharge.

Toddlers tend to develop many colds, which produce thick, green mucus. The nasal passages of infants must be suctioned often to allow normal breathing. Accumulating mucus will cause coughing. The nasal passages close off at night while lying in bed.

Croup with a dry cough, worse when lying down to sleep, is a common complaint. The cough comes when the child is just entering a deep sleep. The half-wakened child coughs deeply and lies back down to enter a deep sleep again, only to cough and start the three- or four-minute cycle over. The sufferer may wake up frustrated and crying due to this syndrome.

Bronchitis is another complaint, accompanied by thick mucus and a wet cough that is aggravated at night when lying down.

Extensive hiccoughing results from nursing. Infants are prone to colic, during which the abdomen distends and rumbling in the intestines can be heard. Colic is ameliorated by being picked up and rocked. Diarrhea accompanies colic; stools are watery and full of mucus. Diarrhea may alternate with constipation.

Boys may be born with congenital hydroceles or develop mumps that metastasize to the testes.

Girls develop strong vaginal odor or a thick, creamy vaginal discharge, especially whenever they develop severe respiratory tract infections.

The extremities are cold to the touch and mottled purple in appearance. This is also true of the skin in general. Any exanthem may respond to this remedy, especially if the condition is accompanied by the appropriate respiratory symptoms and is ameliorated by cool air.

All conditions are helped by holding and carrying the child, and by loving attention, sleep, cool applications, and the morning.

Pulsatilla Outline

I. Mental/Emotional Characteristics
  A. Sensitive and timid
    1. Clingy; close to the mother at all times
    2. Blush easily
    3. Observed behavior in the interview
      a) May not answer
      b) May whisper
      c) Look at a parent for answers
  B. Emotional
    1. Emotions rule the child
    2. Emotions flow easily
    3. All ailments are ameliorated by consolation
      a) Emotional
      b) Physical
    4. Weep easily
      a) Feelings easily hurt
      b) If they feel that the parents do not love them
      c) When mad
      d) When hurt
      e) When tired
      f) Weeping ameliorates all ailments
        (1) Emotional
        (2) Physical
  C. Easy to manage
    1. Mild
    2. Softhearted
  D. Jealous of a younger sibling
    1. Anger directed at the sibling
    2. Obstinacy toward the parents
    3. Physical illnesses may begin at the birth of the sibling
    4. Regression of all skills learned (act like babies)
  E. Irresolute: they cannot decide on any matter
  F. Fears
    1. Abandonment
      a) Desire anything that shows bonding of the

parent to the child
b) Fear and resist any developmental milestone
2. Being alone in the dark
3. Being kidnaped
4. Large animals
G. Sleep
1. Desire parental contact
a) Like to be rocked to sleep
b) Like to lie down with the parent
c) Difficulty falling asleep; will climb into the parents' bed
2. Sleep positions
a) On their backs with the hands above the head
b) On the abdomen
3. Uncover during sleep, especially the feet
4. Nightmares
a) Of the parents leaving them
b) Of growing up
c) Fevered nightmares of black cats
H. Vertigo: orthostatic hypotension in warm rooms such as libraries
II. Physical Symptomatology
A. Head Area
1. Head: headaches
a) In school
b) Digestive, from eating aggravating foods
(1) Ice cream
(2) Sweets
(3) Fat
(4) Rich foods
c) From becoming overheated
(1) Indoors
(2) In the sunshine
d) Menstrual; any time around the flow
e) Sinusitis
(1) Aggravation from lying down
(2) Amelioration from cool air
f) All are throbbing and congestive

   g) Amelioration from cool applications
2. Eyes
   a) Upper respiratory infections spread to affect the
      eyes
      (1) Better with cool applications of water
      (2) Worse with warmth
   b) Discharges resemble those of *Calcarea carbonica*
      (1) Thick
      (2) Yellow-green
      (3) Bland
   c) Styes with the above symptoms
3. Ears
   a) Acute otitis media
      (1) Accompanies any illness
      (2) At night
         (a) Aggravated
         (b) Desire to be rocked
      (3) Weep from the pain
      (4) Discharge
         (a) Thick
         (b) Yellow-green
         (c) Bland
   b) Swimmer's ear
4. Nose
   a) Many colds
   b) Obstructed at night when lying down
   c) Amelioration from cool, open air
   d) Discharge
      (1) Thick
      (2) Yellow-green
      (3) Bland
   e) Epistaxis at night; dark blood found on the
      pillow
   f) Hay fever
      (1) Worse in open air
      (2) At night
         (a) Itching of the palate
         (b) Obstructed nose

(3) Amelioration from splashing cool water on the face

5. Face
   a) Mumps
      (1) Very red face
      (2) Testes may become involved
   b) Flushes with fevers
      (1) Easily
      (2) Occasionally one-sided flushing
6. Mouth
   a) Dry mouth without thirst
   b) White, lacy coating on the tongue
   c) Bad breath, especially in the morning

B. Torso
   1. Lower Respiratory System
      a) Bronchitis
      b) Pneumonia
      c) Croup
         (1) Aggravated at night
         (2) With a feeling that the throat will close
      d) Infections following exanthems
      e) Asthma
      f) All chest problems accompanied by coughing
         (1) Aggravations
            (a) At night when lying down
            (b) In warm rooms
         (2) Ameliorations
            (a) During the daytime
            (b) From cool air
   2. Alimentary System
      a) Food cravings and aversions
         (1) Cravings
            (a) Pastry, cake
            (b) Butter
            (c) Cheese
            (d) Ice cream
            (e) Eggs
            (f) Peanut butter

(2) Aversions
    (a) Meat, especially pork
    (b) Milk
    (c) Fruit (occasionally)
    (d) Bread
(3) Thirstless
b) Stomach
  (1) Frequent indigestion
    (a) Emotions such as grief cause stomachaches
    (b) Aggravating foods
      i) Ice cream
      ii) Fatty foods
      iii) Meat, especially pork
      iv) Candy
  (2) Hiccoughs in infants
c) Rectum
  (1) Colic in infants
  (2) Changeable stools
3. Urogenital System
a) Urinary problems
  (1) Bed-wetting
  (2) Recurrent cystitis in young girls
b) Boys may be born with hydroceles
c) Girls
  (1) Vaginitis with a discharge
    (a) Thick
    (b) Creamy
    (c) Itchy
  (2) Many illnesses begin during puberty
  (3) Menses
    (a) Premenstrual stress
      i) Weepy
      ii) Severe mood swings
    (b) Amelioration of painful flow from cool applications
  (4) Discharge from breasts
    (a) Milky

(b) In nonpregnant girls

C. Musculoskeletal System: extremities
  1. Arthritis
    (a) Migratory joint pains
    (b) Ameliorated by cool applications
  2. Warm feet
    (a) Walk barefoot
    (b) Uncover in bed

D. Skin
  1. Mottled color
    a) Hands
    b) Feet
  2. Foul foot perspiration, like *Silicea*
  3. Hives from strong emotions
  4. Exanthems with respiratory infections
    a) Aggravation from heat
    b) Amelioration from coolness
  5. Aggravations
    a) From warmth, especially the heat of the bed
    b) From contact with wool
  6. Amelioration from cool air

III. Physical Generals
  A. Warm-blooded
  B. Problems from puberty
  C. Symptoms change often
  D. Aggravation from warmth
  E. Amelioration from coolness
  F. Amelioration of illness from weeping and consolation

Pulsatilla Confirmatory Picture

These are mild, timid, pleasant, clingy children whose emotions rule them. They undergo vast mood changes and especially exhibit weepiness. They fear abandonment and are jealous of younger siblings. These states are ameliorated by consolation.

Confirmatory Checklist

- Sleep on the back or abdomen
- Many upper respiratory tract infections accompanied by a cough aggravated by lying down at night
- Avoid fat and meat
- Thirstless
- Vaginitis in little girls
- Symptoms may begin during puberty
- Warm-blooded, warm feet
- Childhood exanthems accompanied by respiratory tract infections
- Infections produce thick, bland, yellow or green discharges
- Changeable symptoms
- Aggravation from warmth
- Amelioration from cool air, weeping, and consolation

Sulphur

Mental/Emotional Characteristics

The First Meeting

Depending upon the remedy type of the doctor, treating the *Sulphur* child will be either nerve-racking or pleasantly interesting; in any case, the *Sulphur* will present as a force to be reckoned with. There are many ways that the *Sulphur* child may present as the doctor enters the waiting room, but typically he or she is **all over the office** exploring everything, touching the pictures, pulling all the toys off the shelves, and generally making a mess of the reception area. Invariably as one observes the scene unfolding, one can hear the mother call the child to her many times. The child's curiosity can easily be deduced from the start.

Sulphur youngsters may commonly be found playing with two toys at the same time, or holding onto one while playing with another. If the child has any fear, it is easily overwhelmed by this **intense curiosity.** This is a very different scenario from that seen with *Natrum muriaticum, Pulsatilla,* or *Lycopodium,* where the children remain timid, bashful, and frightened in the office and therefore stay close to their mothers. The scene is most like what might be observed with *Tuberculinum* or *Medorrhinum* types.

Upon entering the reception area, the doctor may find the child speaking to the secretary, asking about the telephone or the computer, wanting to know how it works and what all the wires are for. One may find that a mother, needing a more subdued remedy herself, such as *Lycopodium* or *Sepia,* is spanking her child or using other disciplining techniques because of her embarrassment at this inquisitive behavior. However, the undaunted

255

Sulphur child is already looking to the next thing of interest even as the mother chastises him. What a contrast this is to a *Natrum muriaticum* or *Pulsatilla* scene in which the child comes to immediate attention and weeps either silently or outwardly with embarrassment if punishments are meted out like this in public!

Another scene that the doctor might find in the waiting room is the *Sulphur* child playing on the floor with others, either siblings or strangers. By watching the interaction it can easily be observed that the *Sulphur* is **in charge of the play**. It is also evident from the interaction with these new children that the *Sulphur* child has **no fear**, but is rather good at clear, easy communication that is rarely attained by many adults.

Looking at the child, one can see that he is not accustomed to being personally neat, as his clothes are **messy**, his shirttails are hanging out, and his hair is flying in all directions.

Already the doctor has formed certain conclusions about this child and, by extrapolation, *Sulphur* children in general. They are curious and without fear of strangers. They can make contact with others quickly and gain their trust. They are messy; but what is more, they do not care a bit about their appearance. Along similar lines, they do not care about their own or the doctor's property. The child may have to be forced by a parent to put all the toys away, to pick them up from the floor in time to go into the exam room. When the child finally does comply, he simply picks up a pile of toys and drops them messily in a heap in the closest repository.

Sulphur children tend to fall into one of **four categories** of temperaments: happy-go-lucky, irritable, hyperactive, or cerebral.

Happy-Go-Lucky Type

Most common is the happy-go-lucky, **smiling** type. I remember eight-year-old Melinda slouching in her chair, chewing gum and swinging her legs back and forth vigorously, as her legs were not long enough to touch the ground. She seemed very relaxed even though it was her first visit to my office. When I asked who the next patient was, the girl volunteered, "Meeeeee! I am the patient," before her mother could answer. Melinda's mother stated that the child was happy and easygoing. In fact, whenever the child seemed angry, the whole family knew she was just "faking it": it was just a show or a joke. "The way she puts her hand on her hip and pouts in front of everyone is just hilarious!"

While some rare children needing *Sulphur* may be shy during the first visit, this shyness will usually only last for a few seconds or minutes at most before their **natural curiosity** takes over and they begin to explore both the office and the doctor.

The doctor and the receptionist usually like this child from the very start. The way the child sits up alertly at the edge of the chair and looks directly at the doctor, smiling and answering, "Ye, ye, ye," is truly adorable, in much the same way that *Phosphorus* can be. With a smile and a winsome personality, and questions that are thought-provoking even for the doctor, the child leaves a **strong, positive impression** in everyone's mind. The *Sulphur* energy, on the verge of exuberance, always shines out.

It is this **exuberance coupled with a strong sense of self-centeredness** that allows a *Sulphur* child to both wish to and truly be able to impress others. This is observed in many ways, from informing the receptionist all about a new toy she just got, to telling the doctor she won an award at school, to directing the attention of other waiting patients to the blocks she just stacked. One toddler would give waiting clients books she had just "borrowed" off my shelf. When I thanked her for giving me one and placed it on the desk, she simply brought another and yet another book until I had to motion to the parent that this behavior was getting out of control.

Another child performed cartwheels in the office. When asked if she did this often, her parents said that she did, and that in the evening before going to bed she performed gymnastics with the whole family in attendance for the ritual nightly performance.

As can be seen, the *Sulphur* child **enjoys being the center of attention.** The girls especially love to speak to others. These children interrupt the doctor's line of questioning without a second thought. Indeed, if the *Sulphur* child is not the actual patient but rather the sibling of one, the *Sulphur* will chime in with the answer whenever the doctor asks the patient a question.

Another may come up and pull at the sleeve of the doctor and say, "You know what?" The doctor may correctly perceive that the child has nothing important to say; he just **does not wish to be left out**. While in most cases this certainly would not be deemed pathological, such behavior does help to differentiate *Sulphur* from more reserved, "closed" remedies and enables the doctor to choose the remedy that will best help the child resolve problems that limit him or her. *Phosphorus*, *Medorrhinum*, and *Tuberculinum* will also behave in a similar fashion, though each for different reasons.

With *Sulphur*, a good way to judge whether or not this behavior has ventured into the realm of ill health is to observe what happens when the child is **interrupted**. *Sulphur* individuals like to do things to impress others and to learn about the world. If one stops them or alters their play or interferes by taking away their audience, emotionally healthy *Sulphur* children simply change gears, take in what has been said or done, and stride onward with a new task. The less balanced children may burst out crying. The weepiness is not from having their feelings hurt, but rather from feeling left out, from being put in a subordinate role, or from being encroached upon by the parent. *Calcarea carbonica* children also cry, but that results from the shock of change, a shock that they are unable to digest and so protest. Clearly, these are not the usual complaints that parents come in wanting to have treated, yet they do help to confirm or dismiss a remedy selection.

The *Sulphur* child may also **stretch the truth** or actually lie during the conversation. This is not the intentional deceitfulness one may find in *Medorrhinum* but rather an outgrowth of getting caught up in their self-importance and in entertaining the audience. These stories are somewhat hard to believe, often fabricated to enhance personal grandeur. If they are challenged on their tall tales, they take it in stride and simply move on to their next adventure without hesitation, nothing and no one dampening their spirits.

As the initial interview progresses or during follow-up interactions, the basically obstinate nature of the child becomes more evident. They have so much energy that it is often necessary to set limits for them while they are in the office. The doctor, nervous about the destruction of sensitive equipment and glassware or about having the office in total disarray, asks the child not to touch this or that, but the child continually tests the doctor's patience. The child will **push against** such **behavioral limits** again and again, attempting to escape their confines. This is especially true of hyperactive *Sulphur* children. They nag at the doctor, asking why they cannot do whatever they wish. This type of obstinacy springs from the desire for freedom and the sense that it is absolutely necessary to let their inquisitiveness run wild. *Calcarea carbonica's* obstinacy, on the other hand, is a direct reaction to whatever is said and is used primarily as a way to "buy time" to categorize and integrate new data.

Irritable Type

This stubbornness is seen even more vividly in the second type of *Sulphur* children: the nasty, irritable sort. These children have a **negative attitude** toward practically everything. They complain that they are made to do too many chores, that nobody appreciates them, and that they are abused. All this whining may result simply from asking the children to clean their rooms. The general feeling conveyed is "I am too good for the rules of the household." They seem dissatisfied with everything the parents do and may criticize them openly at every opportunity.

Twelve-year-old Joey, whose asthma was greatly helped by the remedy *Sulphur*, went shopping with his mother. When they stopped for lunch he saw a shrimp dish on the menu and decided that he had to have it. His mother explained that it would set off his asthma and that it was too costly; she could not afford it. The child protested tearfully and insisted that there was nothing else he wanted. When presented with a delicious but shrimpless favorite dish, he said he was not hungry and refused to touch any of it. This vignette illustrates the *Sulphur* intolerance to encroachment by peons (the mother) and that they know best (haughty).

This irritable type of *Sulphur*, like *Medorrhinum, Tuberculinum, Stramonium,* and *Tarentula hispanica,* sometimes kicks and abuses animals when upset. There is a propensity, especially in toddlers, to become very **peevish** and irritable, screaming so long and loudly that it becomes hard to quiet them down—exactly like *Chamomilla.* I have confirmed this several times in *Sulphur* toddlers during severe fevered states and diarrhea. The parents recount the common scenario that begins when the child asks for something. When the parents show that this is not possible, logically the child should stop demanding and be pleased with an acceptable substitute, but instead he continues to scream and cry.

They become quite **aggressive** and may slap, hit, bite, or pull the hair of the mother, just like *Tuberculinum, Stramonium,* and *Tarentula hispanica.*

These children may also be found to have a peculiar **allergy** in which they become extremely irritable if they drink **milk.** Some children even react to the mother's breast milk if the mother drinks milk, similar to *Tuberculinum.* It should be stressed that this irritable type is the **rarest form of *Sulphur.*** The exuberant, hyperactive, and cerebral types are all much more common. It is important, however, to remember that this type does exist; otherwise the prescriber may be confused when he or she encounters such a case.

Hyperactive Type

The hyperactive child is commonly cured with a prescription of *Sulphur.* The child has a great amount of **energy,** unstoppable by parents and teachers alike. Even the toddler shows this trait. Two-year-old Bobby had so much energy that he would not stay still long enough to allow his mother to change his diapers. This trait seems similar to attempts by *Tuberculinum* to actually stop the changing of the diapers. In *Sulphur,* however, it is due to high energy attached to a grand curiosity, whereas in *Tuberculinum* the child refuses to let the parent change the diapers because he uses this opportunity to control and frustrate the adult. In the office, the *Tuberculinum* child kicks, screams, and bites in typical *Tuberculinum* fashion and forces his legs together until the mother becomes embarrassed and tells the doctor that she will change the diaper at home later.

The hyperactive *Sulphur* **breaks all the rules** of home and school as if he did not listen to or care about the parents or teachers in the first place. Older children come home late after the parents' curfew and claim they forgot all about the deadline. They are worse before lunch, becoming more unruly and disobedient **when the blood sugar level drops,** and again sometime after lunch when the blood sugar, having risen, drops again. They nag to be let out to play. They break down and begin to cry louder and louder, their faces quickly becoming crimson until the parent is forced to concede. They get in between the mother and her chores, not stopping until she hits them or until they win the struggle. It is amazing how quickly this crying stops and the child bounces right back as soon as he has what he wanted and is therefore happy again. The fact that the parent is now in a rage or distraught is meaningless; he has his candy or his toy, which is all that counts. The only good thing that can be said about this child and situation is that the crying child becomes happy very quickly and **does not hold any resentment** toward parents or siblings— once they give in. He becomes his lovable self again in a split second. Similar behavior can be observed in other *Sulphur* children, but in the hyperactive it is much more intense.

Cerebral Type

The cerebral *Sulphur* child is the next type to be considered. These children can be quite different from other *Sulphur* children, **resembling *Natrum muriaticum*** most out of all the remedy types. They tend to be tall and thin, and are the only *Sulphur* individuals who may be shy in the office. Aside from shyness, such children are very **articulate**, answering questions with terse, well-thought-out, direct responses. They are very dapper dressers, although there will often be some telltale casualness or error in dress, such as a shirttail hanging out or a blouse buttoned wrong; errors that would not be tolerated by a *Natrum muriaticum* child.

The cerebral group tends to have few close friends; the big show of gregariousness that other *Sulphurs* put on is of no use to **these more intellectually oriented** youngsters. They can be loners who read about faraway places; indulge in endless science fiction books and movies; or even pore over technical manuals on computers, farm equipment, or airplane mechanics. Boys commonly spend time making airplane models and meticulously arranging baseball card collections or collecting and categorizing other things.

When they become upset they may wish to be **alone and not be consoled**. All of these traits often mislead one to think of

Natrum muriaticum. However, as the patient talks, the doctor may notice a **slouched posture**; the child leans on the office desk, holding her head up with her hand. If the doctor perceives this, right away the challenge may be over, as the doctor realizes this is not *Natrum muriaticum* behavior. Then the doctor elicits the information that the child is **messy** instead of neat, which again contradicts *Natrum muriaticum*. Still, it is an easy mistake to make since most of the physical general symptoms are the same for both. As one delves deeper into the case, another differentiating point to look for is that these children are not overly sensitive to any grief in their lives and that they do not hold grudges at all, forgiving and forgetting easily.

The cerebral *Sulphur* is also more **haughty** than one would find in a *Natrum muriaticum*. One patient liked to read about sports, boats, and space. As I was about to settle on *Natrum muriaticum*, she volunteered that she hated summer camp because she did not like any of the children there. She made this comment with such a haughty flair that I reexamined the case and decided on a *Sulphur* prescription, which nicely took care of her frequent ear infections.

One may also notice that the child is able to **look directly at the doctor** for longer periods of time than could the *Natrum muriaticum*. For example, Alice, a girl of seven, was brought in for vaginitis. Halfway into the interview she began to stare at me over her dangling glasses. Until that point *Natrum muriaticum* seemed to fit the symptoms equally well with *Sulphur*. With this observation, and after hearing the child repeatedly disagreeing with her mother and then producing evidence that indeed the child was correct, the remedy *Sulphur* was decided upon and the case was cured.

Tubercular Type

There is yet another *Sulphur* type described in old materia medicas, though seldom encountered now. These were the children with big heads, open fontanelles, sweaty scalps, eruptions all over the body, slow dentition, many bone diseases, and chronic diarrhea. They were described as often suffering severe weight loss to the point of **marasmus**, even if the child ate amazing amounts

262

of food. All this was combined in a **hyperactive**, out-of-control child. Though it is common to see traces of the above description in *Sulphur* children, this constellation of symptoms was more common when the disease tuberculosis was present; these children developed a miasmatic taint of the disease—what the old books called **scrofula**. Rarely though, one may have a patient like this and confuse him or her with *Tuberculinum*, *Calcarea carbonica*, or *Sanicula*.

Intelligence

Sulphur children are usually born with great natural intelligence: an **ability to quickly perceive and integrate new information**. With this innate intelligence comes the **openness and desire to explore** new situations. As a result, the child appears very bright in comparison to other children who, due to shyness, reservation, or the fear of new situations, are slower to experiment and acquire knowledge. Due to their open natures and the ease with which they communicate with others, they make friends easily when they want to. With strong self-confidence the child can walk up to a complete stranger and begin a conversation.

This intelligent youth often assumes the **leadership** position in a group. While other children may wish to be leaders, it is *Sulphur* children who glide effortlessly into such roles. They love the position and feel secure in it. Other children may marvel at the **quickness** of the *Sulphur* leader, how quickly he or she grasps the game or changes the rules. There is an ability to continually entertain the whole troupe. The *Sulphur* also likes to play complicated games like Dungeons and Dragons, chess, or backgammon. Early on they understand the strategies and are able to think several steps ahead, a necessary quality in order to be good at these pursuits. They may also take a liking to lengthy science fiction games with many rules or other games involving elaborate, imaginative details. It is poignant to see such an intense youngster with perhaps a *Pulsatilla* mother who is surpassed in keenness by the fourth grade.

The child may show the **ability to manipulate new objects and ideas** easily and to utilize familiar objects in new ways, thus showing the highest intelligence quotient test results. These children may receive high grades in school without studying very much, spending more time reading science fiction or other fantasy books that engage their mental abilities to a more pleasurable end.

Their natural curiosity leads them to explore new objects, trying to find out how they work, why they work, and how they can be used. In their curiosity they may tear apart anything in the room. This may seem like *Calcarea carbonica* behavior, but there is one major difference. With *Calcarea carbonica* there is a desire to find out *why* all these things occur, why they are here, as if from a need to categorize them to know where they fit in the world. This is a small symptom that shows *Calcarea carbonica*'s anxieties about the unknown and about the future. With *Sulphur*, however, the desire is to know **how** things **work**, how they can be used to advantage, not out of anxiety but out of the natural inquisitiveness that is distinctly human when not hampered by fear.

In *Sulphur* this may border on **monomania**, although the subject will change from time to time. I remember treating a boy who would habitually ask questions. Whatever the answer was, his next question was why? The answer to this question was followed by scores of Why? Why? Why? Many children go through the "why" phase, which is normal. However, in the *Sulphur* child it often lasts for years, never really ending but rather evolving from asking questions of others to an internalization of curiosity leading them to seek out answers via independent endeavor and study.

Self-Determination

There is a strong degree of self-determination in these children. One seven-year-old interrupted his mother's answer to tell her he had to go to the bathroom. When he did not return, his sister was sent to fetch him. She returned alone with the message that he did not wish to return and that he was bored and would stay in the front office where he had ended up to play. While this was amusing to all of us, it did show the strongly **opinionated** nature of the child, who had the audacity to tell us, if indirectly, what he desired—something that other remedy types just could not do in such a forceful yet unobjectionable manner.

Another child was brought in by a somewhat overbearing mother who would not let her daughter answer independently. While the *Natrum muriaticum* would have gotten upset and the *Pulsatilla* and *Lycopodium* would have appreciated it, the *Sulphur* girl did not like it and acted on this displeasure. She tried again and again to answer to no avail, as the mother continued to interrupt her each time. Finally the exasperated child came up with a plan: every time her mother paused in answering a question, the child quickly and in one breath finished the sentence for her. This was done quite nicely, so as not to be rude or inappropriate. Her exuberance, her self-determination, and her irrepressible enthusiasm could not be held in check when she had something to add, felt suppressed, or wanted to shine forth on her own.

Sulphur children, then, are **fiercely independent**. One finds four-year-olds who demand to wash and dress themselves. *Sulphur* children like to do everything by following their own schedules and on their own terms. This independence can be seen even in babies and toddlers. One twenty-month-old patient refused to let his mother wipe his nose, running away from her and screaming. A three-year-old girl was the only child who talked back to the parents out of a family of four children. She would say no to direct requests and refused to obey. When these children do not get what they want, they begin to cry and or become angry. This type of behavior could also be found in *Calcarea carbonica*, but once again for different reasons: it takes *Calcarea carbonica* children time to change their frames of reference. In *Sulphur* it is the loss of independence that is wept over; the tyranny of parental control that is not tolerated.

This independence was noted in an eight-year-old who was very agitated with his mother. "She always nags me and yells at me," he said. His mother elucidated in a whisper, "I remind him and I do not yell." "She always badgers me to clean my room. Why doesn't she leave me alone?" "He is very messy. His room is a pigsty, and if left to his own devices it would never be clean!" The fight in this family can be distilled into the parents' desire for obeisance and the child's **inability to become subservient, menial, or petty**.

Messiness

The child touches everything, as it is her way of experiencing the environment. It is this **sensual inquisitiveness** that is partially to blame for the "messiness" of the child, who quickly figures out the workings and function of a toy, object, or game and then goes to the next one, perhaps never finishing any activity or puzzle completely. She simply drops what she was working on and goes to the next fascination. Without any restraint, in ten minutes the office floor would be filled with most of the doctor's possessions, tossed about in no particular order; the room would look like a disaster area.

Calcarea carbonica children will also do this, though it may take them a while to warm up and they will not display nearly the degree of **joyful abandon** seen in *Sulphur*. *Phosphorus* is another remedy that may act in a similar manner, though out of excitement. A less commonly prescribe remedy, *Arsenicum iodatum*, also acts like this, but with much more fervor and hyperactivity on the verge of destructive mania. The differentiating point with *Sulphur* is that one feels attracted to this basically **amiable** child, making one feel almost guilty for stopping his or her exploration of the office. This little demolition expert makes the doctor feel like a "stick in the mud" for curtailing the happy child's innocent fun.

After repeated attempts at disciplining the child by the parent, the doctor begins to feel calmly hopeful that his or her office may indeed survive. Then the momentarily repentant *Sulphur* discovers the bookcase full of homeopathy books. It is uncanny how many of these children attempt to drop every book off the shelf, just like *Calcarea carbonica* children. It is both interesting and peculiar that many of these children go directly to the old homeopathy books from the last century. One marvels at how early an age they are attracted to these priceless antiquities. It is as if they have noses so sensitive that they can detect the somehow delightful scent of mold on the pages from a distance of several yards.

Not only do these children tend to be **dirty** and messy, but they **do not mind it**. The mother may state that playing with garbage is a favorite pastime of the child. It is as if the natural grooming impulse and personal hygiene gene is missing from

266

these children. Perhaps they do not care deep down about what others think of them, and so **do not feel that they have to conform to social norms.**

As a point of interest, Kent writes in his *Materia Medica* that *Sulphur* is sensitive to other people's odors and to the odors of his own stools, causing him to be very clean in his anal hygiene. In clinical practice this is not verified in children; in fact, the opposite is more often true. The *Sulphur* child may be filthy, may not wipe adequately after passing stool, and will therefore smell terrible.

They are messy with their clothes, getting them dirty quickly and wearing holes through the knees and elbows of pants and shirts as fast as their mothers can darn them. Unkempt hair framing a dirty face with food stains around the mouth makes for a perfectly **sloppy-looking** *Sulphur* child.

Infants and toddlers will often **not wish to bathe.** Getting them into the tub is a major ordeal; the children scream and kick all the way there. It is not only a possible general aggravation from the water that they resist, but also the imposition upon them of the *need* to wash. Many love to be in the water after the first few minutes and will play with toys or with a sibling for an hour or more. The parent then suffers another travail to get the child out of the tub she so resisted getting into.

Even after bathing, the skin may have a grimy look to it and dirt will still be found under the fingernails. Toddlers can become filthy immediately after hearing the words "go and play."

Teenaged girls may also be quite messy in their rooms and their activities, yet **take great care in their personal appearance.** They want to be included by the "in crowd" and therefore need to look the part. They buy very nice clothes, groom their hair meticulously, and spend much time at the mirror. Deep down, however, they remain messy in nature, not caring as long as no one in their peer group can see it. This type of teenager may be messy at home and often acts disrespectfully to her parents, yelling and arguing with them at every opportunity, refusing requests and lying with ease.

Self-Centeredness

If one looks past the cuteness, past the curiosity, one can discern a child who **does not care about others' feelings or possessions.** The messiness in these children is just one facet of the personality that reflects an attitude that others do not really count. In Kent's *Repertory*, this is described in the rubric: Mind; Disgust. They never say this, nor could they articulate this thought if asked, but the attitude is easily seen in their actions. This is why they can leave the office in a shambles, why they pull all the books off the shelf, why they do not flush the toilet after they are done, or why they can lie down in the middle of the room whenever they wish. This is also why they can be messy and dirty and not care. It is as if they are **above the common rules** of hygiene and the conventions of cleanliness, that these rules apply to the masses of humanity but not to them, and that other people's opinions about their habits do not count.

The child tracks mud into the house—or into the doctor's office, annoying the nurse by putting his shoes, replete with dirty soles, on a chair. The mother yells, "How many times have I told you not to put your feet on the furniture!" What the doctor must perceive is not only how easily the child takes being scolded but how he repeatedly breaks the rules of the house, especially when related to cleanliness. The child just doesn't care about the furniture. *Natrum muriaticum, Pulsatilla,* or *Calcarea carbonica* could never act this way with such disregard toward other people's possessions, if only because of possible disapproval or other repercussions.

These are the children that parents have to constantly **remind to share.** For instance, they eat what they wish from the refrigerator without thought of others. They devour the last piece of cake, drain the orange juice pitcher, or snitch the last candy bar from the cupboard. They do this not out of meanness but rather out of only thinking of their own needs, again showing an attitude that others do not count.

Some of the **habits** picked up by *Sulphur* children can be **disgusting** to others and very specific to *Sulphur.* Younger *Sulphur* children play with their stool, even after the parents tell them to stop. These children, young and old alike, can pick their noses and then eat the mucus in front of the doctor. The first thought one has is likely to be How disgusting! Doesn't this child get embarrassed at anything? The second, more insightful thought that follows is likely to be No—of course he's not embarrassed, he's a *Sulphur!*

Facultative Breakdown

Thus far I have described the sharpness and perceptiveness of the mental processes. However, this is only half of it. Some children needing the remedy *Sulphur* can also enter into the opposite state of **dullness, lethargy, and lack of concentration.** For many, it first begins with a blood sugar problem: just before lunchtime, the children simply cannot apply themselves to their work. They daydream, become hyperactive or lethargic, and find it difficult even to sit up straight. The teacher tells the parent that at eleven o'clock in the morning the child begins to prop her head up in her hands with the elbows on the desk, gazing out blankly with almost crossed eyes due to weakness and lack of concentration. Such droopiness often heralds the beginning of the dull side of *Sulphur.*

They then begin to daydream frequently. They stop doing their chores or do them grudgingly. They come home from school and go to their rooms and lie around, read or listen to music, or, more likely, watch television. This is a very similar state to that reached by *Lycopodium.*

At this stage the *Sulphur* stops doing well in school and begins to **procrastinate.** Now he tells his parents that he hates school, he only wants to stay home and play. This can be found even in a child of seven. He once received top grades in school, but now he does not even care. Such students tell the doctor that they score seventy-five or eighty-five percent correct on tests but they could easily score in the nineties if they wished. They can get these middle grades without pushing themselves; in fact, they may not need to study at all. Since they are still somewhat mentally agile they easily take the tests without studying and receive adequate marks. As they enter the higher grades, the information often becomes too complex for them to be able to pass tests without studying. They still will not study methodically like *Calcarea carbonica*, *Natrum muriaticum*, or *Pulsatilla*, and instead will try to "**cram**" for the test the night before. They no longer do their homework, or they scramble to get it done the morning it is due, perhaps even on the bus to school. They begin to **cheat** from their friends. Anything goes for these once precocious children as long as they do not have to strain their mental faculties.

While this behavior may be mistaken for a school norm, what it really represents is the first step of a facultative breakdown. This information is almost never a part of the presenting symptomatology, so it must be elicited by the doctor.

Eliciting this information may help in differentiating among the more commonly prescribed remedies. Fifteen-year-old Peggy was brought in for acute sinusitis. When asked what else ailed the child, her mother said that she had poor concentration, lacked ambition, and never finished any chores. She procrastinated in school and at home. When asked why the girl was like that, she said she did not know. In the office, Peggy was very witty, making one joke after another like a professional stand-up comedian. These two traits showed the beginning of her mental breakdown; the child was trying to bluff her way though life with a keen sense of humor. The remedy cured her sinusitis, made her schoolwork flow much easier, and even refined her already well-developed sense of humor.

They no longer care about external demands on their mentality, since it has become more difficult to concentrate. Instead, more time is spent on **social activity**. It is important to think of this laziness not as a conscious choice to slack off and engage in other pursuits but as an actual dulling of the mind. At this stage they become more passive, often only sitting around watching television and "spacing out." The next degenerative sign is a poor **memory**. They may forget when they are supposed to come home, what chores they were assigned, and what homework they have to do.

At a later stage they may even forget names and familiar words. This is more commonly found in the *Sulphur* adult, but may be found in advanced cases of *Sulphur* pediatric pathology.

The mentally broken-down state can especially be found in older children who are or were **hyperactive**. A common history is that the hyperactive child was prescribed Ritalin or a similar drug and later, as a teenager, took up recreational drugs such as marijuana. Dullness, forgetfulness, lack of energy, and a tendency to fall asleep whenever they sit too long follows this history. These dull, lethargic children can be intermittently sparked into healthier states if the object or chore at hand fascinates them. For short periods of time they can become leaders of groups again, orchestrating complicated games and reliving a quick and lively pace before returning to a more sedentary mode.

Fears

The most common fear is of **heights**, though this is not as universal in children as it is in adults. *Sulphur* should also be added to the rubrics: Fear of the dark at night, and Fear of insects. In allergic children who look like and can be confused with *Tuberculinum*, the fear of dogs and cats may also be present. As in *Tuberculinum*, this fear is perhaps because they know that the animals aggravate their allergies. Taking these fears as a whole, while they resemble those of *Calcarea carbonica*, they will respond to the remedy *Sulphur* and disappear, though perhaps to appear later with a new picture that points to *Calcarea carbonica*.

Occasionally one elicits in the history taking that the child likes baths but fears **showers**. While this is a common symptom for younger children and for remedy types such as *Stramonium* and *Hydrophobinum*, it is also found in *Sulphur*.

These children may also have the well-known *Sulphur* anxiety about **family members**. If a parent does not come home on time, they begin to imagine the worst and will fret and worry about the parent's well-being.

Sleep

There are several symptoms that point to *Sulphur* in the area of sleep. Like the adults, they may have great amounts of **energy at night** and not wish to go to sleep at all. Jerry, probably echoing what his parents always said about him, put it plainly: "I hate sleep. I don't need much sleep. Let's face it; I have too much energy to sleep." They will be up running around, jumping and doing

271

acrobatics to burn off the last stores of that day's energy. Others rock in bed until they tire.

A few children have a fear of the dark and sleep with the lights on. Many *Sulphurs* twitch and jerk quite intensely as they fall asleep. Children with chronic sinusitis tend to breathe through the mouth as they doze, just as in *Pulsatilla* and *Lycopodium*, and wake up with foul breath. Those who find it hard to fall asleep initially may wet the bed as soon as they do succumb, as their sleep becomes very deep.

Sleeping positions on the **left side or abdomen** are preferred, although a small percent will sleep on the right side. Some children, most notably teenagers, experience nightmares if they sleep on their backs. *Sulphurs* who resemble *Calcarea carbonica* may perspire profusely from the head in their sleep, while others snore or drool. A good number talk in their sleep. They sleep **restlessly**, tossing and turning as the adults often do, and may awaken every hour. A typical story is that they sleep soundly until one or two o'clock in the morning and then begin to sleep in catnaps, drifting in and out of the sleep state. Although this scenario may not be found with infants or young children, it is found with teenagers.

In their sleep they become **warm** and stick their feet out from under the covers or throw off the blankets completely. Another way to observe the heat generated in sleep is that they move their heads from one place to another to find a cool spot on the pillow. Likewise, they may snuggle up to a cool wall. In the early morning hours, however, they feel chilled, and if a parent covers them up again they will usually stay covered.

They may be troubled by many **nightmares**, resembling *Calcarea carbonica* in this regard. A particular nightmare resembles that commonly found with *Natrum muriaticum*: being chased by a monster or by someone with a knife.

Most of the children will be the "**early birds**" in the family, waking up at dawn to read or watch television. *Sulphurs* feel **sleepy after eating lunch**. They may, like *Lycopodium*, come home from school and just passively sit and watch television or lie down because they feel sleepy before supper.

Vertigo

Adolescent boys who grow tall quickly may sometimes have symptoms of orthostatic hypotension in conjunction with vertigo, visual loss, and tinnitus. This is especially noted if they are in a warm place. They may be bothered by dizziness when they arise, sit up quickly, or stand for a long time.

Physical Symptomatology
Head

Eruptions

The head is often the site of skin eruptions, for which *Sulphur* is so well known. Parents often complain of the child's cradle cap or eczema, which can look quite severe and cover the entire scalp. The rash turns an angry **red** any time the child is washed, and the child screams from the irritation of the water.

There are definite **stages to such eruptions.** Soon after it commences, the eruption begins to discharge a yellow, watery pus that later crusts over. While this description fits *Graphites*, one will be surprised by how often the remedy *Graphitis* will not work but *Sulphur* will. The skin easily becomes infected on the head, causing the child to develop impetigo with the above-mentioned symptoms. *Sulphur* children in general do not like to wash or comb their hair, which consequently becomes thick, coarse, and dry, and splits at the ends. The hair and scalp may actually smell bad and need to be washed daily, similar to what is found in *Medorrhinum* children. Quite a bit of dandruff is produced, accompanied by a great deal of itching. The children pick at the dandruff and at little pimples that form under the dandruff until they bleed.

The head is quite **warm** and the child often refuses to wear a hat, as do *Natrum muriaticum, Pulsatilla,* and, during exertion, *Calcarea carbonica.*

Hydrocephalus

Occasionally one finds a miasmatic tubercular *Sulphur* child with symptoms of **failure to thrive**, or marasmus. Less commonly in practice one comes across a *Sulphur* child with hydrocephalus who presents much the same picture as that of failure to thrive. The child is thin, with a big head and belly, open fontanelles, and much perspiration from the head. These children seem virtually identical to *Calcarea carbonica* and may often be mistaken for the latter. While this may confuse the doctor, the physical general symptoms are quite distinct for each. This is a good example of the importance of basing the prescription upon the totality of the case.

Many times, symptoms that are so strongly shared between complementary remedies form a **bridge** between the two. Symptoms remaining behind after the first remedy is given will often be eradicated by the second as the rest of the case evolves. In this case, many *Sulphur* symptoms will disappear; later, the perspiration will return along with a host of symptoms that point to *Calcarea carbonica* when the child needs this remedy, which will finish the case.

Many *Sulphur* children **perspire profusely from the head.** The perspiration has a sour, offensive odor, especially if the child is in the midst of an acute illness. For example, one little girl had acute diarrhea resembling that of *Chamomilla*. She had copious perspiration of the upper body, especially the head. While these local symptoms were shared by *Chamomilla*, the warmth of the child, redness of the anus, offensive odor, and increased thirst helped to differentiate the two remedies. During such attacks perspiration will be noted most during sleep, again necessitating the differentiation from *Calcarea carbonica*, a remedy type that perspires greatly during sleep.

Headaches

A chief presenting complaint is often that of frequent headaches, perhaps to the point of migraines. As in *Natrum muriaticum*, *Phosphorus*, and *Tuberculinum*, such headaches are **preceded by visual disturbances** such as zigzags or, as Kent described, a rhomboid floating figure. More common, however, are flickering lights and halos around objects.

Headaches may occasionally be triggered by **drinking milk**. Another common cause of headaches is **mental exertion**. Some children say that they get headaches from school, that they hate school because it is too hard and they want to stay home and play. The headache tends to throb and may be accompanied by nausea and vomiting. While most materia medicas describe the headache as ameliorated by heat, what will be found in actual practice is that sufferers prefer cold applications. Lying down in a darkened room with the head slightly elevated on a pillow will also offer some relief. With the headache the face becomes flushed, similar to what happens during a *Belladonna* headache.

Eyes

Sulphur influences the eyes, causing **dacryocystitis and conjunctivitis**. Dried, thick, yellow pus coagulates and prevents the eyes from opening in the morning, much like that found with *Calcarea carbonica*. There are, however, a few differences. The inflammatory process in *Sulphur* is very destructive to the mucous membranes of the eye, whereas that of *Calcarea carbonica* tends to be more benign. In *Sulphur* the **eyelids become red, especially at the edge,** resembling marginal blepharitis.

The child may even develop a true **blepharitis** with an oily eczema of the lids that later crusts over into thick, yellow scabs. The tears are acrid and irritating to the eyelid, making the whole area below and above the eye redder than the rest of the face.

The eyes may feel or actually be extremely **hot**, and during infections are almost always **dry and itchy**. If the child is old enough, he may report that it feels as if someone had thrown sand in his eyes. With all this sticky mucus and irritated, dry, hot eyes, one would naturally assume that the child would wish to cover the eyes with a damp cloth. Not so. The *Sulphur* youngster screams and kicks as a warm or cool wash cloth nears the eyes. Instead of soothing the itch, water irritates every little cut; instead of helping the burning and stinging, the water brings as much relief as applying tiny daggers might, causing much additional pain.

A common time to observe this symptom complex is during **summer hay fever season**. Eye symptoms in this case are ameliorated if the afflicted party is in a cool room. The symptoms are aggravated by heat and sun, and, once again, the application of water. *Pulsatilla* types may also be affected with similar eye diseases, but the eyes will not be as irritated as they are in *Sulphur* individuals, and the *Pulsatilla* eye complaints will be categorically ameliorated by cold water applications.

Ears

One usually notices the **redness** of the ears within the first few seconds of observation and wonders why they are so red. This is, of course, only one of the observations that can easily be made when looking at the face.

While the ears are not affected as often in *Sulphur* as they are in *Calcarea carbonica* or *Pulsatilla*, they may still be a weak area in some of these children. The parents state that the child has had very few ear infections, nothing too bad or of great concern. The only problem is that the mucus never did discharge and thickened in the middle ear, preventing normal hearing. At times the cause of this mucus is the indiscriminate use of antibiotics, which kill the offending organisms but leave the child with **fluid in the ears**, as evidenced by a flat reading on tympanometry and the need for myringotomy.

At other times the adenoids are so large that they prevent the emptying of the eustachian tube, causing fluid to remain in the middle ear.

Occasionally one prescribes *Sulphur* during acute **otitis**. The following case describes the classic *Sulphur* otitis. Ricky, a *Lycopodium* child under chronic treatment, developed an otitis with a thick, yellow, offensive-smelling discharge that was streaked with blood. After trying *Lycopodium* to no effect, the intense redness of the ear was noticed and the remedy *Sulphur* was prescribed, successfully ridding Ricky of the problem. This acute otitis announced the constitutional transition of the child into *Sulphur*, as indeed the physical generals indicated.

The *Sulphur* infant, like the *Calcarea carbonica*, *Calcarea phosphorica*, and *Pulsatilla*, may develop otitis **during dentition**. While the *Sulphur* may present similarly to the others with a cough, coryza, diarrhea, and irritability, the easiest way to distinguish *Sulphur* from the others is to notice the discharges and their effects. The nasal effluence of the coryza is excoriating, creating red erosions of the skin. The diarrhea that develops is very offensive and, again, destructive of tissue, causing a bad diaper rash that burns the skin.

Finally, the ears are often plagued by **eczema** either on them or behind them, as is found in *Calcarea carbonica*, *Lycopodium*, and more rarely, *Psorinum*.

Nose

The nose may be affected in a manner similar to the eyes, with **discharges that excoriate and redden the tip**. It becomes raw and red as the child carefully scratches it, trying to relieve the itch without irritating the skin any further. The nose may develop a **staphylococcal infection**, with or without coryzas, that makes the skin so raw and ulcerated that it is painful to squeeze the nostrils together. At first the discharge of the coryza is acrid, burning, and watery, especially when the child is outside. Later the discharge becomes thick, with yellow-green scabs forming inside and outside the nostrils. The child often picks at these crusts, causing them to break open and bleed. What is most peculiar to this remedy is that the child will then eat the crusts unashamedly in public as well as in private. Occasionally a teenager describes a sour, bad odor in the nose, smelling "as if something died in there," although this is heard more from the *Sulphur* adult.

Colds may be more frequent in spring or autumn when the **weather changes**, or they may be associated with **hay fever** as described in the **Eye** section. With these affections, the child may sneeze paroxysmally until the discharge begins to flow from the nose. The nose may be obstructed while indoors, with an accompanying postnasal drip and a congested feeling in the head. This can alternate with profuse, watery mucus whenever the child sneezes.

These symptoms may also be present chronically to a lesser degree. It is possible to find a *Sulphur* child of two years with **chronic sinusitis**. Children like this have what the parents describe as a chronic cold with thick, yellow-green mucus. **Allergies** to mold, pollen, and dust give rise to such coryzas in the "lucky ones," while the unlucky ones develop asthma. The symptoms are similar to those mentioned above for hay fever or acute coryzas.

There is one very unusual thing about *Sulphur* that should be mentioned here. Occasionally I meet a child who **cannot blow his or her nose**, even at eight or nine years old. The child fusses, screams, and refuses, and when finally forced to try, is simply unable to do it. This is not because the nose is blocked, but because of a lack of the coordination needed to blow the nose; the hapless youngster huffs and puffs and tightens the chest, but can only manage to pass a little air through the nose. This is a very strange clue to *Sulphur* children to tuck away in the back of your mind.

Lastly, these children may develop **nosebleeds** that occur once a month from either nostril, whether they are active or asleep.

Face

There are so **many clues** to the simillimum written on the face of a *Sulphur* that it is often tempting not to elicit a full case history at all and just give the obvious remedy.

The first and most striking feature of the face is the **redness of the eyes, ears, and lips.** They do not have to be "ruby red" to warrant the prescription of *Sulphur*, but these parts will often be ruddier than average. At times the face may be pale, but as soon as the child begins to laugh or cry the face reddens instantly. It is interesting to watch how the red glow suddenly radiates when the child becomes excited. This ruddiness has an interesting effect on those around the child. It softens the hearts of people, making them easier to engage, communicate with, and entertain. One look at the pleasingly colored face and the desire to talk, laugh, or play with this person is stimulated.

As mentioned before, the **optimistic, happy nature** of the child can often be **read on the face.** Even if the child becomes startled or frightened, the perpetual smile only leaves for a short time before reappearing, beaming even at strangers in the room.

The next trait one notices is the **skin eruptions** that crop up easily in *Sulphur* patients, especially during **adolescence.** Acne or comedones may cover the whole face, or appear primarily around the nose or forehead, or erupt only on the midline of the face, as they do in *Tuberculinum*. The acne becomes bright red or purplish when the teenager exercises or after taking a hot shower. These are not the little eruptions that one finds in *Natrum muriaticum* or *Silicea*, but resemble angry red boils. The cheeks may become dry and rough from winter winds and smoother in summertime.

In younger children, the main observation to make about the face is dirt. It can prove to be quite a chore to keep *Sulphur* toddlers clean, as they touch everything around them and bring the objects indiscriminately to the mouth and face.

Mouth

The mouth offers a few symptoms for the prescription. The babies may be prone to **aphthae**, and in some it is found as often as one would expect to find in *Calcarea carbonica* or *Natrum muriaticum*. The aphthae become bright red, the color spreading much further than the actual ulcer, perhaps covering a major part of the lip. The skin becomes fragile and bleeds or becomes infected easily. In reaction to what is occurring inside the mouth, the lips become red, chapped, and cracked, and feel as if they are on fire. The mouth is extremely sore, making the child cry out in pain.

Sulphur children, along with *Pulsatilla*, make **clucking sounds** when trying to scratch an itchy upper palate with the tongue, especially during bouts of hay fever.

The **tongue** may guide us to the remedy as well, having a bright red tip in some, while in others, red edges join the red tip, resembling the *Rhus toxicodendron* tongue. During the tongue examination one may also notice **offensive breath**, which may be due to inflammations in the mouth, although it is more probable that they simply did not brush their teeth. The smell could also be due to the presence of food-filled cavities or gum disease because many of these children have quite a number of rotting teeth, as do those needing *Calcarea carbonica, Lycopodium, Silicea,* and *Tuberculinum.*

Throat and Neck

It is not uncommon to have to **decide between *Sulphur*** and ***Calcarea carbonica*** with regard to the throat. The child may have **chronic tonsillitis**, with huge tonsils, swollen glands, much postnasal catarrh, and stuffy sinuses. Since both remedies share all these symptoms, a mistake may easily be made here. The easiest way to tell a *Sulphur* is by **how bad the breath smells**. It is as if the tissue of the throat is dying and decaying, rotting inside the *Sulphur* throat. If one examines the tonsils, one would observe that the **throat and tonsils** have the color that is common to *Phytolacca*: a **dark, reddish**, bloody color in the pharynx. Occasionally, *Sulphur* may be prescribed for acute conditions with the symptoms of pharyngitis plus the modality that the throat feels better after cold drinks and is aggravated by empty swallowing.

Lower Respiratory System

Asthma

The bronchi and lungs are **often involved**; many parents of *Sulphur* offspring bring their children for the treatment of asthma. The asthma may alternate with or follow a skin eruption or, more commonly, follow a cold that has dropped into the chest. It is often found that the asthma and shortness of breath are worse with any exertion, even climbing stairs. When these children are having breathing problems, there is a great deal of perspiration on the face and extreme fatigue that makes them stop their activities. These symptoms greatly resemble those of *Arsenicum album*, a remedy that is frequently called for in acute illnesses of constitutional *Sulphur* patients. Many times, if the attack has begun and is severe, *Arsenicum album* will end it quickly, but to prevent its reoccurrence the constitutional remedy *Sulphur* should be given. The asthma may also be triggered by household allergies, especially set off by exposure to mold or cats. Wheezing and itchy, red, swollen eyes result after contact with those things to which they are sensitive, along with bronchospasm. Rattling mucus is heard low in the lungs.

Pneumonia

Sulphur, along with *Bryonia alba*, *Phosphorus*, *Lycopodium*, and *Tuberculinum*, are the most frequently prescribed remedies for pneumonia, either current or residual. *Sulphur* can be called for at any stage of the infection, although it is more frequently needed toward the end of the bout. The *Sulphur* stage is recognized by the child becoming hot, uncovering the legs or the whole body, panting, and needing ventilation from an open window to be able to breathe easily. The fever attending the infection rises as the day goes on. The child seems to cough incessantly, bringing up green mucus as if there is no end to the supply. Younger children wake up screaming and crying and become very irritable with the fever until they cool off in open air, enabling them to fall back to sleep. A common story is that the *Sulphur* child had pneumonia of the left lung and then recovered slowly, but never totally lost the cough. Even years later, it is found that ever since the pneumonia there has been chronic bronchitis, a chronic cough, or asthma. This is also true with *Lycopodium*, and indeed, they are both listed in bold type under the rubric: Chest; Inflammation; lungs, neglected. Either remedy, when given judiciously, will cure this tendency toward lung problems that developed from the pneumonia.

Bronchitis

Chronic bronchitis may also be generated after a severe upper respiratory tract infection during which the child took many over-the-counter drugs along with antibiotics. Parents and adolescent patients may observe that since the infection the body seems to have been in a lowered state of resistance and frequent bouts of bronchitis now take place.

In this type of bronchitis there is a hard, dry, racking cough, which finally yields a white or yellowish expectoration. The cough is aggravated by lying on the back, **being in a warm room**, or getting warm at night. It is ameliorated in the open air.

Jimmy's case is typical. His parents believed that their child had been much sicker with bronchitis, and more often, ever since a severe episode of tonsillitis. When they discussed this theory with their family doctor, they were referred to a pediatrician. Not knowing what to do for it, this doctor referred them to an allergist who finally threw up his hands and gave up. The pattern of sickness may be eventually understood, but few have the tools to change such a predisposition. With luck such cases are eventually referred to a homeopath who can work well to transform the situation for the better.

One last note about the chest: the perspiration from the axilla can have quite a strong odor. This **offensive perspiration** can be found in young children as well as in adolescents and adults.

Alimentary System
Food Cravings and Aversions

Sulphur children **desire sweets** as strongly as is found in *Lycopodium*, including chocolate and sweet fruits like bananas, apples, and oranges. They also desire **spicy** foods such as pizza, and **meats** such as turkey, chicken, and beef. While most children like the fat on meat, a small percentage are averse to it. Like *Pulsatilla* children, the ones who hate animal fat usually still like butter.

They often **dislike milk**, having the same sorts of reactions to it that *Natrum muriaticum* does. The reaction can be anything from gas, bloating, and regurgitation to vomiting or diarrhea after drinking the slightest amount of it.

They **dislike sour foods** such as lemons, and they strongly dislike **eggs**. This helps to differentiate them from children requiring *Calcarea carbonica*, who predictably love eggs. *Kali sulphuricum*, a remedy that resembles *Sulphur*, shares the dislike of eggs. If a strong aversion to eggs is elicited in what appears to be a *Sulphur* patient, questions should be asked to differentiate these two remedies and make sure that the patient does not really need *Kali sulphuricum*. In addition, about **fifty percent** of *Sulphur* individuals will say that they **do not like vegetables**, especially squash.

Sulphur children tend to be very **thirsty**, drinking large quantities of **cold** or ice-cold water or soda pop. In fact, the *Sulphur* child with any health complaint will remain thirsty, especially for ice-cold drinks. (A rubric that combines the thirsty nature of *Sulphur* and poor appetite is found in Kent's *Repertory*. *Sulphur* is the only remedy listed in bold type under the rubric: Stomach; Appetite; wanting, with thirst. This symptom will frequently be observed in many of the child's acute illnesses and should be remembered as a *Sulphur* keynote.)

Stomach

Stomach symptoms found in practice belong to **two general groups** of children. The first group consists of those who are **thin and hungry** all the time. While they may not like to eat breakfast, they eat voraciously the rest of the day. Because they often skip their morning meal, they are particularly hungry from eleven o'clock until noon, eating with a fervor matching that of *Lycopodium*. The metabolism seems to be quite fast, as they eat a great deal but do not gain weight, just as in *Natrum muriaticum* and *Tuberculinum*.

If older children in this group do not eat regularly, their blood sugar levels get out of balance, causing them to become **hypo-glycemic and hyperactive**. A common scenario is found with the child who does not eat breakfast and then goes to school. During class at ten or eleven o'clock (before lunchtime), she becomes quite hungry and finds it hard to concentrate. She feels faint and begins to slump in her chair with her elbows on the desk and her head in her hands. She begins to fidget and become more difficult to control. Then she eats lunch. While this can only be beneficial nutritionally after such starvation, eating lunch can have varying results. For some, lunch has a calming effect; but for others, the exact opposite is the case: after they eat, they become "hyper" again for an hour or so before drooping once more. Given a chance, they prefer to lie down to rest, watch television, or take a nap, just as *Sulphur* adults do. These *Sulphur* children may behave as *Lycopodium* children do, needing to lie down when they come home from school due to this fluctuating blood sugar level.

The **second group does not wish to eat anything** at all or only small meals at a time. These children eat little snacks throughout the day and then merely pick at supper.

Abdomen

Some of the toddlers resemble *Calcarea carbonica* children with characteristically protruding abdomens. However, at closer inspection one usually finds that the *Sulphur* child is a little taller and a little leaner than the *Calcarea carbonica* of the same age, except for the distended, protruding belly. This distension is only seen in the children who needed *Calcarea carbonica* earlier and have since progressed to the *Sulphur* stage.

Thin constitutional *Sulphurs* who started life needing *Sulphur* tend to be thin throughout their bodies, including the abdominal region. In *Sulphur* children with digestive complaints and

283

abdominal distension, one may find on palpation of the abdomen that the whole abdomen feels sore; any place one presses on will ache. These particular children have gas with rumbling and distension that occasionally causes colic. Such colic precedes the flatus and diarrhea that finally relieves most, if not all, of the aching.

The skin of the abdomen may also have a peculiar symptom that should be added to the repertory. I have used the remedy *Sulphur* with success for several children with **eczema in and around the navel**. Since this symptom cannot be found in the *Repertory*, a new rubric should be made listing both the remedies *Sulphur* and *Phosphorus*.

Rectum

The rectum is the most **ill-affected** portion of the digestive tract, both in children and adults. The healthy *Sulphur* child has very regular bowel movements, sometimes having two, three, or four movements a day. The parents state that when the child becomes ill, even with a respiratory tract infection, diarrhea ensues. Diarrhea also develops quite easily every time the patient is on antibiotics. While this is a common **side effect of antibiotic use**, the ease with which these children develop the diarrhea may point to the remedy.

The diarrhea may be of any color or consistency, but tends toward a watery yellow, brown, or green color with or without mucus. The odor is intense and makes most people aware that the *Sulphur* has walked into the room or has been in the bathroom before them.

While *Sulphur* adults have the keynote of diarrhea upon awakening in the morning, this time modality is not as common in children. Instead, the diarrhea is most frequent from early in the morning until forenoon with the worst time being between five and eight o'clock in the morning, and lessens as the day progresses. The diarrhea may be caused by milk or viral gastroenteritis, or it may simply be an ailment concomitant with another acute illness from which the child is suffering. Common examples include diarrhea that accompanies dentition, chicken pox, or respiratory infections. A parent may notice that the anus prolapses after the diarrhea in some children.

The diarrhea is usually painless in itself except for the excoriated anus it produces. It is so **acrid** as to redden the anus and make the skin raw. The parents of some children report that the child's buttocks are sore and red to the point that sleeping, walking, and sitting are extremely uncomfortable; the only relief to the area is from a cool sitz bath. This rawness may lead the child to such a state of irritability that *Chamomilla* may be mistakenly considered as a remedy. The child is very cross and cries, and does not wish to be talked to, touched, or held. To this peevish and irritable behavior is added screaming before each stool is passed. Let the irritation of the anus, the thirst for cold drinks, and the red lips be the guide in recognizing *Sulphur* in this instance.

While examining the **anal area**, one observes that the anus, the perineum, and the area between the buttocks are all **very red**. The entire area can be messy and **soiled**, even in older children. Personal hygiene is not high on the list of *Sulphur* priorities. The buttocks may also harbor a staphylococcal infection, causing severe diaper rashes to crop up again and again. Children may scratch the pimples of such a rash until they bleed.

In robust *Sulphur* children who resemble *Calcarea carbonica* in appearance, one may find **constipation** rather than diarrhea. The hard stools that are passed with difficulty cause burning, stinging, and itching of the anus afterward. The differentiating point is that in *Calcarea carbonica* the constipation may be painless, and in *Sulphur* it tends to be so painful that the child refuses to move his bowels for fear of the pain it will bring.

Occasionally a mother brings in a little child with a history such as that just described, and as a consequence has developed **hemorrhoids**. There tend to be several at a time, little external ones that do not look inflamed but cause great discomfort. They bleed, itch, or become inflamed whenever an excoriating, watery stool passes over the area. The mother bemoans the fact that she must bathe the child after every bowel movement or the whole area erupts in red, painful rawness.

Urogenital System

Boys

The history elicited may contain many bouts of **inflammation of the penis**, which takes on a red or purple coloration when so affected. There may be stories of phimosis and paraphimosis in which acute swelling of the foreskin temporarily prevents retraction or return of the foreskin. With such infections there will be much attendant pus and inflammation. The genitals, like the anus, may smell bad upon examination. The doctor may be surprised at **how poorly the child maintains personal hygiene.** The mother states that the child tends to develop **rashes** all over the area; *Sulphur*, *Medorrhinum*, and *Calcarea carbonica* are the three main remedies for such a child who is born with a terrible case of "diaper rash."

Young boys seem to have a **weakness of the bladder**, either wetting the bed until they grow older or needing to get up at night to urinate.

Girls

Girls, likewise, tend to develop **rashes and mild infections of the vaginal area.** The vaginitis is not as full-blown as it is in *Calcarea carbonica* or *Pulsatilla*. Most often the worse aspect is the rash, which includes redness and soreness of the vulva. A smelly, irritating, watery discharge that makes the skin raw and makes the girl itch even more can also be present. Improper wiping after stool is the most common causative factor. They must always be reminded to wipe front to back, not back to front, which so easily spreads bacteria to the vaginal area.

Some of these girls **masturbate** as toddlers. One should not automatically jump to remedies such as *Origanum* or *Platina* for this condition. As an example, sixteen-month-old Sheila was seen for recurrent bronchitis. Along with other *Sulphur* symptoms, she vigorously rubbed her vaginal area against toys whenever her diapers were off. While she turned out to have inherited the sycotic miasm, masturbation did indeed cease with the *Sulphur* prescription, as did her respiratory problems.

Before the flow begins, some girls develop **acne** on the face and back, and some desire sweets or alcohol. The **menses** may easily become **irregular**, flowing for a number of days, stopping a day or two, and then starting up again with spotting for a few days more. The flow can be dark or light and may feel a little irritating to the skin or vaginal mucosa if sanitary pads or tampons are not changed frequently enough.

Musculoskeletal System

Back

Back problems in *Sulphur* may be attributed to poor assimilation of nutrients from early childhood on. A good number of earlier homeopaths believed that many *Sulphur* symptoms were caused by **malabsorption**, as reflected in this weakness of the back. It can be predicted that thin babies who seem unable to absorb any nourishment from food despite intense hunger and who develop diarrhea will often develop back problems during adolescence or later. As babies, they may be delayed in the ability to hold their heads up due to the same weakness that later gives rise to **scoliosis**.

While curvature of the spine is not as common in *Sulphur* as it is in *Lycopodium*, *Calcarea carbonica*, or *Silicea* types, in *Sulphur* it produces a great number of symptoms. Those affected begin to stoop slightly, although this is not as pronounced as it is in adults. This is especially seen when they become fatigued or if they are made to stand up for long periods of time. One way this may be elicited is by asking about shopping. Typically, these children tell the doctor that they hate to go shopping for clothes with their mothers because they have to stand for a long time waiting for them in the store. Consequently, they get sore backs and must find a wall to lean against or a place to sit down.

The **slouching** is also seen when they become hypoglycemic before lunch. They must lean on their desks, slouch back in their chairs, or preferably lie down. They have a weakness of the lower lumbar area. They cannot keep the lumbar area stiff, and so they seem to slacken backwards in their seats, adding greatly to the appearance of kyphosis.

Extremities

The extremities are quite **warm**, just as one would expect to find in *Pulsatilla* or *Medorrhinum*. The children walk about barefoot even in winter and stick their feet out of the covers at night, as do *Pulsatilla*, *Medorrhinum*, and *Calcarea carbonica*. They may not wish to wear socks, especially wool ones, because they detest the heat and the itchy feel of wool. Other *Sulphur* children put on a pair of socks and wear them for days at a time, seemingly oblivious to the odor they are generating.

A main *Sulphur* complaint is **eczema of the hands, palms, soles, elbows, and knees.** While the eczema will be described under **Skin** in more detail, that found on the extremities begins with very itchy pimples that become increasingly red, finally burst open, crust over, and then begin anew.

Upon inspection of the hands it is often noticed that the **nails are bitten.** As one takes a closer look at the nails, one can easily deduce the entire hygiene (or lack thereof) of the child by noting how dirty they and the cuticle areas are.

While many of the *Sulphur* toddlers learn to walk by ten months of age, *Sulphur* may also be thought of as one of the four main remedies for **weakness of the ankles.** This weakness causes turning of the ankles or "pigeon-toed" walking, as can also be found in the remedy types *Calcarea carbonica*, *Natrum muriaticum*, and *Silicea*. Another similarity to *Silicea* about which the parents of *Sulphur* children often complain is **offensive foot sweats** in their little ones.

Skin

The skin is perhaps the **most affected body part** in *Sulphur*, as has been previously indicated. Most *Sulphur* children brought in for health problems have an eruption or a history of one. (This fact may be due to the skin being so rich in disulfide linkages.)

The **eruptions can be of any type from scales, boils, and pustules to vesicles and scabs.** While it may be dry, the eruption is almost always wet. If the child gets a scratch or cut, or is bitten by an insect, the skin locally turns purple and often develops an infection. There is a poor recuperative and regenerative ability of the skin that makes both eruptions and surface injuries slow to heal, and leads the child from one skin infection to another.

Impetigo is a common problem for these children. While this can be primary impetigo, *Sulphur* is especially thought of for impetigo that follows a preexisting eruption. The helpless child scratches and scratches an eruption until the skin is torn, making it "open territory" for a bacterial onslaught; and so the impetigo begins. Either streptococcal or staphylococcal strains of impetigo can be cured with the remedy *Sulphur* if the attendant modalities are present.

All these eruptions have some common characteristics. They all itch intensely, especially when the child becomes overheated, as occurs at night in bed. The eruptions also itch upon contact with wool. Such itching and scratching may also be found without any eruption whatsoever. Burning is also a common complaint, found either with the eruptions, after scratching, or after bathing.

Most eruptions do not do well after bathing; this point should be considered a physical general. The rash may feel great while in the water, especially if the water feels almost scalding hot, but ten or fifteen minutes after getting out of the water it begins to itch intensely, sometimes worse than before the bath. Also, rashes and boils tend to turn purple and congested-looking after a bath or shower, most especially any acne on the face or back. *Sulphur* children love to scratch their skin, as if it reaches the nerves themselves and calms them down.

Sulphur is also one of the most important remedies to consider in childhood exanthems. The skin becomes a mottled red and purple and the lips become very red. The rash develops quite slowly or else appears quickly and is about to disappear when another surprise crop surfaces. It often seems to parent and doctor alike that the eruption lasts too long or else does not come out strongly enough to finish off the illness. The child may also develop diarrhea at the same time, as well as an even stronger than usual thirst for cold drinks. These exanthems will, like the other rashes discussed, itch and burn and be aggravated by warmth and bathing.

Sulphur is also the main remedy to think of for suppressed eruptions. For example, if the child had an acute or chronic rash to which a salve or drug was applied, and the eruption disappeared shortly before the onset of asthma, bronchitis, diarrhea, or mood changes, a suppression of the disease has probably been accomplished. If the doctor takes the case and is unable to find a clearly indicated remedy but has discovered a few keynotes of *Sulphur* plus the history of suppressed eruptions, this should be enough to prescribe upon. Although *Sulphur* is not the only remedy that has this history, it should always be considered in such cases. This is such a common occurrence that many parents will not remember it without direct, persistent questioning. Treating diaper rash, eczema, impetigo, and psoriasis with strong topical medicaments is the norm these days, so such histories must be deliberately and carefully elicited.

The remedy *Sulphur* cures **boils and acne** eruptions that look inflamed and have a red or purple circlet around the eruption. When the first crop of boils seems to disappear, the second one quickly begins. The boils never really clear or come to a head except when the child takes a hot bath. These boils will frequently be found on the buttocks.

Urticaria that erupts quickly and is made up of large welts that are very itchy after exertion may also develop. *Sulphur* types may also develop hives from food allergies, just as *Lycopodium* does.

The last keynote of the skin is that all the **orifices turn red easily**. As frequently as this is found in a child, it is often missed by homeopaths who forget to experience the patient visually. It is essential to look at the ears, the lips, and the eyes, as a surprise may await the viewer as to just how very red these orifices are.

Finally, the remedy *Sulphur* should be considered for **neonatal jaundice** as should *Lycopodium*, *Chelidonium majus*, and *Natrum sulphuricum*. The *Sulphur* neonate will have the typical diarrhea described above as well as skin that itches intensely. As they cannot yet scratch themselves, they love to have a parent run a hand up and down the body.

To sum up this lengthy skin section, *Sulphur* should be considered for a child with dry, red, unhealthy skin plagued by many eruptions that itch and burn greatly, especially when the child is hot or after a bath. Profuse and offensive perspiration from the head and feet is another sign of *Sulphur*.

Physical Generals

The general symptoms are varied and quite intense for this remedy. The child is extremely **warm-blooded** and may walk around in shorts and barefoot all year round. Some may be so hot as to walk about comfortably in the snow with no shoes on. They like to play outside and dislike remaining inside a warm house all day.

The next strong *Sulphur* sign is the body type. While some resemble the *Calcarea carbonica* type, being round and plump, they will be much more robust and ruddy than the typical *Calcarea carbonica*. Most of the children become taller and thinner than the rest of their age group, stretching out from the chubby toddler they once were. In this stretching-out process the muscles may not keep up with the bone growth, and may lead to various posture problems. Some of these tall, thin children maintain potbellies, while others completely thin out. Skin eruptions accompanied by intense itching and burning pains, as well as offensive-smelling discharges from practically anywhere on the body, are typically found.

These children hate to get into the bath, screaming and kicking all the way into the bathroom. As can easily be imagined, the children will often be filthy. **Aggravation from bathing** can also be expressed by a chill sustained after swimming.

Another situation where the remedy *Sulphur* can be invaluable is **after vaccinations**. There are some patients who improve quite nicely with a remedy until vaccinated. Then the case begins to unravel. The simillimum seems impossible to find. *Thuja, Silicea,* and *Tuberculinum* may be given to no avail. If one elicits keynotes of *Sulphur* in such cases, it too should be tried; as often as not this will put things back in order.

Sulphur may follow *Aconitum, Arsenicum album, Belladonna, Lycopodium,* and *Pulsatilla*. It may also be indicated to finish an acute disease that lingers, when the symptoms match. One does not need to have the whole picture to prescribe the remedy in these cases. Very frequently the chronic stage will and is shifting into a *Sulphur* picture.

This should not be viewed as "snapshot" prescribing but as

pure homeopathy. It is the nature, the essence, of *Sulphur* to develop subacute disorders with scant or confused symptomatology. For example, while treating Mitchell, a shy *Natrum muriaticum* child, for asthma, it was noticed that after taking the remedy the boy had become messy and disorganized, which was totally unlike his previous neatness. He had also developed loose stools, dryness of the skin, and more offensive perspiration. Now, instead of staying by himself, Mitchell's friends called him all the time to play with them, so he had no time to study. These changes, though not great by any means, do point to *Sulphur* and *Sulphur* alone. It is not necessary to wait in a case like this for the whole *Sulphur* pathology to unfold before prescribing it as a remedy. We must only wait for any complaint or diminution of energy for the remedy to be given with probable success.

Notes on *Sulphur* Infants

Sulphur infants and toddlers show their good-natured curiosity by staring at observers and smiling and by exploring anything put into their hands. Toddlers may become very irritable during illnesses, screaming during high fevers, rashes, and diarrhea.

Sulphur toddlers may not care about being soiled if they have passed stool or urinated. They may actually kick and fight any time a parent tries to change the diapers. They may likewise hate to bathe and will put up a fight until dragged into the bathtub; then they often love it. These attitudes show their innate independence as well as their indifference to filth. One toddler would run away when the mother wished to change his clothes, another if the mother wished to wipe his nose, and yet another if the mother wished to undress him to show me a rash.

Eczema and cradle cap, common problems, are aggravated by water and in the wintertime, which make such dermatitis bright red. Impetigo may develop over an existing rash. While the *Calcarea carbonica* child may be born with a rash located on the forehead and scalp, the *Sulphur* may be born with a rash over the whole face.

The scalp may perspire during sleep and dentition. Loose stools, weight loss, and emaciation may develop with night sweats.

Inflammations of the eyes make them extremely red, and they exude a discharge that excoriates the skin. Water of any temperature will irritate the eyes.

There is noticeable redness of the ears, nostrils, and lips, especially at times when the child has diarrhea or a facial rash.

Aphthae develop easily, which make the tongue and surrounding area bright red.

They may develop colds, bronchitis, or pneumonia, usually of the left lung. Asthma alternates or follows skin eruptions.

Babies vomit milk readily, although yogurt is digested well. *Sulphur* colic is marked by a great deal of gas, rumbling, and abdominal distension; it is relieved by diarrhea that excoriates the anus and perineum, and in boys, the scrotum.

Excoriating, strong-smelling diarrhea is aggravated in the morning and accompanies many illnesses. Diarrhea may also be caused by foods such as milk. The anus may prolapse during or after a bout with diarrhea, as it does in *Podophyllum*. The infant may thin down whenever diarrhea develops. Diaper rashes develop frequently, which are very red and are aggravated by contact with stool.

Phimosis and paraphimosis in boys are treatable with this remedy.

These infants may be chubby or thin.

Some babies are delayed in the ability to hold their heads up or walk.

Skin problems of many kinds are seen in *Sulphur* babies and toddlers. The rashes may be labeled cradle cap, eczema, or childhood exanthems, but they all share similar traits: they are red and itchy, and they are aggravated by heat, bathing, and contact with wool. When scratched, the rashes have a tendency to develop impetigo.

All orifices, even those not affected by an illness, are often red in appearance.

Jaundice accompanied by itchy skin may make the infant love to have a parent stroke the skin for relief. Jaundice is also accompanied by copious, excoriating diarrhea that is worse in the morning.

Babies are warm-blooded and dislike being wrapped up.

Sulphur Outline

I. Mental/Emotional Characteristics
   A. Four types
      1. Happy-go-lucky
         a) Winsome personality
         b) Exuberant "show-offs"
         c) Leaders of groups; hate subordinate roles
         d) Fearless
         e) Curious
         f) Humorous
         g) Answer their own questions
      2. Irritable
         a) Nasty and negative
            (1) Similar to *Chamomilla*
            (2) Kick and scream
            (3) Peevish
            (4) During severe diarrhea
            (5) During fever
         b) Allergic to milk
         c) Rarest type of *Sulphur*
      3. Hyperactive
         a) Break the rules
         b) Messy
            (1) Do not care about objects
            (2) Do not care about the opinions of others
         c) Aggravations
            (1) Before lunch
            (2) Whenever blood sugar fluctuates
         d) Scream until desires are fulfilled
      4. Cerebral
         a) Very similar to *Natrum muriaticum*
            (1) Shy loners; few friends
            (2) Dress well
            (3) Very articulate
            (4) Read voraciously
         b) Slightly messy

c) Haughty
B. Very intelligent
1. Appear very bright
2. Can become leaders easily
a) Due to lack of fear
b) Due to mental capacity
3. Make friends easily
4. Learn how to use new things quickly
5. Explore
a) New objects
b) New places
c) Fearlessly
C. Independent
1. "Rules are not meant for me"
2. Want to do everything for themselves
D. Messy and dirty
1. Lack interest in grooming and personal hygiene
2. Messy rooms
3. Messy work
E. Self-centered
1. Do not care about others
2. Careless with possessions
a) Their own
b) Those of others
3. Must be reminded to share
F. Mental dullness
1. Daydream
2. Socialize instead of study
3. Procrastinate
4. Cheat and "cram" for tests
5. Poor concentration that leads to laziness
G. Fears
1. Heights
2. Welfare of the family
3. Showers (occasionally)
H. Sleep
1. Little need for sleep
2. Excess energy just before bedtime

3. Wake up during the night
   (a) Often
   (b) After the first four hours of sleep
4. Sleep on the left side
5. Nightmares of being chased
6. Perspiration on the scalp
7. Warm at night; throw off the covers
8. Wake up early
I. Vertigo: orthostatic hypotension
   1. In tall, thin teenagers
   2. In warm rooms
II. Physical Symptomatology
   A. Head Area
      1. Head
         a) Headaches
            (1) Visual changes before onset
            (2) In school
            (3) Amelioration from lying down with the head elevated
         b) Skin eruptions
            (1) Red eruptions
            (2) Discharge yellowish pus
            (3) Very similar to *Graphites*
            (4) Skin easily infected; develops impetigo
            (5) Aggravation from washing the scalp
         c) Hair
            (1) Coarse
            (2) Thick
            (3) Smells bad
         d) Warm heads
            (1) Do not wear hats
            (2) May perspire profusely
      2. Eyes
         a) Inflammatory changes
            (1) Dacryocystitis
            (2) Conjunctivitis
            (3) Redness
               (a) In all infections

(b) Due to the destruction of mucous
membranes
b) Hay fever symptoms that are ameliorated in cool
air
c) Aggravations
(1) From heat
(2) From water
3. Ears
a) Otitis media
(1) Chronic, serous
(2) Acute
(a) Red ears
(b) Offensive discharge
b) Skin eruptions
(1) Behind the ears
(2) On the pinna
4. Nose
a) Discharges that excoriate the nose and upper
lip
b) Staphylococcal inflammations, making the nose
red
c) Foul odors in the nose
d) Colds and hay fever
(1) In the spring and fall
(2) Much sneezing
e) Lack of coordination; blowing the nose is
difficult for many of these children
5. Face
a) Red
(1) Eyes
(2) Ears
(3) Lips
b) Expressive
(1) Optimistic
(2) Excited
c) Skin eruptions
(1) Acne
(2) Eczema

(3) Red
6. Mouth
   a) Aphthae that are bright red, especially in babies
   b) Bright red tip to the tongue
   c) Offensive breath
   d) Poorly maintained teeth
      (1) Do not like to brush the teeth
      (2) Decay of the teeth due to poor dental hygiene
7. Throat and Neck
   a) Swollen glands
   b) Postnasal drip
   c) Tonsil problems
      (1) Enlarged to touch each other
      (2) Acute tonsillitis
         (a) Dark red tonsils
         (b) Pain ameliorated by cold drinks
B. Torso
   1. Lower Respiratory System
      a) Asthma
         (1) Alternates with skin eruptions
         (2) Follows infections
      b) Pneumonia
         (1) Copious mucus toward the end of acute cases with fever
         (2) Problems after poorly treated acute pneumonia
            (a) Chronic coughs
            (b) Chronic infections
      c) Bronchitis
         (1) Acute and chronic
         (2) With dry coughs
         (3) Aggravated in warm rooms
   2. Alimentary System
      a) Food cravings and aversions
         (1) Cravings
            (a) Sweets
            (b) Spicy foods

(c) Apple cider
(d) Meat
(e) Fat
(2) Aversions
(a) Eggs
(b) Milk
(c) Sour foods
(d) Squash
(3) Thirst for ice-cold drinks
b) Stomach
(1) Poor appetite in the morning
(2) Hypoglycemic reactions around the noon
hour before lunch
c) Rectum
(1) Prone to frequent or loose stools
(2) Diarrhea
(a) Accompanies any illness
(b) Excoriates the skin
(c) Offensive
(d) Often aggravated in the early morning
(3) Poor hygiene; underwear is often soiled
(4) External hemorrhoids
(a) Bleed
(b) Itch
(5) Itchy anus in teenagers
3. Urogenital System
a) Boys
(1) Inflammation of the penis
(2) Poor hygiene
(3) Diaper rashes develop easily
b) Girls
(1) Redness of the perineum due to poor
hygiene
(a) Eruptions
(b) Vaginitis
(2) Masturbate
(3) Problems with the menses
(a) Premenstrual syndrome

           i) Desire for sweets

           ii) Desire for alcohol

           iii) Acne

       (b) Flow may irritate the skin

C. Musculoskeletal System

  1. Spinal alignment problems

    a) Scoliosis

    b) Spondylolisthesis

    c) Stooped shoulders

    d) Pains in the lower back from standing too long

  2. Extremities

    a) Warm feet

      (1) Go barefoot

      (2) Uncover them in bed

    b) Skin eruptions anywhere

      (1) Red

      (2) Very itchy

    c) Poor hygiene of the nails

      (1) Bitten

      (2) Dirty

    d) Turn ankles easily

D. Skin

  1. Eruptions

    a) Every type of eruption has been cured by Sulphur

    b) Many illnesses develop from suppressed eruptions

    c) Numerous causes will bring on an eruption

      (1) Scratches

      (2) Insect bites

      (3) Drug reactions

    d) Inflammations such as impetigo

      (1) Common

      (2) Often secondary to other infections

    e) Exanthems

      (1) Develop slowly

      (2) Accompanying symptoms

        (a) Red lips

(b) Diarrhea
(c) Thirst for cold drinks
f) Common characteristics of skin disorders
  (1) Itch intensely
  (2) Aggravated by heat, especially the warmth of the bed
  (3) Burning sensation
  (4) Redness
  (5) Discoloration
    (a) Red
      i) Skin in general
      ii) Orifices
      iii) Eruptions
    (b) Jaundice in infants with diarrhea
  (6) Aggravations
    (a) From bathing
    (b) From contact with wool
  2. Foul perspiration of the axilla
III. Physical Generals
  A. Two basic body types
    1. Tall and thin
    2. Stocky like *Calcarea carbonica*
  B. Ill effects from vaccinations
  C. Warm-blooded
  D. Lingering diseases
    1. Recurrent
    2. Never completely disappear
  E. Red orifices
  F. Frequent skin eruptions
  G. Aversion to and aggravation from bathing

Sulphur Confirmatory Picture

These are extroverted, curious children. They tend to be leaders and are independent and perhaps haughty. Occasionally they become hyperactive and break all the rules of the house. Activities are done with exuberance and tireless fun. They can become lazy and procrastinate. The cerebral type is shyer and neater, though still haughty. They fear heights.

Confirmatory Checklist

- Sleep on the left side, uncover, and awaken often
- Crave sweets, spicy foods, and fat
- Avoid eggs and sour foods
- Very thirsty for ice-cold drinks
- Prone to loose stools and excoriating, offensive diarrhea, especially in the early morning
- Many itchy, red skin eruptions accompanied by a burning sensation and aggravated by warmth, contact with wool, and bathing
- Inflammations that turn the area red with an excoriating, offensive discharge
- Very warm-blooded, especially the head and feet
- Poor hygiene, messy
- Lingering diseases or diseases that recur or never completely disappear
- Aversion to and aggravation from bathing
- Aggravation from warmth

Tuberculinum

Mental/Emotional Characteristics

Retardation

Mental and emotional states are often the **leading qualities** that lead a prescriber to consider giving the remedy *Tuberculinum*. The ability to think clearly and act rationally may be disturbed in children needing and benefiting from this remedy.

The range of disturbance is quite wide, with some children expressing a great degree of illness while others show only a very mild imbalance. Be prepared to ask many questions and to discover some challenging familial situations in homes where *Tuberculinum* children reside. As with all remedy types, the state of the mental faculties will often be the first clue that the child needs this particular remedy, although this may not be the reason that the parents bring the child in for a consultation.

A proportion of these children may be born with **mental handicaps** ranging from mild learning difficulties to severe mental retardation. The severely retarded children often have physical developmental problems as well. The most common ones include a host of congenital disorders that range from microcephaly or pectus excavatum to simian creases on the palms and oddly shaped fingers. Some of these children exhibit many symptoms of chromosomal disorders, yet when genetic tests are performed, readings may come back normal.

Tuberculinum children are also born with a preponderance of **midline anomalies**. During the development of the fetus, more specifically during the earlier embryonic period, there is a stage in which the flat cells that make up the embryo begin to round off and encapsulate to form a tube. It is as if there is a breakdown at this developmental landmark, causing any of a number of problems including hydroceles, umbilical hernia, and cleft palate. Many of the children's skulls appear oddly shaped, as if one or more of the sutures closed off prematurely. Most of the deformities involve problems with bone and cartilage development.

These unfortunates were called "backward" children, cretins, and idiots in the old materia medicas. *Tuberculinum* should be added in italics or bold type to all rubrics that mention this state of **retardation.**

It may also be noted that these children, even when more or less normal, develop quite late mentally and lag behind at all developmental milestones.

The descriptions that parents give may lead the doctor to prescribe the remedy *Baryta carbonica*. A helpful hint to aid in **differentiating** the two remedy types is that the *Baryta carbonica* child is rarely found to exhibit all the physical anomalies that are commonly found in *Tuberculinum* backward children. In contrast to the child needing *Baryta carbonica*, where the most striking features of the case involve mental or emotional retardation, the ***Tuberculinum* child has many other disorders** or physical deformities as well.

Another clue that helps to guide one to prescribe the remedy *Tuberculinum* rather than *Baryta carbonica* is that those requiring the former often have an impish quality to both their faces and their natures, as opposed to the heavier, more languid-looking *Baryta carbonica*.

Fear of new situations and of new people are two of the strongest symptoms that point to *Baryta carbonica*. Clinically, the *Tuberculinum* child who has some degree of mental retardation can also exhibit similar symptoms, centering mainly on the **fear of new situations** and less so on the fear of new people. Because this information has not been taught about these children before, a strong expression of these fears on the part of a patient may be confusing to the prescriber.

Slow *Tuberculinum* children also show an **aversion to being observed**, as do *Baryta carbonica*. Like some *Medorrhinum* children, they may hide during an office visit or tell the parent not to answer the doctor's questions. Since these symptoms have not been known before to be major symptoms of *Tuberculinum*, the mistake has often been made that after prescribing *Baryta carbonica* or other remedies that seem to reflect the simillimum and finding little or no change, the homeopath proclaims the case incurable. Many of these children would be greatly helped by the remedy *Tuberculinum*.

Within the **wide range of retardation,** on the less affected side of the spectrum we find children who are merely slow at comprehension. This is commonly seen when the children are in new situations or when they are given new directions. The weakness in their mental abilities has a peculiarity: they find it **exhausting to apply themselves** to a lesson or a project. Though the mental aptitude to work at a certain level may be there, the child has only a weak ability to concentrate on the task at hand. The strain of focusing on the task, of sitting and doing the job, is too great.

Some develop **headaches from studying** or concentrating for too long. In this sense there is some similarity to other remedies such as *Natrum muriaticum* and *Calcarea carbonica.* Because of this mental strain from concentrating, which can easily lead to physical aggravation, the child becomes averse to taking on mental activities.

Thirteen-year-old Tyler became "lazy" after a case of acute bronchitis. He procrastinated at his work and began to receive failing grades. Because of this lack of concentration, he developed an aversion to studying and even fell asleep during class. This description, along with the physical general symptoms, called for the remedy *Tuberculinum.* It was remarkable to see just how quickly after the remedy was given that Tyler "buckled down and began to study hard" with a newfound ability for lengthy concentration.

Homework is an agonizing topic for many *Tuberculinum* youngsters, and if asked to do it they will typically respond in one or more of the following ways. They lie to their parents that they have finished their homework when actually they have not yet begun. They develop physical aggravations from the work such as fatigue, headaches, or eye aches. They refuse to do the work out of a strongly disagreeable nature: "If they want me to do my homework, I won't do it," is the unconscious response to such parental orders. Finally, they may not do any work because, they claim, they are too restless and "hyper" or that the work is boring. In this case, the parents may exclaim that the child absolutely cannot sit still long enough to do an assignment. These are often the *Tuberculinum* children who have been diagnosed with an attention deficit disorder.

Another common scenario is of the *Tuberculinum* child who is quite bright and excels in school until befallen with a severe physical illness. Then the spark with which she studied and concentrated flickers out and she begins to behave in the ways just enumerated. The parental description is that "ever since she had pneumonia, she just cannot study," or "she needs to read and reread the material, not being able to concentrate or comprehend the way she used to." These broken-down youngsters may leave home for school but instead take a private holiday to play in town.

The **memory becomes affected**, forcing them to read a chapter or learn numbers or the alphabet over and over again. Some of these children wind up in special education classes simply because of a poor memory. They make mistakes in reading and writing, omitting letters and even writing the word from top to bottom instead of from left to right. After taking the proper remedy, the child will be able to concentrate and learn much more easily.

It is common for teachers of such children in the special education system to write letters to the parents stating, "I don't know what has changed, but your child is suddenly learning much more, does not need to be pushed as much to study, and can comprehend and remember things for the first time." All this can be offered spontaneously without the teacher's knowledge that the child is now taking a homeopathic remedy.

It is important to note here that parents of mentally handicapped children often report that the child is learning much more effectively and has changed a great deal since the remedy was prescribed. The doctor must analyze the answers carefully, as this type of parent is often overly optimistic and may see great improvement where there is little or none. It is a bittersweet aspect of pediatric homeopathic practice. These parents, who may have been offered no other hope for their child's improvement, all of a sudden see some change for the better and start to feel that their child now has a chance to become normal. While a doctor wants to be encouraging, and can in fact expect real improvement, the **degree and depth of amelioration varies greatly**. Parental optimism should be tempered with conservative realism.

One often finds that the best measure of improvement comes from the special education class reports. In general, the teachers of these children are both objective about and quite sensitive to their pupils' progress. They eagerly reward any advances. Special notes to the child and gold stars for achievement as well as notes to the parents will show that the teacher, unaware of the homeopathic treatment, has noticed an improvement in learning.

Finally, one should make a note that children can be found with these types of mental symptoms who improve greatly from the administration of this remedy, yet who have none of the other key symptoms of the *Tuberculinum* personality such as aggression or irritability.

Restlessness/Hyperactivity

Restlessness is an important feature of the *Tuberculinum* child's behavior. There is an odd **dissatisfaction with whatever he is currently doing**, which leads the child to become restless.

It is good to note here that equipping one's office with a wide array of toys, books, blocks, crayons, paper and so forth, appropriate to the various ages of the children one treats, can greatly assist one in finding the right remedy. Watching children at play is often the key to finding the remedy because actions speak much louder than their or their parents' words.

Tuberculinum children **desire to move**, to change positions, to ramble from room to room and from toy to toy. They move all over the office, changing from one seat to another, quickly moving through all the books, toys, and games one has for them. They may take a particular liking to bouncing on a couch in the office or rocking a nonrocking chair back and forth.

Young Daniel was brought in for enuresis. In our office we have a wooden straight-backed chair. It is loose-jointed and creaks when one first sits down or shifts one's weight about in it. It has been interesting to see how many of the *Tuberculinum* patients, and this one in particular, quickly found this seat. In a second Daniel moved into the chair; and hearing the creaking, began to rock back and forth, farther and farther, harder and harder. Even though the chair could have broken, even though the chair scraped the wall, even though the noise was clearly irritating to his parents, the boy was thrilled by the motion, the sound, the whole experience. Many other remedy types would not have rocked in the chair out of embarrassment or the fear of breaking the chair or of falling. This behavior shows not only the restless nature of the child but also the reckless abandon with which the typical *Tuberculinum* youngster plays.

Such restlessness may escalate to the point of **hyperactivity**. This high-energy child is hard to keep still and quiet. In church the parents must struggle to keep the child well behaved. It is common for little children of five, six, or seven to run and spin faster and faster in a circle during the office visit.

These hyperactive children are noisy, repeating things over and over, louder and louder. Not only do they scream when they desire someone's immediate attention, but they also like to be loud in general. These children come right up to their parents' faces to get their attention and speak very forcefully with an unnecessary urgency to their statements. These hyperactive children may have **rages** in which they become physically very demonstrative, striking out at siblings and parents alike and hurting even those larger than themselves, while continuing to scream throughout the episode.

Tuberculinum constitutes the main group of hyperactive children that responds to changes in the **diet**. Like *Lycopodium* and *Sulphur* types, they **react intensely to sugar**. But for *Tuberculinum* children, it is **especially dairy products** that trigger impulsive, restless, and malicious behavior. After eating cheese or drinking milk they often end up breaking objects and hitting others.

Many times parents proudly state that their hyperactive child has become much better since the diet was changed. As the dietary control of hyperactivity is in vogue these days, and as parents may try it with varying degrees of success, a homeopath may make the mistake of not taking such information too seriously. The doctor *should* pay careful attention here, eliciting what the child was like before the dietary modification. It should also be noted which foods the child usually reacts to and the strength of those reactions. While in many situations the kind of food causing an adverse reaction will not be very clear, *Tuberculinum* children strongly react to dairy products and experience great ameliora- tion from their removal from the diet. Fruit may also cause the child to become more aggressive, as is true of *Medorrhinum* hyper- active children.

The hyperactive *Tuberculinum* child is also very affected by **outside stimulation**. As found in *Phosphorus*, when the *Tuber- culinum* child goes into a store that he likes, for example a toy store, he touches everything and wishes to play with everything. He slowly begins to go wild and finally is not able to control himself any longer. This happens only in stores that are considered desir- able. As a differentiating point, when these youngsters do not wish to go to a specific store; for example, the grocery store; they whine and complain the whole time until they return home. *Phos- phorus* children are excited by all outside stimulation and will in comparison continue to behave well in any store.

Parents of such children complain that they run at top speed all day and evening before finally exhausting themselves and falling asleep. However, even in their sleep they continue to discharge energy via the restless movement of tossing and turning. A way to observe this energy is to note that these exhausted children often **grind their teeth** voraciously, as well as burrow their heads into the pillow, in their sleep.

Many parents can tell the moment their *Tuberculinum* off- spring is at all under the weather because the amount and inten- sity of basic energy being expended is greatly reduced. During a respiratory illness she may become lethargic and weak. She will need to sleep long hours or lie in bed all day long—almost the opposite energy expression of her usual self. While the parents may like this because they can get so much more done, they are usually happy when the little one is back to her usual "hyper" self because then at least they know that she is well.

These restless juveniles, just as do adults, may crave a change of locale. Like *Tuberculinum* adults, they may **love to travel**. The parents of such a child state that he likes to go to new places all the time, with or without the accompaniment of an adult. This is a good differentiating point because remedy types such as *Calcarea carbonica*, *Lycopodium*, and *Pulsatilla* will not wish to explore new places, especially not alone.

The most common way this is elicited is by asking about car rides. A usually nasty, irritable *Tuberculinum* child may become quite agreeable, attentive, and playful during a ride in the car. This is due to the fact that the ride fulfills an inner desire for change.

There is a small subset of *Tuberculinum* children, however, who hate car rides and become obnoxious, fighting and yelling and demanding attention in the back seat during the entire outing. For this segment of the population, the outburst is primarily caused by the fact that they do not like the crowdedness and tight quarters of the automobile. Once they have arrived at the destination and are out of the car, they generally behave much better.

Irritability

Many *Tuberculinum* babies seem to be **born irritable** and angry, crying and being very fussy, especially upon first awakening. Others may be born placid and sweet, but the parents notice that the older they become, the more they "act out" and the more they need discipline and even punishment.

Tuberculinum children exhibit **irritability, contrariness, or destructive tendencies early and to an extreme degree.** Parents bemoan the fact that one or more of these behaviors is so strong that if it can be stopped, the doctor does not even have to cure the child's asthma or headaches; they will learn to live with it. This shows how much the family can suffer from the presence of this *Tuberculinum* member.

There is often a total disruption of family life when this child enters the picture. These strong negative tendencies may remain hidden until the child develops an acute illness. For example, during dentition or diarrhea the child will become destructive. The child with a high fever may become totally uncontrollable in the office. He becomes nasty: kicking, screaming, hitting, and pushing the mother or father away. " This is unusual," apologizes the mother for a usually well-behaved child.

Irritability is easily observed in these children. A very good symptom that should become a keynote for *Tuberculinum* is **irritability in the morning upon awakening**. If elicited, this little-known symptom should point to *Tuberculinum* just as often as it points to *Lycopodium*. The child may wake up in a bad mood and yell at or fight with a parent.

Alternately, parents may state that the child wakes up in a good mood unless awakened earlier than usual, at which time the child becomes a terror. It is also common to find that the child may be in a good mood if she wakes up by herself and goes to the parent when she wants to as opposed to being awakened by a parent before she is ready. She also becomes irritable when tired or if a naptime is missed, quickly becoming angry and yelling, throwing things, and refusing to budge in any discussion.

Irritability is quite marked in these children whether it is continuous or intermittent (as is more usually the case). They have fits of irritability that lead to **temper tantrums**, which are common. The child so seized becomes violent, kicking and scratching others, throwing himself on the ground, and shrieking so loud that it is impossible to get anything accomplished until he gets his way. Parents say they have to physically control the child, using a good deal of strength, or lock the child in a room until the fit is over. During these tantrums it is common for the child to pound his fists and feet on the floor or strike his head on the floor, wall, or door.

This "head-thumping" is very characteristic of the remedy, as is the strong aversion the child has to being touched when having one of these attacks. It is a remedy type that will also curse when in this state with all the oaths and obscenities commonly uttered by the remedy types *Anacardium*, *Stramonium*, and *Hyoscyamus*.

The intensity of the problem runs the gamut from irritability to full temper tantrums and from frequent whining to general negativity in children who typically tell parents that everything they are doing is wrong. A lesser form of irritability is capriciousness, expressed in criticism of the parents or fits of peevishness and mild crankiness in which the child bursts into tears of rage when upset.

311

This range of reactions indicates the **unpredictable** nature of the *Tuberculinum* child. At his least intense the child may still be whiny, as if he *must* complain about every little thing and put up a fight every time the parent tries to take the child anywhere against his will. At this lesser intensity the nastiness may resemble *Lycopodium* and the obstinacy may resemble *Calcarea carbonica*, yet at the more intense levels there is little confusion among these three remedies.

Contrariness

Contrariness is also noted with great regularity; the child is **negative!** Any time someone suggests an activity to this child, he says no. "Let's pick up the clothes." "No!" "Let's go shopping." "No!" This sort of behavior may be very similar in appearance to that of the controlling *Lycopodium* child.

Another point that is shared with *Lycopodium* is an **intolerance to contradiction** that makes the child violently angry, even to the point of weeping from the anger. These children cry and scream from contradiction and yell warnings such as "hands off me!" if parents attempt to console them. They may even hit the parents if the parents do not heed the warning and try to touch their children.

This contrariness leads to the quarrelsome nature for which this remedy type is well known, which in turn leads to the aggressive fighting behavior often seen in these children.

When corrected, the *Tuberculinum* child may tighten his lips, clench his fists, and then explode. This type of child opposes another's every decision. This is the child who disobeys for no apparent reason, deliberately doing what is not allowed. The contrariness as well as selfishness is seen in the interview when the doctor has to ask the child a question six or seven times before an answer is forthcoming. It may seem as though the child is averse to answering questions, but all it really shows is contrariness.

Opposition to taking directions from others also leads to reactivity and violence with the child responding in kind: if pushed, he pushes back; if hit, he hits back.

Another example of contrariness can be observed in the office; younger children often **refuse to take the remedy**, just like *Cal-*

carea carbonica. One has to pry the mouth open while the child kicks and yells and puts up a fight. I have come to be surprised if the child takes the remedy without putting up a fuss. To illustrate, I once treated Annette, a four-year-old girl, for failure to thrive. At a certain point in the interview she started hitting her father and the door, saying she wanted to leave. Dismayed, I said I wished to give her a remedy. She said okay. I got the *Tuberculinum* and put one dose in her mouth. She took it gladly, but then spit it back onto the floor and turned to her father, saying, "Let's go!" *Tuberculinum* children also put up a fight while the doctor attempts to perform a physical examination.

An example of the contrariness, taken to extremes, is seen in the child who does just the opposite of what he is told. This can be illustrated by the case of George, who was about to break some office furniture. When George's mother yelled at him to stop playing on it, this only encouraged him to play harder.

Parents may complain that it is a constant power struggle over every issue at home, with the child kicking and crying continuously for half an hour or more before giving up. "It does no good to punish him. If I spank him, he slaps me back." Or, "If I punish him, he seems to be unaware of it and continues to act the same way. He is so obstinate." These children talk back to the parents and threaten them with violence when they are disciplined.

Changeability

Mood and behavior can change quickly. Children can switch from being obedient to becoming very obstinate and difficult to satisfy. They might ask for one thing, refuse it, and then immediately ask for something else. This emotional changeability is found in Kent's *Repertory* under the rubric: Mind; **Capriciousness.**

A parent often describes the child as unpredictable, expressing a wide range of behaviors even in very similar situations. If the child is not particularly "hyper" or irritable, she can obey a request. Yet the same order given at a later time may trigger the child to throw a temper tantrum. This unpredictability can drive a parent to distraction.

This inconsistency occurs for two reasons. First, the child suffers internally, **not really knowing what she wants**. Yet she knows that she needs something; something other than what she has. The other reason is that the child **enjoys being contrary** and derives pleasure out of letting the parents know that they are doing a poor job. The *Tuberculinum* child cannot help but torture the poor parents to do more and better all the time.

Destructiveness

Destructiveness and violence should always make one think of *Tuberculinum* in a differential diagnosis. One finds both self-destruction and destructiveness toward others.

The **self-destructive** tendencies are seen in the child who hits his head on the floor or wall, pulls his hair, or picks at his scabs. He is also **destructive to others.** "He is slaphappy," as one parent put it.

These children get into many fights with siblings or schoolmates, provocatively poking them in the chest or hitting them. If they themselves suffer a blow, they automatically hit back and will even hit teachers and parents. The parents say that there is an instantaneous lashing out, as though anger and violent reaction precede thought.

This **violence** may begin **after** a bout with **an acute disorder**, most frequently acute diarrhea or a respiratory infection. "Now," one mother reported, "my son Nate is whiny and nothing seems to please him. He has become strong willed, wanting everything his way. If he does not get it, he quickly becomes angry, making fists and hitting people for little reason." Such dramatic changes in the ability to deal with authority, especially after an illness, should always make one consider the remedy *Tuberculinum*.

The mother may wait until she and the doctor are alone before breaking down and confessing that as hard as she might try to feel otherwise, she simply hates this child.

Another mother may complain that her child has many illnesses in the chest, head, or nose, but when finally asked point blank what is it that she most wants to change, what limits the child most, she talks about the behavior and states that the child is an absolute terror at home. If the child is in the room during the interview, he or she often demonstrates these traits. The *Tuber-*

culinum may begin to yell, throw toys, or actually hit the parent if he or she does not attend to the child immediately.

This strong feature of violence is exemplified by the following incredible scene with Rory, a boy of five. After careful questioning, *Tuberculinum* along with three other remedies were chosen for consideration.

Questions were then aimed at confirming one of the remedies as the prescription. As each question was asked, the child playing on the floor would turn around and give his father a searing, disgusted, and somewhat lethal look.

These expressions on the part of the child quickly cued me to explore *Tuberculinum* more closely. The father was asked if the child hit him. He said yes. Further along in the interview the boy turned around before every answer and made a fist that he shook threateningly before his father's face. Still further into the interview the child began to throw toys at the parent and at one point even spat in his father's face.

Once the remedy *Tuberculinum* was given in the office, Rory wished to take the whole bottle at once! When his father told him that he could not, the boy began to rage. He first began to cry and, throwing himself on the carpet, began to hit the floor with his hands, feet, and head while screaming for several minutes. He then stood up and began to hit his father with his fists, screaming, "Give me! Give me!" while punching his father in the thighs with all his might, back and forth, quicker with every punch. Rory finally began to kick the defenseless parent with his sharp, booted foot, not on the calf or any part of the thigh but on the shin, obviously the most sensitive part of the leg.

Not being able to bear this scene any longer, I gave a bottle of blank pellets to the parent to give to his son. He handed the bottle to Rory, who nevertheless continued to hit the parent with the same intensity as before. After a minute the child began to laugh heartily; holding the bottle up in the air, he repeated gleefully, "See, I did it! See, I did it!" He then turned around to his father and kicked him in the shin one last time for good measure.

This type of scene has been reenacted many times over during interviews. However, the intensity of the violence toward the contradicting person was exceptional in this case.

Lodged deeply within the psyche of these children is an eye for an eye mentality. If they are hit, they hit back as a matter of course. If they are forbidden to do something they wish, they lash out at the forbidding person directly or indirectly. Indirect methods are those in which the parents are controlled, such as by having to watch the child or being slowed down by the child. The child on purpose will wait, dillydally, and waste time dressing just to perturb the parents by ruining their plans.

Another method of irritating offending persons is by intentionally ruining their belongings. They destroy jewelry, presents, favorite plants—in short, anything that is cherished by the other. The **malicious character** is easy to see in this type of *Tuberculinum*. If one asks the parents, they often confess that, yes, they think the child really enjoys tormenting them.

Some of the more intellectual parents barely notice any of these negative characteristics. "This is normal for their age," the mother might offer. The parents might only note that "if the child becomes ill, he becomes reckless and uncaring." As an aside, to show the genetic component of this behavior, many parents, especially fathers, chuckle when asked about their child's behavior, as their mothers have told them that they were exactly the same way as youngsters.

These destructive children **break things** easily, repeatedly, and with enjoyment. Breaking things is one of the major ways they release tension. This relief from pent-up neurologic energy is analogous to that seen in patients needing the remedy *Zincum*, who have an uncontrollable need to move their bodies in order to attain some peace from an inner irritation. *Tuberculinum* children seem driven to destroy objects, as can be recognized in the child rocking the chair almost to the point of breaking it.

With similar destructive energy they **lash out at** their parents, teachers, or older siblings; that is, at **anyone who has some authority over them.** These aggressive tendencies may be more manifest in the home. The parents might say that the child hits and chokes her siblings or does more devious, even meaner things to them. Young Diana would even put thumbtacks in her sister's shoes. This acting out may be within their control; in a day-care or school setting their behavior may remain within normal limits.

Younger children love to sit and destroy a magazine or newspaper in the middle of the waiting room. They open one page after another and clip with scissors every square inch of the page before going on to snip up the next one. Alternately, they may not be so refined and simply tear up the papers with their hands and throw them all over the office floor.

Another type of destructiveness is more spontaneous and mean. If a sibling builds a model, the *Tuberculinum* will break it. It is as if they are relieved of some mental anguish when they demolish something. In the office they may play with cars, making them crash into each other violently and very noisily with sound effects. They may play with toys that allow them to pound and jam a peg into the wrong hole just to see what will happen.

While walking at the seashore, if they see a just finished sand castle, they may run and throw themselves on top of it and completely demolish it. The sardonic grin on the child's face may make parents think that their child has periods of demonic possession that cause this destructive type of "play." When this "possession" is over they may be very remorseful and apologetic, but the memory for such apologies is usually short.

It is interesting to read about the remedy *Tuberculinum* in older materia medicas and published cases from the early part of this century. While there was no well-defined chronic picture of the remedy at that time, one occasionally reads about the case of someone who was afflicted with tuberculosis of the nervous system. Many doctors described these patients as becoming so causelessly violent that they seemed to be possessed. Just as chronically violent people can now be cured with the remedy *Tuberculinum*, so too were the acute violent episodes described long ago attributed to the disease tuberculosis.

The family pet commonly takes the brunt of a *Tuberculinum* child's anger. As mentioned under **Fears**, the child may be **afraid of and/or mean to animals**. If the child is raging, he may go directly to the animal and treat it cruelly. It is very common to hear that the child tortures the cat or dog of the house. The child enjoys choking the animal, pulling the tail, pulling the fur a little too roughly while petting, dragging the pet on the ground, throwing it against the wall, or even putting the hapless creature in the washing machine. Ten-year-old Frances put her cat in the clothes dryer and watched it spin until the horrified parent rescued it.

In another case, Bruce would fish in a small, well-stocked pond, catch a fish, and then kick it back into the pond. The child gleamed with joy as he caught and returned many fish in a short period of time. All this aggressiveness seemed to be without thought or control. Bruce seemed to do these things without having the inhibitions that keep the rest of humanity from acting this way.

Combining Traits

The *Tuberculinum* child is contradictory and obstinate, just as *Calcarea carbonica* can be. But to this one must add selfishness, aggressiveness, irritability, and the tendency to be extremely demanding. It is this combination of symptoms that points to the remedy *Tuberculinum*. **Selfishness** shows itself in many ways. *Tuberculinum* individuals demand this and that but never consider other people's feelings or plans, and can easily be hurtful or destructive to friends and foes alike.

They also deliberately **demand** things that are contrary to others' wishes. If the parents want to go out to the park at sunset, it will be the *Tuberculinum* child who throws a fit and makes them miss it. Strangely, it is not that the child did not wish to see the sunset; rather, it is a combination of contrariness (since the others wish to do something), selfishness, (in that he controls the outcome of the family decision), and destructiveness (of others' happiness). In this particular example, intangible plans were destroyed instead of objects. Again, the child seems to receive amelioration from this perverse behavior even if he, too, wanted to see the sunset.

The selfishness may also be observed in the lack of consideration for others. During the interview the child may spit or throw things at, or even physically abuse, the parent. I recall a child who would mess up her mother's hairstyle and then grab her by the chin and move it up and down as she threatened her mother with the other fist. This child was only seven years old! The parents commonly fear for their child's future. "What will he be like when he is sixteen?" is a frequent anxious comment.

When these children want something, they want it NOW! They demand to be heard NOW! They are very loud whenever they want anything. They demand to get their own way or else they become peevish, upset, and angry, and will not forget the topic until they succeed. This is behavior similar to that of *Calcarea carbonica*, but much meaner. They throw things, stamp their feet, and demonstrate. "I'm not going to go! I'm not going to do it!" they shriek in high-pitched screams.

Impishness

The children may also be quite **playful, teasing,** and impish. They like to play with many toys. Somehow they always wish to play with the toy someone else has. They do this just to "get at" the playmate, to pick a squabble, though not out of jealousy as in *Hyoscyamus* or *Lachesis*.

The desire to **tease siblings** comes out in many ways, often with an edge of destructiveness as described above. The child may hide toys or books that a sibling wants. He then watches with amusement as the sibling is driven mad by the search for the object. He may race ahead of a sibling into the bathroom because he knows that the brother or sister desperately needs to use it. He may also try to get his siblings in trouble with the parents or with teachers. Again one observes the vindictiveness of the child, the "get at them" feeling to this supposed playfulness.

Tuberculinum children can also be liars, lying about such things as beating up siblings or pets, claiming they did not even though they did.

The impish character can also be seen in the smiling, coy, **mischievous** face while they ask what everything in sight is during the interview. One such child was particularly difficult to find the simillimum for as I tried to decide between *Tuberculinum* and *Natrum muriaticum*. The child sat rocking his legs back and forth in a seat three feet away from me, his interviewer. While I was concentrating, looking up rubrics in the *Repertory*, the child's foot gently touched mine a number of times. With that motion, I decided upon the remedy *Tuberculinum*. Still staring at the *Repertory*, it was easy to observe out of the corner of my eye the pleasure the child derived from that gentle kick. *Natrum muriaticum* could never have made such a "mistake," and definitely would not have smiled with enjoyment.

Tuberculinum children who are not aggressive or mentally slow tend to be **leaders**. With their individualistic manner they usually get what they want. They talk others into doing what they wish. Some may have many friends and talk easily to adults. They, like *Sulphur*, try to take over the conversation, even during the interview while one tries to elicit the history from a parent.

This type of child is **extroverted** and easily communicative. She looks around all over the office, like *Sulphur*. The child is an "up" person—active, wriggling about in her chair, asking, "What's an MD? What's an ND? What's this pill? What's that?" She shares with others and often has many toys. She does not fight and only becomes irritable if she is hungry or uncomfortable. She tends to be quite competitive, never giving up or quitting when she plays.

Artists

Tuberculinum children who are not destructive can be quite sensitive and artistic. In the office they are somewhat timid, shyly sitting on the floor playing quietly with their toys but answering questions with more confidence than would *Lycopodium*. The children may show interest in and ability for artistic or musical endeavors at an early age and benefit emotionally from such activities.

These children often experience a slight lack of self-confidence, as may be evident by the way they answer questions. They may also refuse to answer questions altogether. This is the kind of child who becomes peevish and introverted most easily. They sulk and become antisocial and wish to be left alone. They are very sensitive to pain, crying with it as do *Chamomilla, Pulsatilla, Lycopodium*, and *Hepar sulphuris*. These children sometimes push their mothers away or hit them if they try to touch or console them.

Materia medicas describe *Tuberculinum* dreamers who enjoy being by themselves, making up imaginary friends or inventive tasks and greatly enjoying solitude. This is seen more in teenagers and adults and less often in children.

As a final comment on the artistic type of *Tuberculinum*, I would like to say that it is very **rarely seen in pediatric practice**; the nasty and slow types are much more common. One should not wait to elicit this behavior before deciding on the remedy; otherwise, many correct prescriptions will be missed.

Fears

The fears of *Tuberculinum* are **few but very strong**. Materia medicas describe an apprehension, a worrying over trifles, just as is seen with *Calcarea carbonica* children. This apprehension is not a common finding in general pediatric practice.

The strongest fear to be seen is a **fear of animals, especially cats and dogs and all their wild derivatives** such as lions, tigers, wolves, and bears. A minority will be afraid of chickens or insects as well.

Unlike other remedy types who have a fear of animals, the *Tuberculinum* child may try to bluff by ascribing negative attributes to these animals. They state that they are gross, ugly, and disgusting. They claim to hate these animals because they carry germs and diseases like rabies.

I recall the case of John, a child who had always loved animals. During an acute infection when he had pneumonia, he developed a strong fear that his own pet dog would bite him. Strong fears like these may be translated into violent outbursts against the animal in question. Strangely enough, many of these children are also allergic to the very animals they despise, experiencing urticaria or asthma whenever such an animal is nearby.

Fear of being alone is often found in the retarded *Tuberculinum* children. They feel that something bad will happen to them if a parent is not around, similar in this to *Lycopodium*. For this reason, if one treats a mean child who has difficulty concentrating and is assumed to be *Lycopodium* type, but who takes a dose of the remedy *Lycopodium* with no effect, one should next consider *Tuberculinum*.

Fear of being alone is heightened when they are in the dark. Like *Lycopodium* types, *Tuberculinum* children may whine, ask not to be left alone, and hang on to the mother or father for dear life at these times.

They may also have a strong **fear of new situations**. Fear arises when they first attend a new school or a new classroom and meet new children, or, in our case, meet a new doctor. The fear of the unknown comes through in any novel situation.

Thunderstorms and monsters may also appear high on the list of fears.

Sleep

The sleep of *Tuberculinum* has many keynotes to offer. If the child has a fear of the dark, he may wish to sleep with the parents. Even though the child is tired he may find it **hard to fall asleep** both from physical restlessness and an inability to calm the mind. He may need to rock to sleep or bang his head on the pillow or bed rhythmically until he fades away.

Once *Tuberculinum* children do fall asleep they usually sleep quite deeply—so deeply, in fact, that they often lose the inhibition against **wetting the bed** and urinate. This is a common symptom for *Tuberculinum*, as mentioned in the section on the **Urogenital System**; some children urinate several times during the night. The sleep may be so deep that the child does not wake up when a parent carries him to the bathroom or even while urinating there. After administration of the remedy, the sleep state becomes lighter and the child is able to wake up during the night and get to the bathroom by himself.

Almost all of these youngsters **grind their teeth** during sleep. Many also develop severe **night sweats**, especially of the face and scalp, with or without an accompanying fever.

Upon questioning, one finds that a good many of these children sleep on their backs, at times with their hands above their heads, just like *Pulsatilla*.

Others sleep on either side, on the stomach, or in the knee-to-chest position, like *Medorrhinum*. Indeed, the knee-to-chest sleeping position is found especially in those children who later need the remedy *Medorrhinum*. The symptom disappears with the first prescription but returns with a host of *Medorrhinum* symptoms that crop up.

Some *Tuberculinum* sleepers may go back and forth between

chilliness and overheating, staying covered until they feel hot and then throwing off the covers until chilled and needing warmth again.

Sleep may be **restless**, punctuated by tossing back and forth, bruxism, and talking or screaming. Loud verbalizing may be due to nightmares of being chased or threatened by monsters.

Tuberculinum children often **wake up slowly and unrefreshed**, but eventually they feel okay. However, if one wakes them up or if they are pushed in the slightest in the morning, one will find their tempers very difficult to handle. After a few weeks of this, parents will be trained to leave the child alone when he or she first wakes up. I consider this to be a keynote for prescribing the remedy, and is as commonly found with *Tuberculinum* youngsters as it is with *Lycopodium* or *Nux vomica*. If the child is allowed to approach the parent first, then everything is fine.

Some children need to be rocked by the parent in perfect silence until they awaken fully. Younger children also often benefit from a nap in the late afternoon, preferably from three to six o'clock in the evening. If they cannot take their regular nap they become very irritable, reminding one of *Lycopodium* or perhaps *Calcarea carbonica* in this regard.

Physical Symptomatology
Head

The head provides a number of clues to this prescription. The first clue is that these children are **often born with a large amount of long hair all over the scalp and on the back.** This can be thick, dark hair long enough to cut at birth. Most parents remember this hair, as it is not very common for babies to be so hirsute, especially down the center of the back. However, most parents do not report this spontaneously, so if one is thinking about *Tuberculinum*, be sure to ask about it.

The second clue is that these children develop **ringworm** on the scalp very easily. The eruption causes circular patches of hair to fall out. This may be a presenting complaint or simply an occurrence that one hears about in the taking of the health history.

The third clue is that these children often strike their heads against objects, being what used to be called "**head thumpers.**"

Some strike their heads against the wall or the floor when they are mad. Others do it during a headache or sinusitis attack. The most common time, however, is during attempts to sleep, when they burrow their heads into the pillow or hit their heads against the pillow or mattress as a way to relax. The remedy *Tuberculinum* is much more frequently needed for children who do this than are other remedies such as *Helleborus*.

The fourth clue is that the head may also be **misshapen** or out of proportion with the rest of the body. While some *Tuberculinum* heads seem appropriately sized, one also finds children with true microcephaly or skulls that seem as though some of the sutures closed too early, giving the head an unusually lumpy or irregular look. Others will appear hydrocephalic.

Tuberculinum children **perspire profusely**, as much as or more than *Calcarea carbonica* children. They have night sweats that include the head, especially the the hairline and forehead. With all this wetness, it is easy to see why they may develop **moist eruptions** on the scalp that resemble those of *Calcarea carbonica*.

Headaches

The fourth clue to *Tuberculinum* in the head area is found with headaches. These children develop headaches as often as *Calcarea carbonica* or *Natrum muriaticum* children. Like *Natrum muriaticum*, *Calcarea carbonica*, *Calcarea phosphorica*, or *Pulsatilla*, the headaches can be **caused by studying** or by fixing the attention on books or television for too long at a time. It may perhaps be due to **poor eyesight**, as in *Natrum muriaticum* or *Calcarea carbonica*.

The headache may in fact begin with **visual disturbances** like those found in *Natrum muriaticum*, *Sulphur*, and *Phosphorus*: flickering, zigzags, and lights. Occasionally, the child notices that everything he looks at just before a headache strikes has a **blue tinge** to it. This is very confirmatory of *Tuberculinum*.

Also, as in *Phosphorus* and *Lycopodium*, the headache may be preceded by a feeling of severe emptiness of the stomach and an **intense hunger**.

Tuberculinum must be added in italics to the rubric: Stomach; Appetite, increased, headache, before.

Since the child realizes that every time he applies himself

mentally he develops a headache, he stops trying to excel in school. He may begin to seem dull, lazy, or uncooperative. Other types of overwork also bring on a headache. Some children develop headaches when they exert themselves too much. Others suffer when they are overtired. Girls may suffer with them just before, during, or after their menses. Yet others develop headaches related to the weather. Whenever a low pressure front passes through the area bringing a big change in humidity, they develop a chill and then a headache, like *Calcarea carbonica*.

The headaches are **severe**, with so much pain that it typically leaves the little patient ravaged for days afterward. The most common description of this is that they feel pressure above the eyes along with tension; a tightness like a band pressing across the forehead. Younger children unable to describe the pain fully only point to the forehead and describe a type of pain that fits sinusitis. Other pains are described to be "as if knives are cutting the scalp," or "like the headache is deep in the skull behind the eyes." These headaches may also be periodic.

When they develop such headaches, they need to stop whatever they are doing and lie down in order to try to bear with the pain. They are just as, or even more, **irritable** than *Lycopodium* patients become during a headache, and desire only to be left alone.

An interesting, though rare, observation is that these children sometimes **sweat profusely**, especially from the scalp and forehead, during a headache. This is peculiar to only a few remedy types and so may be used to confirm the remedy. Other modalities are that headaches are aggravated by motion and ameliorated by rest, lying down, and being in the cool air with a cap on for warmth.

Eyes

The eyes can be used as a confirmatory area for symptoms indicative of *Tuberculinum*. Just as these children are often born with long hair on the head, they are also born with **long, full, beautiful eyelashes**; this is a symptom common to all remedies that are strongly tubercular, such as *Phosphorus*. The child has a **twinkle** or brightness in the eyes like that found in *Phosphorus*. This sparkle can easily turn into a gleam of aggression or a fiendish look, as if the child has suddenly become possessed.

The **sclera** may have a **blue** hue or may actually be blue to the point of being deeply discolored, as is found in *Carcinosin*. These children are often born with **strabismus** or astigmatism. It is interesting to find that in Kent's *Repertory*, only *Tuberculinum* is listed under the rubric: Eyes; Astigmatism. They are born with **weak eye muscles** that give rise to weaknesses of accommodation such as myopia, all of which cause the child to develop headaches from reading too much.

Besides the visual disturbances mentioned, *Tuberculinum* should be thought of when there are **visual changes** that occur before a headache, especially if the child states that everything has a bluish tint. Looking at the eyes, one may see that the pupils are quite dilated.

There may be occasional problems with styes. Like *Sulphur*, *Natrum muriaticum*, and *Thuja*, **eczema** may occur on the eyelids. The children who develop upper respiratory infections also develop blue allergic "**shiners**" around the eyes.

Many old materia medicas state that *Tuberculinum* is a specific against ulceration of the cornea. This has been confirmed several times in my own experience, but only in adults—most interestingly by an elderly man with this problem who had contracted tuberculosis in his youth.

Ears

The **adenoids enlarge easily**, as they do in *Calcarea carbonica*, *Calcarea phosphorica*, and *Sulphur*, causing *Tuberculinum* children to develop chronic **fluid** in the ears. These children also develop **recurrent ear infections** in which the ear becomes red and painful, making the victims cry before the eardrum finally and inevitably ruptures. The ear then discharges thick, yellow pus. Some children are originally brought to the homeopathic physician because the discharge mentioned develops into a chronic condition with a thin, white discharge that lasts for months.

Tuberculinum children who perspire a lot on the head often develop eczema behind the ears, much like *Calcarea carbonica*.

Nose

The nose is affected in two ways. **Nosebleeds** develop from over-heating, exertion, fevers, sleep, or from the slightest blow to the nose. The other problem is the ease with which *Tuberculinum* children contract colds. These frequent colds begin when cold, wet weather passes through the area or when the child becomes exposed to the cold wind. Others develop chronic coryzas after they drink milk products.

The child who has allergies wakes up with a stuffy nose that stays stuffy until he goes outside to play. Then the nose begins to discharge clear mucus, just as it does in *Calcarea carbonica*. Authentic coryzas begin with the production of thick, yellow mucus that extends to the ears, sinuses, and lungs.

Finally, the old materia medicas often mention that the *Tuberculinum* patient perspires profusely on the nose. Actually, he may perspire freely anywhere on the face.

Face

The face is often **pale**, or pale with **patches of ruddiness**, especially on the cheeks. Occasionally the entire face or just the cheek area becomes bright red; this happens during fevers, exertion, or excitement. The materia medicas describe the face becoming red in the afternoon. This is actually caused by the afternoon fevers that develop (see **Fevers**). The cheeks may also develop dry, red patches that occasionally lead to eczema.

Looking at the face, one may find that the child has an "adenoidal" look along with swollen, puffy skin and allergic "shiners." This is especially apparent upon awakening in the morning.

The face may exhibit terrible **acne** in the teenager, almost to the point of boils. The central line of the face (the nose, chin, and central forehead) is most affected. This is somewhat peculiar to *Tuberculinum* and *Sulphur*. Finally, *Tuberculinum* **perspires** quite easily on the face, noted most during exertion or sleep.

Mouth

The mouth is almost always affected in *Tuberculinum*. The child may be born with **anomalies**, such as a cleft palate or a small dental arch, that will cause many problems with the teeth.

The **teeth are greatly affected**. First is the curious fact that the child may be born with **too many sets** of teeth; natal, neonatal, or supernumerary teeth may all be present. This will force early dental treatment to extract some of the teeth in order to let the others erupt. In most, the teeth are too **crowded** and will not align properly along the dental line, so that some of the teeth will lay in front of or behind the others. It is interesting to note in provings and old materia medicas the elicited *Tuberculinum* symptom of feeling as if the teeth were all jammed together and that there were too many for the head.

Some children may have **tardy eruption** of their permanent teeth, becoming six or seven or eight years old and still not having any of their second set. Dentition may occur very **early in life** and may be slow and painful as well as accompanied by fevers, diarrhea, sweats, and colds that remind one of *Calcarea carbonica*. Unlike the *Calcarea carbonica*, however, this child grinds her teeth violently during dentition. During this time the child becomes intensely irritable and appears as though she needs the remedy *Chamomilla*.

Looking at the mouth, one may observe many **cavities** at the base of the teeth, like *Staphysagria*. Even more commonly seen are teeth that are severely **serrated**, as in *Syphilinum*.

These children **grind their teeth** in their sleep; if a child is old enough to have worked at it for awhile, the teeth may be ground down and perfectly flat!

Throat and Neck

The throat may show large tonsils from repeated or chronic **tonsillitis**. During acute tonsillitis, children complain of sharp pains that shoot up to the ear while swallowing solids, much like *Hepar sulphuris*. With tonsillitis or any respiratory infection (even if the child does not currently have an infection but tends to contract them), one will be able to palpate all the cervical lymph nodes, as they will be enlarged and indurated. The nodes of the neck will feel like a chain of marbles. This is even more pronounced than is found in *Calcarea carbonica* or *Silicea*.

Lower Respiratory System

Chest

The chest is greatly **affected** in these children, just as might be expected from the remedy's namesake. Afflictions vary from physical deformities to acute or chronic infections.

The chest may be narrow and long or take the form of a pectus carinatum (pigeon chest) or a pectus excavatum (funnel chest). The **shape** of the chest and rapid growth during adolescence often lead to chest pains, felt as stitches whenever there is exertion. The shape of the chest is a good indication of the weakness of the lungs.

Weak Lungs

Lung problems may begin from the first day of life. Some of these children are born with **fluid in the lungs**. Most catch colds frequently that drop into the lungs and settle into a **persistent cough**. The health history commonly reveals **repeated and frequent bouts of bronchitis, croup, whooping cough, pleurisy, or bronchopneumonia**. The parent may also let it slip out that all her children have these problems, showing the inherited taint or weakness of the lungs.

They tend to develop these infections when the weather becomes **damp** or when they are around smoke or other airborne **pollution** for very long. A child seems to recover from one attack, retaining perhaps only a lingering cough, only to suddenly develop a new infection.

There are a few **symptoms common to all** these respiratory infections. The child has a high fever in the evening that is accompanied by a red face, profuse perspiration, and very swollen, hard cervical glands.

The child may also have a dry cough at night, even during sleep, without any expectoration. In the morning there is copious mucus that is thick, yellow, and puslike. If the child is old enough, he may notice and report that the expectoration tastes salty or sweet.

Tuberculinum children develop **chronic coughs** due to a little **tickle in** the back of the throat, similar to that found in people needing the remedy *Rumex crispus*. Weakness of the lungs precludes the ability to recuperate completely, and so the children maintain this cough. Parents might add that it is always there but that sometimes it gets worse. Such a cough becomes more noticeable after playing outside awhile exposed to the cold. The child then develops a fever and has to lie in bed for several days with yet another acute illness, taking yet another course of antibiotics. Once an acute cough has developed, it is aggravated in a warm room and ameliorated somewhat in the fresh, open air.

Pneumonia

Tuberculinum is one of the best remedies to give during **pneumonia** with chills, nausea, vomiting, and high fevers of one hundred and three degrees or more that recur in the afternoon, and where there is a distinctly red face. The coughing fits that accompany the pneumonia typically begin from two or three o'clock in the afternoon and continue on into the evening, and consist of dry, painful coughs that make the child cry. Headaches also prevail at these times.

The lungs of the pneumonia patient are full of **mucus** that makes breathing difficult, causing shortness of breath and wheezing. The child must use all of her accessory breathing muscles. This is especially the case when lying down at night. Anxiety and restlessness go hand in hand with the shortness of breath, as may be found in *Arsenicum album* individuals with similar disorders. While much mucus can be heard in the rattling breathing, the child may not be able to bring it up easily. Sufferers cough and cough, moaning with the pain of each spasm. The expectoration may be difficult to bring up in the evening and easier in the morning. The expectoration is, as in *Phosphorus*, often reddish or tinged with visible blood.

They perspire profusely all over with this illness, most especially on the face. As is also found in *Phosphorus*, they desire ice-cold water during coughing fits. Diarrhea develops, as well as bone aches throughout the body.

The key factors pointing to *Tuberculinum* here are the great amount of sweating, a high fever that may even lead to unconsciousness, moaning with discomfort, and the constant grinding of the teeth caused by neurological irritation. In my practice, I have noticed that there is a slight predilection for the left upper lung field to be affected in the same area where a Pancoast tumor would develop, but any part of the lungs may be involved.

The remedy *Tuberculinum* is also helpful for children who have had pneumonia that never fully resolved and left them with the type of ongoing cough described here and a tendency for recurring bouts of bronchitis.

Asthma

These children may also develop asthma quite easily. It may be the allergic variety, set off by domestic animals such as cats, dogs, and horses, or by pollen and grasses. It may follow an acute infection such as pneumonia or come on during a simple upper respiratory tract infection.

Exertion may also be the inciting factor. Running around outside during hay fever season is particularly troublesome.

Alimentary System

Food Cravings and Aversions

Their food cravings are distinctive. They strongly **crave cold milk**, drinking up to gallons a day, and **spicy meats** such as ham, bacon, sausages, and salami, especially if these are **smoked** or **soft**.

They may also crave other **delicacies**, sampling a little at a time from sauces, candy, and sardines.

Many have very strong desires for **sweets, salt, spices, eggs, butter, peanut butter, and yogurt, as well as macaroni and cheese**. This set of food desires should be added to the *Repertory* in italics or bold type, as *Tuberculinum* is not mentioned there.

It is interesting to look at the foods just mentioned and analyze the case solely from that list. Most of the foods fit *Calcarea carbonica*, yet the desire for fat goes strongly against that remedy. The desire for fat, butter, and meat points to *Sulphur* quite strongly, yet the desire for eggs and milk goes against that remedy. The desire for eggs, butter, peanut butter, and sweets may also point to *Pulsatilla*; but again, the craving for fat rules out that remedy.

Before discovering from experience these food cravings of *Tuberculinum*, one might disregard half of any reported cravings because other materia medicas do not mention them, and take into account only those cravings that would lead one to a particular remedy even though the child exhibited other contradictory cravings strongly.

Reviewing mistaken prescriptions, it came to light that often only the food cravings that would confirm the assumed remedy were paid any attention. This is a common mistake in prescribing. The doctor only looks at the aspects that he or she recognizes and disregards the rest as unknown or irrelevant to the case, even though the case may very well rest on the material being thrown out. One must always work inductively, eliciting all the particulars of the entire case first and later matching a remedy to the case, not making a case fit the remedy.

If one were given the chance to review many *Tuberculinum* cases, one would be shocked at how many of the cases have these particular food cravings. If we look at the cravings as a group, it is worth noting that **there is no other remedy type that has all of these cravings.**

About a third to a half of *Tuberculinum* children are **averse to eating meat as well as vegetables.**

In *Tuberculinum* cases the **main clue** in the food section is the strong **desire for cold milk**, some children drinking gallons a day.

They also have a high thirst for cold water, like *Phosphorus* and *Sulphur*, even if they themselves are chilly.

Occasionally one may find in the child who loves to travel (or who has a general dissatisfaction ingrained in her) a particular method of eating in which she keeps her **foods separated.** She eats one bite from the first portion, then the second, the third, and finally back to the first to start the cycle again.

Stomach

Children who need the remedy *Tuberculinum* tend toward **poor nutrient absorption or a fast metabolic rate.** This can be recognized by the fact that they can eat as much as an adult but not gain any weight; in fact, they may even lose weight, similar in this way to *Natrum muriaticum* and *Sulphur.*

Like *Psorinum*, *Phosphorus*, and *Lycopodium* children, *Tuberculinum* youngsters may have an **increased appetite before or** during a headache, feeling an emptiness in the stomach that must be filled with food. They also tend to get stomachaches and become irritable if they are hungry, and holler at the mother to bring them some food quickly—or else.

Rectum

The rectum is affected in two major ways. While materia medicas describe stools that alternate between constipation and diarrhea, in practice most of the children experience one or the other, most commonly diarrhea.

If present, **constipation** is usually quite severe, with the stools becoming very hard and consisting of little balls. It is accompanied by colic that is reminiscent of *Plumbum* stools. These children may develop hemorrhoids that bleed due to such great straining at stool.

The **more common complaint**, though, is **diarrhea**. First, the thin *Tuberculinum* child may suffer from lactase deficiency, causing profuse diarrhea every time milk is taken. The common history elicited from the parents is that the child has recurrent bouts of diarrhea that last for one, two, or even three months; for some children this type of stool gets to be the norm.

In other children there may appear to be no reason for the diarrhea. The food is mild, the child does not appear to be ill, and yet the diarrhea persists and the child loses weight. This diarrhea may accompany any illness, but especially respiratory diseases and fevers. The loose stool often persists long after the illness has ended. The specific symptoms of the diarrhea may remind one of *Sulphur*. It occurs mainly in the **morning** when the child wakes up, forcing the child to run to the bathroom or stain his clothes or sheets. The stool is painlessly and explosively expelled without effort.

While this is common with *Sulphur* and may in fact lead the doctor to mistakenly prescribe it, after the remedy does not work and the case is reanalyzed it will be realized that the stools do not have the characteristically strong *Sulphur* odor, nor do they excoriate the anus as one would expect to find with that remedy. These two points should lead one away from considering *Sulphur* and toward *Tuberculinum*.

Urogenital System

Enuresis

The remedy *Tuberculinum* is the best friend that parents of a bed wetter can have. This remedy has cured more children of the embarrassing, socially stigmatizing disorder than any other remedy in the materia medica. The problem may be lifelong or have only begun after an acute illness such as an upper respiratory infection or a fever. A statement such as: "After receiving the treatment for the illness, he began to have bed-wetting spells," is a common tip-off to *Tuberculinum*.

The bed-wetting may occur at any time from the first sleep of the evening to the deep sleep of the early morning; or more typically, several times during the night, some urinating every hour. The urine has a very **strong odor** that can remain in the bedding long after the child quits the habit.

It is common for parents to tell the doctor that they took the child to the bathroom to urinate during the night but that it accomplished nothing, as the child wet the bed later anyway. It can be difficult for parents to awaken the child. They may pick the child up from bed, carry him to the bathroom, hold him over the toilet, and tell him to urinate. The child often remains asleep during this whole procedure, grinding his teeth or thrashing about, but will urinate profusely when bidden.

For most children the cause of the problem is that they **cannot rouse themselves from a deep sleep** to get up and go to the bathroom. This is especially true with *Tuberculinum*, but it is not the only reason: there is a **lack of inhibition** that makes urinating in bed a meaningless event to the child. It is commonly found that after the remedy has acted the sleep is not as profound and the child will awaken if needed.

Boys

The boys tend to **masturbate** from the early age of four or five years. Embarrassed parents mention that the child either masturbates or is always touching his genitals and can maintain an erection. This can be quite bothersome to the parents. A few may tell the doctor that the child rubs his genitals against his mother's leg or other body parts, even in public, "just as a dog might."

Girls

Even from menarche the girls develop **dysmenorrhea** before the period, complaining of severe cramps, backaches, and swelling of the breasts. It is of interest to note that the pains increase with the flow. This is unusual as most women experience relief of the pains as the flow becomes heavier. The flow may be bright red or contain dark clots that pass after a colicky pain. It may also be quite heavy and last a week or more.

Some thin, **emaciated-looking girls do not begin to menstruate at the normal age.** They can get to be fourteen or fifteen years old and still not show any sign of approaching menarche. These girls begin to lose weight in their teens, have slow comprehension, and develop one respiratory disease after another. The problem is not so much the menstrual cycle or the lack of it, but rather a deep constitutional disorder that may first make itself known at the expected time of menarche.

Musculoskeletal System

Back

In some children the back is covered by **long hair at birth.** In others the hair may only cover the spine.

Along with pectus excavatum or carinatum, there may also be **scoliosis.** Teenagers may complain that their backs hurt whenever they stand too long and feel better if they walk about or play. While this may seem like a *Sulphur* keynote, during the physical exam one can find the differentiating point: in *Sulphur*, the lower lumbar vertebrae have slipped forward, causing pain in the lower lumbar area when the child stands; whereas in *Tuberculinum*, the examination shows that the child has a lateral curvature of the spine, and frequently a severe case of it, that causes the pain.

Extremities

One may observe out of the corner of an eye that the feet and legs are restless during the interview. The child **kicks the legs** vigorously from the knees down. Occasionally the mischievous child kicks the doctor's foot or the corner of the desk or other furniture during this restless motion, apparently by accident. This is typically restless, provocative *Tuberculinum* behavior.

The child may have quite a few **deformities of the limbs.** He or she may have abnormally **slow bone growth.** There may be no apparent problem during the first few years. However, as the child continues to grow older, X-ray examination will reveal that the child is falling behind in bone development.

Tuberculinum children are at great risk of falling prey to rickets, even nowadays. The children may be bowlegged or have ankles so weak that they frequently turn them. Bone development may not be equal in all joints. Looking at the fingers and toes, one may notice that they are deformed and crooked, turned medially or laterally. It is incredible to watch these crippled digits straighten out over a period of months with the prescription of *Tuberculinum.*

Alternately, the child may undergo **rapid bone growth** accompanied by many problems in overall health. With every growth spurt, the tall, thin person grows weaker and experiences lethargy and problems such as a runny nose, swollen glands, tonsillitis, and aching joints. The child just lies around watching television until the growth reaches a plateau. The remedy *Tuberculinum* can be helpful in the treatment of Osgood-Schlatter disease when these symptoms are present.

Fingernails and **toenails** may be quite a problem as well. They may split or peel easily, be plagued by hangnails, or become ingrown.

As described, the child **perspires from the feet,** especially at night, occasionally giving off an offensive odor.

Arthritis

Tuberculinum is one of the common remedies for **juvenile rheumatoid arthritis.** The symptoms may seem to be very similar to those found in *Rhus toxicodendron,* with pains and stiffness aggravated by many factors: damp weather, a change of weather, sitting for too long, rest, standing too long, and first motion after rest. They are ameliorated by continued motion and heat (especially hot baths); these relieve the great stiffness. One good differentiating point between *Rhus toxicodendron* and *Tuber-*

culinum is that the pains of *Tuberculinum* arthritis are aggravated by all types of weather change: from hot to cold, but also from cold to hot, especially if it is wet and hot; whereas in *Rhus toxicodendron*, the pains are aggravated only by the change from hot to cold and damp weather.

In arthritis, the joints of the **legs** are the most affected in this remedy type. The pains wander and are accompanied by acute swelling, heat, and redness. After the fluid enters a joint and the acute inflammation stops, the joint remains large but becomes externally pale looking. This apparent cessation of the arthritic process only seems to prompt another joint to go through the same sequence of events. This is a very similar arthritic progression to that of *Pulsatilla*, *Kali sulphuricum*, *Kali bichromicum*, and *Formica rufa*.

Children with arthritic bone inflammations wake up stiff and feeling crippled until they move about. This may also describe an acute rheumatic attack or other joint disease in which exacerbations come on periodically.

Skin

The skin gives few but very important keynotes for *Tuberculinum*. As mentioned before, the health history may contain the fact that the child was **born hirsute**. This is a big keynote for the remedy. The hair is fine and smooth and usually straight but sometimes curly, and may grow on the head, face, spine, shoulders, or entire back.

Looking at the child's skin, one finds qualities similar to the skin of those needing the remedies *Silicea* or *Phosphorus*. It is **pale**, **thin**, delicate, and has a translucent quality.

This type of skin is very susceptible to **ringworm**, making *Tuberculinum* the main remedy for this condition. While the infestation can be anywhere on the body, it tends to be on the head and the extremities. On the scalp, the lesion takes the form of a perfectly circular patch of baldness. On the extremities, it causes the skin to dry out and crack and become slightly discolored to a dark red tint. *Bacillinum* shares these symptoms.

The overall **allergic predisposition** of the child may show itself on the skin as well as in the respiratory system. The child may develop **hives** all over the body, especially on the face and neck, that can be aggravated by animal fur touching the skin.

Eczema also readily develops. Some *Tuberculinum* children have eczema from birth, as do some *Medorrhinum* infants. The most common locations of the rash are the head in general, including the eyelids and cheeks; and the calves and forearms. The eczema and the hives have common modalities: the itching is intense at night, as it is in the cold air or during cold, wet weather; and is especially intense when the child is taking off his clothes at night. The eczema may be very dry, cracked, and flaky, as is found in *Phosphorus* types; or very wet on the face, as is found in *Calcarea carbonica*. In this case the child scratches the rash to the point of making the skin bleed. The most beneficial palliative for this condition is dry heat.

The skin of some children, especially those with birth defects, has a very sour, offensive, **cadaverous odor** to it.

In general, the *Tuberculinum* child **perspires easily**, especially if he or she plays hard, as do the remedy types *Calcarea carbonica* and *Sulphur*.

Fevers

These children **develop fevers very easily**. *Tuberculinum* is the main remedy to consider for a **fever of unknown origin**. The fevers usually begin or rise at **three or four o'clock** in the afternoon and continue into the night, dropping in the morning and rising once again in the afternoon. **Perspiration** is evident all over the body, but especially on the head. The face becomes very red.

Diarrhea and weight loss occurring at the same time may make one assume that there is a malabsorptive syndrome operating, yet the results of conventional tests for this will probably come back negative.

A great **thirst for ice-cold water** may develop during the fever, reminiscent of *Sulphur* and *Phosphorus*.

The whole pattern here described may also be seen accompanying any infection of the digestive or the respiratory tract.

Physical Generals

The remedy *Tuberculinum* must be considered and applied in a slightly different manner than the other remedies discussed in this book except for *Medorrhinum*. The remedy may be called for in the case of a child exhibiting only a few symptoms of the remedy picture, be it one or two keynotes plus a family history of tuberculosis; allergies such as hay fever, asthma, and eczema; scoliosis; rheumatoid arthritis; or birth anomalies.

This remedy may also be considered for cases in which a disease recurs over and over again and when the child manifests appropriate keynotes. One may repertorize a case to find that *Tuberculinum* comes up in a few rubrics and that there is a strong family history that supports this finding. A keynote or two coupled with a chief complaint that fits the remedy, and one may feel the obligation to try it.

Most commonly found will be the child who becomes a *Tuberculinum* type having only the recurrent symptoms of colds, diarrhea, and a stuffy nose. As can be discerned from this, there is a weakness that not only prevents acute conditions from ending quickly but also brings out constitutional symptoms with every acute attack. It is this underlying weakness that forms the basis for understanding the remedy and the constitutional type *Tuberculinum*, similar to that discussed in the chapter on *Medorrhinum*.

The generalities are numerous in *Tuberculinum*. The child is negatively affected by changes in temperature such as those common before a storm; at the onset of cold, wet weather; and in fog and drafts, all of which aggravate respiratory and rheumatic complaints.

Ironically, the child tends to be chilly yet prefers the cool air even though it aggravates physical complaints. Children who are not disposed toward respiratory tract infections may be "warm-blooded," refusing to wear socks and shoes and walking about wearing fewer clothes than others around them. They prefer to be in cool, dry, mountain air and may have complaints such as asthma that are aggravated by seaside conditions.

While the child's state seems to be aggravated by changes in atmospheric conditions, he or she desires and is benefited by other environmental change. Mentally, the child is restless and desires change. Conditions of the musculoskeletal system are also aggravated by rest and ameliorated by motion.

The **changeful nature** of *Tuberculinum* is a very important concept to grasp in order to understand this remedy type. Along this line one may find two corollaries. First, the complaints often change location from one body system to another. Second, the complaints are never really completely eradicated from the body. The children do not have the requisite strength or stamina to completely conquer these diseases, and so they suffer relapses.

In this sense, an illness may change symptomatology within the same system, yet still remain essentially the same disease. As an example, one may find a child who develops bronchitis followed by sinusitis followed by pneumonia and so forth, none of these ailments ever leaving the respiratory tract but running the gamut of all the diseases that can affect that system. This is especially true of children who cannot seem to recuperate from upper respiratory tract infections and who have a chronic cough with swollen glands and weight loss. These are what the old materia medicas termed "scrofulous children."

Tuberculinum should also come to mind for the **congenital anomalies** and illnesses that seem to be plaguing humanity ever more frequently. Besides skeletal deformities, there are deformities of the extremities, cleft palates, strokes in utero, pneumonia at birth, retardation, and other birth defects or crippling childhood diseases; especially those that may be traced to a calcium deficiency or a thyroid disorder.

These children are also prone to slow and irregular growth and its attendant problems, often remaining small in stature, failing to develop teeth on schedule, and having a fontanelle that remains open too long.

One commonly finds retarded *Tuberculinum* children with large heads, swollen glands, and bone anomalies who have constant upper respiratory tract infections and other keynotes of the remedy. After taking the remedy they seem to brighten up and become healthier.

Notes on *Tuberculinum* Infants

The remedy *Tuberculinum* should be considered for the congenital anomalies that seem to be increasingly plaguing humanity. Besides major skeletal deformities, there are deformities of the extremities, cleft palates, strokes in utero; and neonatal pneumonia, hydroceles, hernias, and many other defects, especially those that may be traced to problems with calcium metabolism or thyroid function and those that are midline anomalies. Toddlers who respond to the remedy *Tuberculinum* may have had a sibling who was born anencephalic.

Irritability is common in babies and toddlers, especially during dentition, when waking up in the morning, and when hungry. The irritability may lead to nasty behavior in young children. Some may bite others, while some may show it by putting up a fuss and preventing parents from changing the diapers.

Babies and toddlers burrow their heads into the pillow, grind their teeth, and perspire at night.

Babies are often born with long hair on the scalp and along the spine, and have long eyelashes.

Teeth erupt too soon. Teething is painful and causes fevers, respiratory tract infections, and irritability. There are many problems with the number and position of the teeth. Babies grind their teeth as soon as they erupt, and some infants are born with already erupted teeth.

There are many respiratory tract infections of the ears, nose, throat, and lungs. Infants may be born with or develop fluid in the lungs or pneumonia in the first few days of life. Respiratory infections occur especially when weather changes to cold and wet and after drinking milk. With such infections they perspire profusely at night, have fevers that increase in the afternoon, develop diarrhea, and become brightly red faced and irritable. Toddlers have many swollen and indurated cervical glands.

They like milk. Diarrhea accompanies many illnesses, especially in the lactose intolerant who drink milk. They often lose weight with diarrhea, even if they nurse and eat often.

Tuberculinum babies are typically born thin or are born plump and suddenly thin down in early childhood to become tall, frail, anemic children, even if they eat as much as adults. It is hard for these children to gain weight. They may grow quickly and gain height easily, but they wind up paying for it with bones that cannot keep up with this fast-paced growth; the unfortunate children may suffer from scoliosis, rickets, or Osgood-Schlatter disease, and often from "growing pains." These thin, wiry, anemic children may be hyperactive, but they tire more easily than do *Medorrhinum* or *Sulphur* hyperactive children.

The opposite is also true: they may also grow very slowly and remain small in stature, fail to develop teeth on schedule, or have a fontanelle that remains open too long.

Perspiration is characteristically profuse, and in the congenitally ill child, cadaverous and sour smelling.

In general, infants may be retarded in all their mental acquisitions and have large and misshapen heads, swollen glands, bone anomalies, and constant upper respiratory tract infections.

Tuberculinum Outline

I. Mental/Emotional Characteristics
  A. Retardation and slowness
    1. Difficulty in comprehension
      a) Poor concentration
        (1) Physically tires them
        (2) Makes them ill
      b) Averse to mental activity; will not do homework
      c) Memory weakens; must read and reread
    2. Often accompany physical birth anomalies
    3. Dullness may occur
      a) After illness
      b) Even in bright children
    4. Fears
      a) Strangers
      b) New situations
      c) Like *Baryta carbonica*
  B. Restlessness
    1. Intense energy
      a) All day long
      b) Still energetic at night: restless in sleep
        (1) Grind teeth
        (2) Toss about in bed
      c) Like to leave the home, go with the parents on errands
    2. May lead to hyperactivity
      a) Love to run, spin, and shout
      b) Strike others
      c) Aggravated by eating dairy products
    3. Restlessness in the doctor's office
      a) Play with many toys
      b) Bounce on the couch
      c) Move around
        (1) From one object to another
        (2) From one chair to another
  C. Irritability
    1. Can be born irritable

2. Especially worse upon awakening
3. May be continuous or intermittent
4. Become violent with anger
    a) Hitting or biting others
    b) Throwing fits, striking the head on the ground
5. May be more mildly irritable: peevish

D. Contrariness
  1. Say or do the opposite of what others wish
  2. May refuse to take the remedy

E. Destruction and violence
  1. Self-destructive: strike themselves, especially on the head
  2. Toward others
    a) Hit them: "slaphappy"
    b) Threaten parents in the interview
    c) Break things that others value
  3. May be episodic with apologies afterward
  4. Love to sit and cut paper with scissors
  5. Violent toward pets

F. Selfishness: uncaring
  1. About others
    a) Their persons
    b) Their property
    c) Their plans
  2. Enjoy ruining all of the above

G. Teasing; impish character in some

H. Fears
  1. Animals
    a) Dogs
    b) Cats
  2. Being alone
  3. New situations

I. Sleep
  1. Restless
    a) While falling asleep
    b) During sleep
  2. Sleep very deeply; cannot be awakened easily
  3. Nocturnal enuresis

4. Almost all will grind their teeth

5. Night sweats

6. Sleep positions

    a) Knee-to-chest

    b) On the back with the hands above the head

7. Very irritable upon awakening

II. Physical Symptomatology

  A. Head Area

    1. Head

      a) Born with hair

        (1) Much

        (2) Long and dark

      b) Ringworm develops easily

      c) "Head thumpers": they strike their heads against objects

      d) Severe headaches

        (1) Due to eyestrain from study

        (2) With visual distortions

        (3) Accompanied by intense hunger

        (4) Very irritable with the pain

        (5) May perspire during the headache

      e) Perspire

        (1) Profusely

        (2) Easily

      f) Misshapen skull, as if sutures had closed too early

    2. Eyes

      a) Born with long eyelashes

      b) Sparkle

        (1) With mischievousness

        (2) With aggression

      c) Discoloration

        (1) Blue sclera

        (2) Blue rings around the eyes

      d) Physical problems

        (1) Astigmatism

        (2) Strabismus

        (3) Weak accommodation of the eye muscles

3. Ears
  a) Adenoids enlarge, causing hearing impairment
  b) Recurrent otitis
4. Nose
  a) Nosebleeds develop from the slightest
    provocation
  b) Many colds
    (1) Frequently begin with a change of weather
    (2) Due to milk allergies
  c) Profuse perspiration on the nose
5. Face
  a) Color
    (1) Pale
    (2) Patches of ruddiness
    (3) Blue circles around the eyes
    (4) Bright red face during afternoon fevers
  b) Eczema on the cheeks
  c) Severe acne
    (1) To the point of boils
    (2) On the midline
  d) Perspire easily and profusely
6. Mouth
  a) General structural anomalies
    (1) Cleft palate
    (2) Small dental arch
    (3) "Tongue-tied"
  b) Dental problems
    (1) Born with too many teeth
    (2) Teeth can erupt during the first month of
      life
    (3) Teeth may be crowded and misaligned
    (4) Primary teeth may not fall out and must be
      pulled to make room for the second set
    (5) Dentition accompanied by many illnesses
    (6) Many cavities
    (7) Serrated teeth
7. Throat and Neck
  a) Frequent tonsillitis

b) Enlarged cervical lymph nodes
    (1) Many
    (2) Hard
B. Torso
  1. Lower Respiratory System
    a) Distorted shape of the chest
        (1) Long and narrow
        (2) Funnel chest
        (3) Pigeon chest
        (4) Painful
    b) Infections
        (1) Begin at birth
        (2) Repeated bouts of infection
        (3) Various types
        (4) Accompanying symptoms
            (a) High fever in the evening
            (b) Red face
            (c) Copious perspiration
            (d) Swollen glands
            (e) Dry cough at night
        (5) Cough
            (a) Chronic
            (b) From a tickle in the throat
        (6) Pneumonia
            (a) When all the above symptoms pertain
            (b) Additional symptoms
                i) Shortness of breath
                ii) Thirst for cold drinks
                iii) Diarrhea
                iv) Grinding of the teeth in sleep
    c) Asthma
        (1) From allergies to animals
        (2) With respiratory tract infections
        (3) Worse with exertion, such as running
  2. Alimentary System
    a) Food cravings and aversions
        (1) Cravings
            (a) Cold milk

       (b) Soft meats
         i) Ham
         ii) Bacon
         iii) Salami
         iv) Processed sandwich meats
         (v) Especially if smoked
       (c) Salt
       (d) Spicy foods
       (e) Sweets
       (f) Cheese
       (g) Eggs
     (2) Aversion to mixed foods
   b) Stomach
     (1) Greater appetite before a headache
     (2) Very irritable if hungry
     (3) High rate of metabolism
       (a) Eat much
       (b) Do not gain appropriate weight
   c) Rectum: Chronic diarrhea or frequent loose
     stools accompany every illness
 3. Urogenital System
   a) Frequent bed-wetting
     (1) During deep sleep
     (2) Accompanies acute respiratory tract
       infections
   b) Boys masturbate from an early age
   c) Girls are prone to severely painful dysmenorrhea
     (1) From an early age
     (2) Worsens as the flow increases
C. Musculoskeletal System
 1. Back and spine problems
   a) Born with hair along the spine
   b) Curvature of the spine with pains from standing
 2. Extremities
   a) Restless legs in the interview
   b) Deformed joints anywhere in the extremities
   c) Slow growth
   d) Osgood-Schlatter disease from too rapid growth

of the long bones

   e) Nail problems

     (1) Deformed

     (2) Weak

   f) Offensive foot perspiration

   g) Rheumatoid arthritis

     (1) Aggravations

       (a) First motion

       (b) Any change of weather

     (2) Ameliorations

       (a) Continued motion

       (b) Warmth

D. Skin

   1. Much long hair at birth

   2. Pale, thin, delicate-looking

   3. Recurrent ringworm

   4. Urticaria due to animal dander

   5. Eczema from birth

   6. Lesions

     a) Itch

       (1) At night

       (2) From exposure to cold

     b) Better from dry heat

   7. May have an odor

     a) Offensive, sour, cadaverous

     b) Especially found in retarded children

E. Fevers

   1. Of unknown origin

   2. Recurrent

   3. Begin around three o'clock in the afternoon

   4. Red face with a great deal of perspiration

   5. Accompanied by diarrhea and weight loss

   6. Thirst for cold water

   7. Accompany any illness

III. Physical Generals

  A. Respiratory tract infections

   1. Chronic

   2. Recurring

B. Family history of lung problems
    1. Tuberculosis
    2. Hay fever
    3. Asthma
    4. Infections
C. Congenital anomalies
    1. Thyroid gland malfunction
    2. Calcium metabolism problems
    3. Midline deformities
D. Aggravations
    1. From contact with animals
    2. From change of weather
        a) To cold and damp weather
        b) Before storms
E. Amelioration from motion

Tuberculinum Confirmatory Picture

These are restless children who are mean and irritable. They throw fits and wantonly destroy the possessions and plans of others. They are contrary and violent toward themselves and others. There is often an impish or aggressive glitter in their eyes. They may have mental difficulties and so be classified as retarded. They fear animals.

Confirmatory Checklist

- Grind teeth during sleep
- Irritable upon awakening
- Strike their heads
- Born with much hair on the scalp and down the spine
- Misshapen skulls and other birth anomalies, especially on the midline
- Long eyelashes
- Recurrent upper respiratory tract infections
- Many dental problems, especially too many and badly aligned teeth
- Swollen and hard cervical glands
- Chest and lung problems
- Crave cold milk and soft, smoked meats
- Avoid mixed foods
- Big appetite without weight gain
- Frequent diarrhea
- Bed-wetting
- Early masturbation
- Recurrent fevers
- Family history of tuberculosis or lung problems
- Aggravation from exposure to animals

INDEX

Abandonment, 153, 215, 218, 228; dreams of, *Puls.* and *Nat. mur.* compared, 154; fear of, *Puls.* and *Lyc.* compared, 70

Abdications, to keep social status, 57

Abdomen, bloated, in teens, 121; colic, 30; cramps, from milk, 159; cramps (vomiting and diarrhea), 199, 238; hard, and cramps, 160; large, 29; lower pains < emotions, 200; pain, at menses, extends to thighs and knees, 161; pain > bending and eating, 72; protruding, *Calc.* and *Sul.* compared, 283–284; rippling with gas bubbles, 240; sleeping on, 190, 231; sore everywhere, 284; tympanic, 76

Abstract thinking, difficult, 151

Abuse, of animals, 259

Acceptance, intense desire for, 219

Accidents, dreams of, 231

Accolades, reception of, *Nat. mur.* and *Phos.* compared, 179

Achievement, inner drive towards, 144

Achilles tendonitis, 162

Acid, stomach, 159–160

Acidophilus supplements, 34

Acne, 290; before menses, 78, 161; *Med.*, *Tub.*, and *Nat. mur.* compared, 117; midline of forehead, *Tub.* and *Sul.* compared, 278; on midline of face, 327; premenstrual, 286

Addiction, to feeling of power, 59

Adenoidal appearance, 70, 327

Adenoids, enlarged, 276, 326

Adopted, telling other siblings they are, 219

Adult/child, dichotomy in *Lyc.* types, 49

Adult-like, 52 (see also Mature)

Aesthetics, 186

Affectation, flat, 57

Affection, craved , 201; gives and receives, 205; instantaneous feeling of, 185; shows and needs, 217; physical and verbal, 177

Age 4–6, often, before *Nat. mur.* pathology develops, 166

Agglutination of eyelids, yellow pus coagulates, 275

Aggression, 260, 307; against younger sibling, 220

AIDS, fear of, 188

Alcoholism, in families, 148

Alienating parents, fear of, 219

Allergens, producing cough, 27

Allergies, in childhood and return of candida rashes, 34; eczema, and asthma alternate, 126; environmental, 156; food, and hyperactivity, 228; predisposition to, 337–338; shots for, 56; to animals despised, 321

Allowance, spends completely, 180

Alone, fear of being, 151, 186–187, 321; *Nat. mur,. Lyc.*, and *Puls.* compared, 50; esp. in dark, 12, 64; *Med., Lyc., Puls.*, and *Phos.* compared, 109

Aloofness, 146

Alopecia, 163

Alternating cruelty and sweetness, 96

Alternation of asthma, eczema, or allergies, 126

Anal fissures, 160; painful, 30

Anal sphincter, tightens, 76

Anchovies, aversion to, 159

Anemia, 236; chronic, 244

Anencephalic, 341

Angels, talks about, 14

Anger, faking, 256–257; from jealousy, 220; *Nat. mur., Nux.*, and *Tub.* compared, 150

Animals, afraid of and/or mean to, 317; chokes, 317; imagines in dark, 244; dreams and fear of, 231, 321, *Med.* and *Tub.* compared, 110; large, fear of, 64, 229; love of, 107; nightmares of, 190

Ankle, moves in circle, an emotional gauge, 141; turns, 162; swollen, 123–124; weak, 32–33, 288, 336

Anonymity, desired, 148

Anorexia, 121; and bulimia, 121; *Med., Cinch.,* and *Ign.* compared, 108

Antibiotics, abuse of, 281; unwarranted, 24

Anticipation, and apprehension, 54; illness from, 182

Antihistimines, detrimental, 24

Anus, red, excoriating, *Calc.* and *Sul.* compared, 31

Anxiety, about family members, 271; expressed on face, 70; felt in stomach, 56, 74; fraught dreams, 153 –154; from over conscientiousness, 145; and nausea in teen girls, 121; > passing flatus, 74

Apologies, short-lived, 317

Appendicitis-like symptoms, 239

Appetite, good without weight gain, 283, 332; loss/nausea in headache, 155; wanting, with thirst, 282; small, 74; voracious, 74

Apples, craved, 119, 282

Apprehension, 12, 50; before event, 111

Apthae, 166, 279; < acidic foods, 158; ulcers, 25

Arches, aching, 124

Arthritic inflammation, and fears and irritability, 56–57

Arthritis, *Lyc.* and *Rhus,* compared, 78–79; *Phos., Tub.,* and *Rhus* compared, 203

Articulate, 261

Artistic, 146, 186, 320

Arts, visual, 144

Asthma, 27, 101, 114; after birth of sibling, 221; after respiratory infection, 73; allergy related, 277; allergy related, < spring and fall, 197; *Ars.* and *Sul.* compared, 280; and candida rashes, 34; and eczema, 18, 125; < exertion, 158; < exertion, *Lyc.* and *Calc.* compared, 73; from birth, 117; from dust or pollen, 238; from nearby disliked animal, 321; from suppressed eruptions, 290; *Nat. mur.* and *Ars.* compared, 158; tight, high in chest, 117; triggered by allergies, 331; < 1–5 a.m., 118

Astigmatism, from birth, 326

Attention deficit disorder, 306

Attention span, short, 183

Attention, center of, 178–179; *Puls.* and *Phos.* compared, 218; craved, 217–218; desire for, constant, 220; diverted easily, 179; embarrassed by being, 145

Attentiveness, 141

Attracts others like magnet, 176

Autonomic nervous system response, 189

Average, desire to be considered, 179

Awake, at night, concern about things to be done, 153; unrefreshed and irritable, 66, 150, 310 –311; *Lyc., Nux.,* and *Nat. mur.* compared, 154; staying, obstinately, 9

Babbling, in sleep, 66; like baby, 221

Baby-like behavior, 221

Backache, at menses, > lying on hard surface, 161; premenstrual, 335; sleep on back, 231

Baldness, in areas, in bronchitis or pneumonia, 191

Bananas, allergic reaction to, 156; craved, 119, 282

Band tight around chest, 197

Barefoot, 123, 165; in winter, 243

Bargains with parents, 180

Basement, refuses to bring things up from, 52

Bathing, hatred of, 291; in cool water, 128

Bathroom, hanging out in, 202

Beans, aversion to, 120

Bears, fear of, 321

Bed wetting, 78, 322; see Enuresis, 202

Beef, craved, 282

Bees, fear of, 187

Behavioral limits, pushes against, 259

Beliefs, does not stand up for, 226

Belladonna, complementary of *Calcarea,* 22–23, 26–27

Birth anomalies, 77, 82, 338; trauma,

as etiology in early seizures, 35; illness from, 91, 129

Bites, 260; siblings, 341

Bitter foods, aversion to, 159

Bladder, disease, 202; small, weak muscles, and thirstlessness, 241; weakness, 286

Blaming, and lying, *Tub.*, *Med.*, and *Tarant.* compared, 101

Blankets, buries self in, 153; kicks off, 231

Bleeding, between menses, 202

Blepharitis, 113, 233, 275

Blinking, repeatedly, 189

Blisters, bright red, 125; tiny, after citrus, 115

Blood sugar level, 73, 269, 283; and unruliness, 260–261; sugar problems, under 5 in age, 200

Bloody discharge from ear, 193

Blue rings around eyes, 193

Blue tinge to everything, 324

Bluffs way through situations, 55

Blushes, 216; easily, 25

Boils, 290, 327; angry, red, 279

Boisterousness, in small groups, 139

Bone, and cartilage, deformity, 37, 304; disease, 262; from suppressed eczema, 126; growth (slow and rapid), 336; injuries, 3; problems, 32; pain < pressure, 124

Bossiness, 220

Bow-leggedness, 33, 336

Bowel movement, 7–10 days, 30; incontinence, 227; painful, 30

Brain injury, from birth, similar etiology of *Nat. mur.* and *Nat. sul.*, 152; sides, not integrated, 62; tumor, 193

Brassica family, aggravates, 73

Bread, aggravates, 73; aversion to, 198, 238; desired, 27, 159

Breaks things, 98, 316

Breast-feeds, forcefully, greedily, sucking air, 75

Breasts, swelling, premenstrual, 335

Breath control, and emotion control, 158

Breath, bad in morning, 195; foul, 237; foul, wakes with, 272; offensive, 279–280; shortness of, < exertion, dust, evening, dry, cold air, 158; through mouth, 23

Bribes parents, 180

Brilliance, 4

Bronchitis, 27, 72–73, 81, 237, 281–282 329; from colds, 194, 196; from suppression, 24, 290; sequela, 238; with rash, 244

Bronchiolitis, 72

Bronchopneumonia, 229

Bruxism, 328, see Teeth grinding

Bubble gum, craved, 198

Bucktoothedness, 70

Bulimia, 121

Burning sensation, in pneumonia, esp. inhaling, 197; tender, soles and heels, 124

Butter, craved, 238, 331

Buttocks, in air, in infants, 129; sore and red, 285

Cabbage, aggravates, 73

Cakes, craved, 238

Calamity, fear of, 12

Calcium, assimilation poor, 35; imbalance, 32; metabolism, 338

Calendula, for rashes, 34

Candida rashes, 34

Canker sores, 25, 166, 195; < acidic foods, 158; from citrus, 119

Capriciousness, 311–313

Car exhaust, breathing of, 93; and headaches, 192

Car rides, like and dislike of, 310

Carbohydrates, desired, 27

Cardiac sphincter, improper function, 28

Casseroles, aversion to, 159

Catamenia, 242

Cataracts, congenital, 22

Catarrh, albuminous, clear or white, 157; postnasal, 156

Categorizes things, 10, 15, 261

Cats, and allergies, 280, 331; black, dream of, 231; fear of, 271, 321

Cavities, at base of teeth, 328

Celiac disease, 30; celiac sprue, diar-

rhea-like, 161
Cellophane-like strips on skin, 67
Cerebral types, *Nat. mur.* and *Sul.* compared, 261
Cervical glands, swollen, tender, 71
Cervical nodes, palpated, 23
Chalk, appetite for, 28
Change, desire for, 310
Chapping, of lips, 71; of skin, 80
Character, strength of, 9–11
Charisma, lack of, 57
Charm, natural, 176
Chase scenes, in dreams, 153, 190
Checks beds, to see if everyone in correct one, 51
Cheeks, one flushed, one pale, 236
Cheese, aggravates, 73; aversion to, 159; desired, 27, 238, 231
Chest, tightens, 158; inflammation, lungs neglected, 73; perspires profusely, 204
Chicken, craved, 282; fear of, 321
Chickenpox, 244
Childishness, 217
Chilliness, 80, 205
Chips, desired, 159
Chocolate, desired, 159, 198, 282
Chromosomal abberation, as if, 102
Cigarettes, 107
Circles, dark blue, at eyes, 70, 72, 156; puffy under eyes, "shiners," 195
Citrus, craved, 119; skin problems <, 126; aggravates allergies and asthma, 115; aggravates dry skin, 80
Claustrophobia, 151
Cleanliness, 141–143, 145
Clears throat often, 196, 198
Cleft palate, 304, 327–328
Clenches fists, 312
Clinginess, 215, 221; during illness, 13
Closed-in place, fear of, 110
Clothes, aversion to, 245; changing, embarrassment about, 144; *Nat. mur.* and *Puls.* compared, 226; messy, dirty, 267; trying on, *Puls.* and *Phos.* compared, 181; wears excessive, 140
Clucking sounds, 235, 279

Cognitive difficulties, 102–106
Cold and wet weather aggravates, 35
Cold drinks, >, 238; desired, 120, 196, 282
Colds, 114; go to chest, 196; chest, from birth, 117; extend to ears, 129; repeated, with mucus and sneezing, 234; sensitivity to, 105; to eyes, with purulent, yellow-green discharge, 233
Colic, 73, 75, 81, 240; alternates with Coryza, 23–24; in babies, 112–121
Colon, as if grasped by fist, 160
Color coordination, *Nat. mur., Phos.,* and *Puls.* compared, 186
Comforts ill parent, 189
Communicates, easily, clearly, 256
Communicative, 175
Company, aversion to, yet dreads being alone, 51
Competitive, 320
Complains, as if atrocity committed, 61
Compliments, unacknowledged, 145
Comprehension, slow, 3, 5
Concentration, deep and lengthy, 11, 35; lack of, 269, 305
Concepts, forgets, 94
Conceptualizing, weakness in, 102
Concern, intense, for parent, 189
Condemnation, fear of, 54–56
Condescending, 60
Confidence, decrease in, 106
Confusion, inability to focus, 104; that people are observing her, 14
Congenital disorders, 303
Conjunctivitis, 113, 233; with rash, 244; *Sul.* and *Calc.* compared, 275
Considerateness, affectation of, 57
Consolation, aggravates, 149; and bonds of love, 224; >, 205, 228, 238; aversion to, *Nat. mur.* and *Sul.* compared, 261–262; desires, but does not request, 149
Consonant exchange, 104
Constipation, 56, 76; cheerful in, 30; *Calc.* and *Sul.* compared, 285; from birth, 121; *Lyc.* and *Calc.* compared, 77; with colic, 333;

stool, long thin or pellets, 201; tendency, dry hard stool, straining, cramping, 160

Contradiction, intolerance of, 7–8, 60, <, 95

Contradictory behavior, 107, 313–314

Control, of events, attempts to, 150; of adults by child, 49; of situations, 58

Conversation, loses thread, 103

Coo, in sleep, 66

Cool wall, snuggles up to in sleep, 272

Corneal ulcers, 22, 326

Corpus callosum, as if severed, 62

Correction, intolerance of, 60

Corrects parent, 60

Coryza, 327; frequent, *Calc.*, *Puls.*, *Dulc.*, and *Lyc.* compared, 24; with gastroenteritis, 238

Cough, allergic, progress to asthma, 158–159; chronic, with tickle, 329; *Calc.*, *Bell.*, and *Puls.* compared, 27; < cold air, lying on left side, excitement, eat, drink, talk, morn. and eve., 196; < by damp, cold, oranges, running, spring, 118; medicine, 93; dry except loose, wet, on waking, 237–238; dry, loose, no appetite, *Bell.*, *Puls.*, and *Calc.* compared, 27; dry, < lying, 72; fears to, 196; harsh, 196–197; mucus rattling in chest, *Kali.*, *Sul.*, *Ant. t.*, and *Lyc.* compared, 72; severe, *Med.* and *Spongia* as complementaries, 118; sounds like dog's bark, 158; tickling, night, 235; with retching and vomiting, 237

Covers self with blankets in summer, 66

Coyness, 96, 153, 319

Crabbiness, 56–57

Cradle cap, 25, 34, 273, 292; sour, thick, white-yellow exudant, crusts, 18

Cramping, at menses or ovulation, 122; in calves, 33; severe, premenstrual, 335

Crankiness, 27, 59, 61–62, 81–82, 311

Crawling, incorrectly, 82

Creases, under lower eyelids, 156

Creativity, priority of, 146

Crippled feeling, wake to, 337

Criticism, of parents, 311; not tolerated, 60; sensitive to, 146

"Cross crawling," 62

Croup, 237, 329

Cruelty, 94–96

Crying, continuously, 216; easily, 106 –108; from shame, of enuresis, 240; little, infants, 166; when lights go off, 81; and consolation, 187; uncontrolled, 98

Cucumbers, craved, 198

Curiosity, 175, 257, 268; intense, 255; *Phos.*, *Sul.*, *Tub.*, and *Med.* compared, 183

Cursing, 98, 311

Cuteness, 268

Cystitis, recurrent, 241

Cysts, ovarian, 123

Dacryocystitis, 233, 235, 275

"Daddy's girl," 220

Dairy foods, trigger destructiveness, 308

Damp weather and respiratory infections, 329

Dandruff, 204, 273

Dark shapes, amorphous, in dream, 231

Darkness, fear of, 11, 151, 186–187, 228, 271–272, 228; fear of, esp. when alone, 51–53, 56, 321

Deafness, 23, 114, 234; gradual, 68; fear of, 188; in family, 145–146

Deceitfulness, 107

Decision making, faulty, 226

Defending, opinions or self, incapable of, 227

Delicacies, craved, 198, 331

Delirium, during fever, 244

Demanding, 318

Dennys' lines, 156

Dentition, 3, 25; and destructive tendencies, 310; and digestive upsets, 28; early, *Calc.* and *Tub.* compared,

328; epilepsy in, 35; slow, 262
Despondency, and drugs, 107–108
Destructive tendencies, 314; *Nux.,*
Tarant., Tub., and *Med.* compared,
97–98
Detachment, extreme state of, 184
Development, slow, physical or mental, 151
Developmental delays, 3
Diabetes, 73
Diaper rash, from birth, 286; yeast
infection, 31
Diarrhea, 240, 333; chronic, 262;
chronic, with flatus and cutting in
lower abdomen, odorless, 161; explosive, *Podo., Sul.,* and *Calc.* compared, 30–31; from birth, 129;
from fear, 189; from milk, 159,
282; from suppressed eruptions,
290; *Med.* and *Tub.* compared,
121; on awakening, 284; painless,
watery, gushing, offensive, 201;
recurrent, 227, (in infants, 201);
recurring after illness, 205; yellow-
green, excoriates, 121; and destructive tendencies, 310; and
strong emotions, 201
Dictatorial, 59–60, 107
Die, desires to, 108; and wants to see
angels, 14
Diesel exhaust, headache <, 156
Digestion, slow, 28
Directness, in response, 92
Disappear, desire to, 108
Disasters, dreams of, 153
Discharges, suppressed, 24
Discoloration, face and abdomen,
pale, circular, 126
Discouraged, easily, 225
Disease, and depression linked, 146
Disgust, attitude of, 268; feeling of
elicited, 111; for certain objects,
221; expression of, 315
Dissatisfaction, 307; with own abili-
ties, 145
Distractability, 183
Distrustful stare, 50
Divorce, and separation, 145–146
Dizziness, from bending, 231

Doctor, fear of, 187
Dog bones, appetite for, 28
Dogs, allergies to, 331; black, dream
of, 231; dream and fear, *Med.* and
Tub. compared, 110; fear of, 12,
229, 271, 321; fear of, in fever, 246
Dolls, boys play with, 106
Domineering/fearful, needy nature,
59
Doubling over, due to ovarian pain,
123; from abdominal pain, 160
Dracula, dreams of, 153
Dress, coordination, 143; *Nat. mur.*
and *Puls.* compared, 217
Drinks, cold, aversion to, 74; warm,
desire for, 71
Drooling, in sleep, 115, 195, 231, 272
Drugs, 107; and suicidal thoughts,
108
Dullness, 269, 271, 325
Dusk, <, 205
Dwarfing, physical and mental, 102
Dyes, in food, especially red, and hy-
peractivity, 228
Dyslexia, 62–64, 82, 104, 151
Dysmennorhea, 335; and grief, 162;
similarity of *Nat. mur.* and *Bell.,*
161

Ear, as if something crawling out of,
234; itching, 114; red, 276
Ear discharges, thick, yellow, smelly,
23; bloody, 205; yellow-green dis-
charge, *Puls.* and *Kali sul.* com-
pared, 234
Ear infections, (recurrent), 326
Ear wax, increased, 156
Earaches, 36, 220; *Bell.* and *Calc.*
compared, 23; somaticized, 221;
Eardrum, ruptured, 193
"Early birds," 27
Eating disorders, 108–109
Eats often, 199–200
Echoing sounds, 193
Eczema, 114, 163; at genitals, per-
ineum and anus, 121; behind ears,
68, 326; flaking, itching, < heat,
154; from birth, 34, 79, 125, 130,
338; in and around navel, 284; on

scalp, 67; life threatening, 18; on palms, soles, elbows, knees, 288
Effeminate, 226
Eggplant, aversion to, 120
Eggs, aversion to, 198, 282; craved, 27, 238, 331; softboiled, aversion to, 120
Ego, deflates, 63
Eleven a.m., aggravation, 269; hunger, *Phos.* and *Sul.* compared, 200
Emaciation, 162; babies, and pneumonia, 196–197; girls, late menarche, 335
Embarrassed by parents, 147
Embryonic period, and birth anomalies, 303–304
Emotions rule, 4, 226
Emotional, avoidance, 140; causes and asthma, 158; intensely felt, 147; involvement without emotional vulnerability, 147; rewards, seeks, 218; shut down, in severe illness, 178; situations, fear after, 182; stress, and hives, 244
Encephalitis, 192
Enemy lines, behind, in dreams, 153
Energy, lacks, 271; swings, 94
Entertainers, 92
Entertains others, 258
Enthusiasm, 179
Enuresis, 122, 202, 228, 286, 307, 334; and sleep walking, 153; < lying on back, 240
Environmental sensitivity and headaches, 192
Epilepsy, 35; and teething 25; attack, after irritation, 15–16
Episodic, ominous dreams, 190
Epispadias, 77
Epistaxis, see Nosebleeds
Erotic play, 93
Eructations, 239; empty, sour, 28
Eruptions, angry, red, 273; discharge, yellow, crusts, 273; hairline margin, behind ears, 154; head, *Calc.* and *Sul.* compared, 19; itches, oozes yellow, 125; oozes yellow-white discharge, 67; over whole body, 262; < bathing, 289

"Estrogen rash," 15
Etheric children, 204
Eustachian tube, catarrh, 23
Evening news, sensitivity to, 51
Evening, fear in, 229
Events, upcoming, anxiety over, 106
Evil, fear of, 150
Exaggerates, 61
Exams, dreams of, 153
Exanthems, 289; childhood 244
Excitability, 175, 179–181, 182; irritates, 150
Exhaustion and sleep, 230
Expectoration, difficult, 119
Experience altering substances, 92–93
Explores everything, 255
Expressive, 175
Extremities, spindly, 81; warm, 243, 288
Extroversion, 175–176; 320; extreme, 91; and introversion, transformation, 185
Exuberance, 257
Eye, as if sand in, 233, 275; contact, lack of, 141; itch, bloody green mucous discharge, 194; mucous, yellow-green exudant, 21; symptoms, < warm, > cold, 233; swelling, red, with thick green pus, 113;
Eye for eye mentality, 316
Eye muscles, weak, 326; *Nat. mur.* and *Calc.* compared, 21
Eyebrows, eczema or seborrheic dermatitis, 193; pencil thin, 117
Eyelashes, falling out, *Sul.* and *Med.* compared, 113; long, 192; long, born with, 205; long, full, and beautiful, 325
Eyelids, agglutinate, 223, 246

Face, fine featured, beautiful, 195; pale, 236; pale with ruddy patches, 327; perspires, redness, 278; round, 25; scratching, in infants, 34; *Tub.*, *Ign.*, and *Phos.* discussed, 195
Facial hair, minimal, 117
Facultative breakdown, 269–271

Failure, fears of, 54, 63–64, 144, 225; feelings of, 225;
Fallopian tube, scarring, 123
Family history of sycosis, 128
Family members, anxiety over, 271
Fantasy, addictive, 147
Fat, aggravates, 73; aversion to, 159, 238; craved (butter), 120, 282; cysts, 126; desire/aversion, 198, *Calc.*, *Sul.*, *Tub.*, and *Puls.* compared, 331; disliked, 28; *Phos.* child, 204
Fault-finding, 60–61
Fear, disappears, if parents near, 64; of dark, alone, *Nat. mur.* and *Phos.* compared, 187–188; *Stram.*, *Caust.*, *Phos.*, *Puls.*, and *Lyc.* compared, 52; rival drug games, 189
Fearful, 215; behavior, chronic 13; /dictatorial, types in *Lyc.*, 49
Fearless, 256
Febrile state, eggs craved, 28
Feet, as if not touch ground, 191; perspire, 336; perspiration ice cold, 33; perspire, profuse, if excited, 203; purple and cold, feel warm, 243; sway gently, 203; turned in, 32, 153; warmth, 123
Feigning illness, for attention, 218
Fever blisters, 115, 117, 157; of unknown origin, 338; produced for attention, 218; somaticized, 218, 221; "spiked" at will, 244
Fidgety, 76, 180
Fifth disease, 244
Fight or flight reaction, 189
Fighting, 95; of parents and acute illness, 182
Fine features, 141
Fingers, in others eyes, 96; oddly shaped, 303; tips and soles as *Med.* keynotes, 126
Finish tasks, compelled to, 6
Fire or fire drills, dreams of, 153
First word, "Dog," 107
Fish, aversion/desire, 198; scale skin, 204
Fissures behind ears, *Lyc.*, *Sul.*, and *Calc.* compared, 23

Fist through door, 97
Fistulas to thyroid, 27
Flaky skin, 204
Flatus, better by, 82
Floaters, 192–193
Fluid, in lungs, at birth, 341; lactose intolerant, 342; retention, in menses, 33
Flushing of face, premenstrual, 236
Focusing eyes, impossible, 155
Follower, a, 217; only with bigger kids, 60
Fontanelles, delayed closure, 17; open, 262
Food, cool or cold craved, 28; cravings, *Med.* and *Sul.* compared, 120; craved, yet aggravate, 238; mixed aversion to, 28; unreasonable aversions, 220
Foot placed on foot, coyly, 216; sweats, offensive, 282
Foreboding, 188
Forehead, center, acne and rashes, 157; wrinkled, 70, 73, 80
Foreign accent, as if, 105
Forgetfulness, 4
Forgive, and forget, 262; but not forget, 148
Forgotten, fear she has been, 223
Four in p.m., < time, 62; four to eight p.m. aggravation, 62, 65
Freckles, 71, 79, 157
Friends, many, 92; moving, 145; only one or two, 146
Frowns, 50, 62
Fruit, and aggressive behavior, 309; aversion to, 238; craving after self starving, 108; desires, 159, 282; unripe craved, 119
Frustration and crying, 98
Funnel chest, 329
Furfuraceous skin, 204
Future, fear of, 12; world, talks about, 14

Gait, jerky, 103
Games, love of, 178; orchestrating complicated, 271; sexual role reversal, 93; slow at, 5

Ganglions, inflamed, 162
Garbage, plays with, 266
Garbled speech, 105
Gas, 73, 75; abdominal, 160; from milk, 282; > hot compresses and abdomen massaged, 76
Gastroenteritis, 225, 238
Gaunt, 80, 205
Gaze, away, when speaking or questioned, 148; direct, 262; staring, 292; strong, 21
Generosity, from sympathy, 182–183
Genetic weakness, 91
Genital, handling, 227; rashes, 31; rashes in infants, 125
Gentleness, 215
Gestures, hand, eye, whole body, 181
Ghost, dreams of, 153; fear of, 12, 64, 109–110, 186–187, 229; imagines with eyes closed, 16; interest in, 15; nightmares of, 190; stories, sensitivity to, 51
Giggles, nervously, 52, 140
Glands, enlarge, and indurate easy, 35; swollen, palpated, 26–27
Glaucoma, juvenile, 22
Gloominess, 107–108
Glue, appetite for, 28; fumes, 93
Goblins, perceives, 187
God, interest in, 15
Gonorrhea, effects in newborn's eyes, 113
Gout, 77
Grapefruit, craved, 119
Grasses, allergic to, 331
Gregariousness, 261
Grief, 58; and clinginess, 13; and peptic ulcers, 200; as etiology, 146; not great sensitivity to, 262; reaction from, 222
Grieved, 141
Grin, sardonic, 317
Grooming, meticulous, 141; preoccupation, 55, 61
Group leaders, *Phos.* and *Sul.* compared; 178
Growing pains, 342
Growls, when hypoglycemic, 62
Growth, difficulties 3; resistance to, 221; slow and irregular, 341; spurts, 3, 32
Grudges, from ridicule or sadness, 149–150; holding, 97–98, 148
Grumpiness, 154
Guilt, 148
Gums, bleed easy, 195; grinds, 17
Gurgling, abdominal, 240

Hair loss, 163; at eruption site, 18
Hair, dry or oily, 154; long, over scalp and back, at birth, 323, 325; on back and spine at birth, 335; pulling, 260; pulls own, 314
Hairline margin, eruptions, 154
Halos around objects, preceding headache, 274
Hand washing, all day, 141
Handling, toddlers resent, 149
Hands, in sleep (under abdomen, above head), 231; perspire profusely, if excited, 203
Handshake, weak, 57
Hang nails, 163
Happen, fear something bad will, 150
Happy-go-lucky, 256–259
Happy, from birth, 205
Hardened, 220
Hats, aversion to, 154; love/hate, *Sil.*, *Puls.*, and *Calc.* compared, 20, 26; off in cold weather, 232; on, 233; earaches >, 23; refuses to wear, 273; wearing, 80
Haughty, 259, 262
Hayfever, 78, 114, 277; symptoms from dust, molds and pollens, 156; < hot days, season change, sun in eyes, 236; *Sticta* and *Phos.* compared, 194; with itching nose, 115
Head, large, 81; large for body, *Lyc.*, *Calc.*, and *Sil.* compared, 66; large, round, *Calc.*, *Lyc.*, *Calc. phos.*, *Sil.*, and *Sul.* compared, 17–18; thumping, 311, 323; perspiration, profuse, 26, 204; perspires easily, 19
Headache, at school, with digestive upset, 232; before menses, 155; congestive, before headaches, 20; from anticipation, 182; from

studying, 324, *Nat. mur., Calc., Phos., Puls., Tub., Calc. phos.,* and *Sul.* compared, 20; from missing meal, 73, *Phos., Lyc., Tub.,* and *Sul.* compared, 67; in grief, 222; *Nat. mur., Bry., Phos., Calc., Tub.,* and *Sul.* compared, 154–155; *Nat. mur., Phos., Tub., Sul.,* and *Bell.* compared, 274–275; *Phos., Nat. mur., Tub., Lyc., Puls., Bry.,* and *Sul.* discussed, 191–192; periodic, visual loss, 154; sinus related, 113; throbbing, with nausea and vomiting, 274; with appetite, 333; with menses, *Puls., Sil.,* and *Bell.* compared, 232

Hearing, muffled in colds, 193

Heart palpitations, 189, 198

Heartburn < spices, pumpkins, seafood, cinnamon, and much salt, 160

Heaven and hell, interest in, 15

Heaviness in chest, 197

Heels, dry cracked skin, 79; painful, 124

Heights, fear of, 4, 12, 151, 271

Held, aversion to being, 148; aversion in colic, 160; desires to be, with fever, 27; needs to be, 245

Hemorrhoids, 285; in pregnancy, 55; *Lyc., Nux.,* and *Mur. ac.* compared, 77; painful, 30

Hemorrhages, 204

Hepatitis, in young, 201

Hereafter, interest in, 15

Hernia, 56; right, inguinal, 78; strangulated, 29; umbilical, *Calc.* and *Nux.* compared, 29

Herpes, 115

Herpetic eruption, cheeks, < sun and fevers, 117; sores, 157

Hiccough, after eating, in infants, 29, 239; after nursing, *Lyc., Nux.,* and *Calc. c.* compared, 75; in utero, 75

Hips, wide, with thin neck and torso, 78

Hirsute, born, 323, 337

Hitting, 16, 220, 260; playmates, *Lyc.* and *Tub.* compared, 60

Hives, 79, 242, 290, 338; recurring, 34; < sun, 157, 164

Hoarseness, painless, 27; < talking and coughing, 196

Holding breath, to not cough, 196

Holds chest, *Bry.* and *Phos.* discussed, 196

Homeostasis, and genetic flaws, 127; mechanism and natural modalities: strong medications, 165

Hormonal treatment, for irregular menses, 202; of pituitary dysfunction, 242–243

Horses, allergy to, 331

Hostages, household, to child's irritability, 62

Hot head, and cold extremities, 27

Hot-blooded children, *Med., Sul.,* and *Puls.* compared, 128

Hugs, readily returned, 176

Human voice, difficult to hear, 193

Humanity, distant from, 106

Humidity, and asthma, 197

Hunger, after big meal, 200; at 11 a.m., 159; on rising, 66; precedes and with headache, 155

Hurriedness, 93–94

Hurt, expressed openly, 185

Hurting, even larger persons, 308

Hydrocele, 31, 241, 304

Hydrocephalus, 273–274

Hygiene, poor, 286

Hyperactivity, 64, 94, 220, 228, 263, 270–271, 282, 307–309; in children, 259; boys, and toilet training, 122; *Med., Sul.,* and *Tub.* compared, 340; *Sul.* and *Tub.* compared, 260

Hyperextension, of fingers and ankles, 33

Hyperthyroid, 26

Hypnotizing, 182

Hypoglycemia, 73, 198–200, 283; and headaches, 192

Hypospadias, 77

Hypotension, and vertigo, 231

Hypothyroid, 26

Hysterical, near, 223; describing fears 186

"I am a bad person.", 108
Ice, chewing, 120; compress, cubes, craved, 198; desired in headaches, 19; drinks, craved, 197
Ice cream, craved and <, 238; desired, 27, 73, 159, 198
Ice-cold drinks, abdominal pains >, 200
Ichythosis, 204
Illness, acute, inability to shake, 91; behavior, *Nat. mur.* and *Phos.* compared, 177–178
Imaginary friends, 320
Imagination, wild, 188
Immaturity, for age, 216
Immobilized, in trance-like state, 184
Immune system, damage from birth, 114
Impatience, 61, 95
Impetigo, 273
Impetigo, following pre-existing eruption, 289
Impishness, 304, 319
Implacability, 95
Impressionability, 176
Inarticulateness, from grief, 222
Inconsolability, 222
Indecisiveness, 57–58
Independence, 9–11; fierce, 265
Independent endeavor and study, 264
Inertia, incapacitating, 94
Infection, acute, with diarrhea and vomiting, 205; viral, 199
Influenza, sequela, 238; with nausea and vomiting, 199
Information assimilation, slow and systematic, 3, 4–6
Ingrown nails, 336
Inhibition and introversion, *Staph.* and *Med.* compared, 109
Initiative, lack of, 53, 216
Insects, bites and allergies, 126; fear of, 11, 65, 187, 229, 271, 321; large mandibled, fear of, 151
Insecurity, 50; concealed, 149
Insignificant things, irritable over as manipulation, 61
Insolence, 150
Insomnia, from anticipation, 65; go-

ing over day's encounters, 152
Insulin, increase, and headaches, 192
Insults parents, 60
Intellectual, 261
Intelligence, innate, 263
Interruption, reaction to, 258
Intestinal rumbling, 76
Intolerance of contradiction, 98
Introversion, 96, 146–147; extreme, 91; *Nat. mur.* and *Med.* compared, 106–108
Inward, turning, 5
Irresoluteness, 226
Irritability, 50, 76, 95, 259–260, 307; from birth, 310; from jealousy, 220; if not obeyed, 59; intense, 61; waking, 73; weepy in headache, 156
Irritable bowel syndrome, 160; from anticipation, 182
Isolation, *Med., Cannab., Thuja,* and *Plat.* compared, 103–104
"It's not my fault.", 100
Itch, intense, 289

Jaundice, at birth, 70, 79; neonatal, 290; with itchy skin and diarrhea, 293
Jealousy, and lying, 101
Jellyfish, fear of, 110
Jittery, 198
Joints, as if tightening, 123; hyperextend with ease, 37; pain and stiffness, *Tub., Med., Rhus, Thuja,* and *Lyc.* compared, 124; swelling, 124
Journal and diary-keeping, 147
Joyful abandon, *Sul., Phos.,* and *Ars. iod.* compared, 266
Judgmental, *Nit. ac., Lyc.,* and *Nat. mur.* compared, 61

Kicking, 311; of parent, 315
Kidnap, fear of, 151, 153, 229
Kidney, disease, 202; infection, 241; stones, right side, 77
Killer bees, fear of, 151
King, acts like, 60
Kleptomania, in jealousy, 219
Knee joints, tighten, 203

Knee to chest, position in asthma, 101; sleep position, 322
Knives, as if cutting scalp, 325
Kyphosis, 287

Labored breathing, 196–197
Lacrimal duct, fistula, 21
Lacrimation, profuse, 233
Lactation, in non-pregnant girls, 242
Lactose intolerance, 30, 159
Laparoscopy, 122
Laryngitis, 196
Larynx, irritated, 196
Lasagna, desire for, 27
Lashes out, 316
Laughs in sleep, 66
Laughed at, aversion to being, 14
Laughing, /crying alternating, 148; involuntarily, 149
Laziness, 325
Leaders, 320
Leadership, 263
Learning difficulties, mild to severe, 303
Left shoulder, tendonitis, 162
Legs, thrashing in night, 112; restless motion, *Nat. mur.* and *Lyc.* compared, 79; restless, kicks vigorously, 335
Legumes, allergic reaction to, 156
Lemons, aversion to, 282; craved, 119, 198; desired, 159; <, 238
Lethal expression, 315
Lethargy, 27, 269; chronic, 6
Letters omitted, 306; used wrong, 63
Leukorrhea, thick, creamy, offensive, 241
Lichen sclerous and atrophicus, 164
Licks lips, 71
Light, and shadow patterns in dark, startle, 190
Light headed and dizzy, 191
Lightning flashes, perceives, 192
Lights on, going to sleep with, 109
Limbs, deformities of, 336
Limestone, appetite for, 28
Lions, fear of, 321
Lips, dry, cracked, peeling, 115; fissure in center, 157; lower mid-dle, cracked, *Phos.* and *Nat. mur.* discussed, 195; tightened, 312; upper, protrudes, 25; red, dry, cracked, 195, 236
Lip-biting, 195
Lipomas, 126
Lists, makes, 4
Little old people, infants, 25
Liver, tenderness, 79
Locomotion, twitches forward, 103
Loner, 106, 146, 261
Long bones, weakness of, 33
Looked at, aversion to being, 148
Looking up, fear of, 229
Loss, illness from, 229
Love, fear loss of, 230; of others, 178; fear of being unworthy of, 225
Low blood pressure, on rising, 191
Low spirited, 14
Lumbar weakness, 287
Lungs, inflammation neglected, 281; lower lobes, in pneumonia, 197
Lying, 100, 319; *Med.* and *Sul.* compared, 258; on left, <, 205

Macabre dreams, 190
Macaroni, desired, 27, 331
Made fun of, See: Ridicule, fear of
Malabsorption, 332; and back weakness, 287; syndrome, 70, 76
Male strangers, fear of, 189
Maliciousness, 316
Malnutrition, babies, and pneumonia, 196–197
Malposition of tissue or organs, 82
Manipulation, 101, 220; of objects and ideas, 263; of possessions, 60
Manners, good, 175
Marasmus, 18, 120, 262; *Calc.* and *Sul.* as complementaries, compared, 273–274
Marijuana, 271
Marry, will not, 220
Masturbation, 93, 122–123, 286, 334–335
Mathematics difficult, 151
Maturity, of attitude, 140, 144
Meal, missed, and headaches, 192
Meanness, 94–96

Meanings of words forgotten, 102

Measles, 234, 244

Meat, aversion/desire 198; craved, 282; disliked, 28, 159, 238, 332; spicy, smoked, craved, 331

Melancholy, 14

Memory, declines, 105; weak from babyhood, 102

Memory problems, 306; *Calc.* and *Baryta c.* compared, 4, 270

Menarche, at early age, 162; late, 78, 242, 335

Menses, abnormally short periodicity, 202; heavy, and light headedness, 191; bright red, with anemia and dizziness, 202; irregular cycle, 242, 287; pain, doubling over, > cold, < flow, 242; profuse, long-lasting, 32

Menstrual blood, *Nat. mur.*, *Lyc.*, *Puls.*, and *Ign.* compared, 162

Mental, confusion, 98; disconnectedness, *Plat.*, *Cannabis ind.*, and *Med.* compared, 104; exertion, headache caused, 274–275; focus, lack of, 183; handicap from birth, 303; strain, 4

Messiness, 256, 266; yet preoccupied with looks, 55; in hyperactive child, 64; irritates, 142; *Med.* and *Sul.* compared, 94

Metabolism, high rate, 332; rapid, *Phos.*, *Iod.*, *Sul.*, and *Tub.* discussed, 199–200

Miasmatic treatment, 91, 127

Mice, fear of, 12

Microcephaly, 303, 324

Middle ear infection, 81

Midline anomalies, 303

Migraines, 191–192; from fear of abandonment, 228

Milk, aggravates dry skin, 80; allergic reaction to, 156; allergy, and extreme irritability, 260; and colic, 160; aversion to, 159, 238, 282; causing nausea, vomiting, colic, and diarrhea, in infants, 166; cold, craved, 198, 331–332; cold, thirst in active girls, 158; craved or aversion to, 28; hot, and stomach aches, 201; intolerance of, 28; triggering headaches, 274; vomited, 129; < or > in *Tub.*, 95

Mind ahead of mouth, 105

Mischievous, 175; face, 319

Mistakes, fear of making, 60, 64; unbearable, 151

Moaning, in sleep, 191

Moles, 79, 125

Monomania, 264

Mononeucleosis, 72

Monosyllabic, in grief, 222

Monsters, fear of, 12, 64–65, 322; fears, sees, *Med.*, *Calc.*, and *Phos.* compared, 110; imagines with eyes closed, 16; nightmares of, 190; perceives, 187

Mood swings, 107, 185

Moping, 6, 217, 225

Moroseness, and suicidal thoughts, 222

Morphea, 163

Mother, as child's peon, 259

Mothers, of *Sul.* children, 255

Motion sickness, 160, 239

Motor skills, anomalies, 103; poor, 82

Mouth, always slightly open, 70–71; dry, 236

Moving, desire to and change positions, 307

Movie, as if all is in a, 184

Mucus, blood-tinged, thick, green-yellow, excoriating, 194; eats, 269; hard crusts, picks all day, *Lyc.* and *Kali b.* compared, 69; in stool, 121; membranes, dry, 157; rattling, lower lungs, 280; suction, in infants, 81; white, salty or bad taste, 157; yellow-green clumps, 114, 119

Mumps, metastasized to breasts or testes, 236, 241

Murders, dreams of, 190

Music, 144, 186

Musicians, 146

Myopia, 326; at early age, 156

Nail biting, 79, 124, 130, 163, 189, 288

Nails, brittle, cracking, ingrown, 33, 336; cracked and disfigured, 243; deformed, *Thuja* and *Med.* compared, 125; slow growth, 33

Names, forgets, 270

Narrow spaces, fear of, 12

Nasal, crusts, 235; obstructions in babies, 68–69; polyps and hayfever, 194; problems, *Puls., Med., Tub., Lyc.,* and *Sul.* compared, 115

Nastiness, 61; *Calc., Lyc.,* and *Tub.* compared, 312

Nausea, 199; before menses, 160; from anticipation, 182; from milk, 159; in headache, 192

Neatness, 217; /messiness in teen girls, *Sul.,* 267

Necklace of cervical lymph nodes, *Calc., Sil.,* and *Tub.* compared, 328; of swollen glands, 32

Needle pain, feet to ankles, 124

Negative attitude, 259

Negative self-image, from ridicule, 143

Nervous, 198; appearance, 140; tension, *Ign.* as acute complementary of *Nat. mur.,* 150

Neurodermatitis, 79, 126

New, environments relished, 179; group, nervous in, 12; situations, fear of, 64, 304, 322; things, fear of, *Lyc., Baryta c.,* and *Calc.* compared, 52–53

Niceness, affectation of, 57

Night person, 112

Night terrors, 16

Nightmares, 13, 190; from family stress, 231; in dark room, 11; sleeping on back, 272

Noise, 308; fear of, 205; sensitivity to in headache, 67; striking offender, 104

Nose, lacking in coordination to blow, 278; stuffed, chronic, 56

Nosebleed, 115, 194, 278; and sneezing, 194; before menses, 203; in a.m., 25; in sleep, winter, summer,

red and gushing, 194; night, 235; summer, 70

Nostrils, alternate from clogged to flowing, 157; flaring, 69–70, 73, 81, 181, 195–197; flare, obsessively, 189; left and nosebleed, 194

Novel reading, 152

Nursing, reaction to mother's milk, 260; regurgitates undigested milk, 28

Obedience, from other siblings, 60

Obedient, 139

Obscenities, 311

Observed, aversion to being, 14, 106, 304; fear of being, *Thuja* as *Med.* complementary, 111

Obstinacy, *Calc.* and *Tub.* compared, 318; in jealousy, 9, 35; 219; *Med., Lyc., Calc.,* and *Tub.* compared, 97

Ocean, fear and love of, 110

Odor, cadaverous, skin afflictions, 338, 342; offensive, any part of body, 244; putrid, sour, from nose, 235; sensitivity to, 267; strong, and headaches, 192, 194

Offended easily, 143, 224; and cries easily, 63

Oily skin, 116

Okra, aversion to, 120

Omissions, lying by, 100

One-to-one relating, 146

Onions, aggravate, 73; aversion to, 120

Open air, craved, 205

"Open" type, *Med.,* 92

Openness, 176–178, 181, 263; personality change to, 178

Opinions of others, concern with, 143

Opinionated, 220

Opposite sex, repulsion to, 220

Optimistic, 278

Oral fixations, 71

Orange juice, meanness < or >, 95

Oranges, craved, 282

Orderly, 145

Orifices, turn red, 290

Orthostatic hypotension, 273; and vertigo, 231; on rising quickly, 191

Osgood-Schlatter disease, 33, 336, 342
Osteogenesis imperfecta, 33
Others don't count attitude, 268
Otitis externa, 234
Otitis, acute, *Sul., Calc., Calc. ph., Puls.,* and *Lyc.* compared, 276–277; from suppression, 24; media, 22, 225, 234; with rash, 244; recurrent, from colds, 245; right side, with cracks behind ears, 68
Ovarian pain, 122; right side, 78; sharp pains, cramping, doubling up, 203
Oysters, as poison, 73

Pain killers, 93
Pain, feigned, 64; physical, irritable from, 62; threshold low, 62–64; sensitive, screaming, 245; sensitivity to, 225, 320
Painting, 186
Pajamas, not tolerated, 231
Palate, itches, 156; upper, itching, 235
Pancoast tumor, 331
Panic attacks, before exams, 145
Papilledema, 193
Paralysis of optic nerve, 193
Parasites, 204
Parent/child dynamic, reversed, 49
Parents, neutral or negative to *Lyc.* child, 57; under child's control, 58
Parties, fear of, 143
Passing stool, painful, 76
Passive, 220
Pasta, desired, 27
Pastry, craved and <, 238
Pathognomics and ultraviolet light in skin lesions, 165
Pathos, appealing, 177
Peacekeeping child, 148
Peanut butter, craved, 238, 331
Peanuts, allergic reaction to, 156
Peas, aversion to, 120
Pectus carinatum, 329
Pectus excavatum, 303, 329
Peevishness, 259, 311
Pelvic inflammatory disease, 122

Penis, inflamed, red or purple, 286; yeast infected, 37
People, approaching quickly, fear of, 12; fear of in children, *Lyc.* and *Baryta c.* compared, 50; loud-voiced, fear of, 12
Peptic ulcers, in adolescence, 200
Perfectionism, 141–143; obsessive, 143
Performance, anxiety, 74; fear of, *Nat. mur., Lyc.,* and *Sil.,* compared, 145
Perfumes, and headaches, 192; headache <, 156
Perineum, red and blistered, 122
Peripheral vision, rapid motion perceived in, 114
Personal grandeur, 258
Perspiration, foul, feet, *Sil.* and *Puls.* compared, 243; head, at night, 67–68; offensive, 281–282; profuse, offensive, sour, 274; sour, and cadaverous, 342
Perspires, night, 341; profuse, 327
Persuaded, easily, 227
Pestering, obstinate, 220
Petit mal, state verging on, 183
Pharyngitis, 118; right, < morning and 4 p.m., 71; sequela, 238; *Sul.* and *Phyt.* compared, 280
Phimosis, 122, 129, 286, 293
Phonographic memory, 152
Photophobia, 156, 162, 192, 233; and headaches, 192; *Calc.* and *Nat. mur.* compared, 21–22
Physical contact, craved, *Puls.* and *Phos.* compared, 188
Physical developmental problems, 303
Physical problems and emotional changes, 56
Pica, 28, 37
Pickles, craved, 198
Picks on family members, 60
Picky eaters, 29, 153
Pigeon chest, 329
Pigeon-toed, 288
Pillow, buries face in to stop cough or asthma, 118; burrows head in,

324, 341
Pimples, itchy, 288; red or hard white papules, 157
Pinching, in soles and arches, 124
Pineapple, headache <, 113
Pinkeye, with pus accumulation, 113
Pinned down, fear of being, 110, 151
Pizza, desired, 27, 282
Plantar warts, 164, 203; right heel, 79–80
Play, and excitement, almost uncontrollable, 179; and self-control, *Phos.* and *Tub.* compared, 175; independent and contented, 35; takes charge in, 256
Playfulness, 319
Playmate, older, as possession, 223
Plethoric, face, 236
Pleurisy, 329
Plums, craved, 119
Pneumonia, 72–73, 81, 237, 280–281; from cold, 196; neonatal, 341; with flared nostrils, red face, labored breathing, 205; *Tub., Ars.,* and *Phos.* compared, 330
Poetry, 144, 146
Polarity of behavioral extremes, 96–97
Pollen, allergy to, 331
Pollution, and respiratory infections, 329
Popping neck muscles, 163
Pops joints, 123
Pork, and stomach aches, *Phos.,* and *Puls.* compared 201; <, 238
Possessed, as if, 317, 326
Possessions, manipulative with, 60
Possessive, of parents' attention, 101–102; in jealousy, 219; only appears, 142
Postnasal catarrh, 196
Postnasal drip, 55, 117–118, 235
Posture, slouched, 262, 269, 287
Potatoes, even raw, desired, 27
Pouts, 217
Power struggle, parent/child, 96; with parents, 313
Power, desire for, 50
Power, external, internally weak, 59

Praise, embarrassed by, 145
Premenstrual, feelings all month, 242; irritable, appetite increase, sweets craved, 78; syndrome, 161; tension and suicidal thoughts, 108; tension, sad, weepy, suicidal, 123; vaginitis, coryza, and headaches, 32
Presence, unseen, fear of, 109–110
Procrastination, 3, 106, 269–270; *Lyc.* and *Sul.* compared, 63
Profound emotions, 145–146
Promiscuity, 93
Proper, 141
Pseudoambidextrous, 105–106
Psoriasis, at genitals, perineum, and anus, 121; pustular, rapid spread, with chills, 164; very painful, and burning, 164
Puberty, as cause of regression, 221
Public failure, fear of, 54
Public rest rooms, anxiety in, 76
Public speaking, anxiety over, 151
Pummels parents, 96
Punishment reinforces resentment, 148
Pus, offensive smelling, 71–72

Quarrels, 95
Questions, asking and answering many, 176; *Phos.* and *Med.* compared, 183

Rage, 58, 61, 308; weeps from, 148
Rape, fear of, 189
Rapport, easily established, 177, 184
Rash, along jaw line, 157; as homeostatic mechanism, 34; especially on face, 338; from birth, *Sul.* and *Calc.* compared, 292; on penis, 122
Raspberries, craved, 119
Rational faculty effected, 303
Rattling in chest, 81
Razors, cutting self with, 108
Readers, voracious, 147
Reading, excessive and headaches, 155; mistakes, 63, 306
Reality, discontinuous, 100
Recall of what was to be done, 184

Reckless abandon, 308
Redundant colon, 201
Regression, from major stress, 221
Regurgitation, from milk, 282
Relationship, problems in dreams, 224
Remedies that follow, *Calc.*, 16
Remedy, cycle: *Calc.*, *Lyc.*, and *Sul.* discussed, 80; refuses to take, 312 –313
Remedy order, related to *Sul.*, 291; *Calc.* after *Puls.*, 229; *Sul.* after *Puls.*, 229–230
Remorse, 148; at over generosity, 182–183; lack of, 95; short-lived, 317
Reprimands, and reprisals, 95; as if longs for, 99
Resentments, 97–98
Reserved, 139
Respiratory infection, 59, 70, 72, 107, 235; and grief, 146; and leukorrhea, 241; and stuttering, 105; chronic, 23
Respiratory problems, from suppressed eczema, 126; < cold, wet, and draft, 339; > lying on abdomen, 128
Respiratory, upper tract infections, become asthma spasms, 197
Restlessness, 64, 307; from excitement, 179–180; *Phos.*, *Tub.*, and *Lyc.* compared, 180; in sleep, 190; with fear, 189
Retardation, 303–307; *Baryta c.* and *Tub.* compared, 304–305
Rheumatic pains, *Lyc.* and *Rhus* compared, 78–79
Rheumatoid arthritis (juvenile), 57; migratory, < morning and warmth, 243; *Rhus* and *Tub.* compared, 336–337
Rheumatoid arthritis, sharp pains, rapid spread, follows grief, 163
Rhomboid, floating patterns, 274
Rich foods, <, 239
Rickets, 32–33, 336, 342
Ridicule, 143–145; avoids, *Nat. mur.* and *Calc. c.* compared, 5; fear of, *Nat. mur.*, *Lyc.*, and *Puls.* compared, 54–56; reinforces negative self image, 143; refuge from in fantasy, 147
Right-side, sleeps on, 190
Rigid behavior, 221
Rinds, relishes, 119
Ringworm on scalp, 323
Ritalin, 103, 180, 271
Robbers, dreams of, 153; fear of, 64, 151, 228
Rocking, 221, 238; babies like, *Calc.* and *Puls.* compared, 16; desired, 230; gently, >, 245
Rolls back and forth and screams, 75
Roseola, 244
Round pellet, bowel movement, 121
Rubbing, desired, 177; >, 205
Rudeness, around strangers, 58
Rules, above, 268
Rumbling, abdominal, 240
Runny noses, in health, 23–24

Sadness, 14, 106–108; and irritability, before menses, 161; and bonds of love, 224; as etiology, 146; predisposed to, 145
Salt, craved 119, 159, 198, 311
Sand, sensation of in eyes, *Sul.* and *Med.* compared, 113
Scabs, picks at, 314
Scalp, dry, 114; eruptions, 18; perspires profusely, 191; sweaty, 262
Scarred skin, after eruptions, 79
Scary movies, 13, 17, 51; with violence, 99
Scary something around corner, 151
Schizophrenic, as if living with, 225
School, as stress, 223; beginning, and enuresis, 240; dislikes, 269, 274; dreams of, 224; fear of, 223; stress, causing regression, 221
School/home behavior, *Med.* and *Tub.* compared, 94
Scoliosis, 32, 287, 342; *Sul.* and *Tub.* compared, 335
Scowling, 75
Scratching, 311
Screaming, 7, 75–76, 95, 308; wakes

up, 17; wakes, and dentition, *Cham.* and *Calc.* compared, 26
Scrofula, 263
Sea bathing, 128
Searing expression, 315
Secondary sexual characteristics, late, 78
Secrets revealed in sleep, 153
Security, craved, 217
Seizures, before menses, 32
Self, plagued by feelings of power-lessness, 58–61
Self-blame, 108
Self-centered, 257; *Phos., Puls.,* and *Calc. Carb.* compared, 179
Self-concept, fragile, 146
Self-confidence, lack of, 50, 63
Self-conscious, 143–145
Self-denigration, 146
Self-destruction, from self-blame, 108–109; tendencies toward, 314
Self-determination, 264–265
Self-esteem, low, 107
Self-importance, 258
Self-recrimination and condemna-tion, 144
Self-reliance, 5
Self-restraint, impossible, 181
Self-willed, 7
Selfishness, 101–102, 318; in jealousy, 219
Sensitivity, 141, 144; and oversensi-tivity, 216
Sensual inquisitiveness, *Sul., Phos.,* and *Ars. iod.* compared, 266
Sentence, begins in middle, ends at start, 181; structure, 105; or thought incomplete, 103
Separation and divorce, 145–146
Sequela, influenza, bronchitis, phar-yngitis, 238
Sequelae of colds in middle ear, 114
Serious, 14, 149; takes self too seri-ously, 61
Sexual experimentation, early, 123
Shadows, fear of, 11; moving, fear of, 231
Sharing, not natural, 268; selfish re-action to, 102

Shin pains, 33, 203
Shiners, blue, around eyes, 326–327
Showers, fear of, likes baths, 271
Shrieking, 311
Shyness, alternates with anger, 107; *Med.* children and fathers, 109; of *Nat. mur., Puls., Lyc.,* and *Phos.* compared, 184; states, 100, 139, 144, 223
Sibling, birth of, and regression, 221; new, shock of, 219–224; older, as possession, 223; "Siege mentali-ty," and perfection anxiety, 143
Silence, in order to concentrate, 104
Silicea as *Puls.* complementary, 216
Simian creases on palms, 303
Singing, 186
Sinus, colds, 20; infection, chronic, 4, 196
Sinusitis, and eczema, 18; or asthma from colds, 115; chronic, 272, 277; chronic, after hernia, 78; severe and headaches, 192
Sissy, 227
Skeletal deformities, 340
Skeletons, fear of, 64
Skin, bite or injury turns purple, 288; cracks behind ears, 81; dry, cracked, red tinted, 337; eruptions suppressed, 289–290; greasy and greenish, 157; pale or gray, *Med., Tub.,* and *Sil.* compared, 116; pale but flushes easy, 195; purplish, mottled, 243; tags, 125
Skull, oddly shaped, 304; sutures, closed early, 324
Sleep, alone, averse to, 190; refusal to, 218; deep, 322, 334; difficulty going to, 230; difficult, after ex-citement, 182; hates, 271–272; if emotions high, 190; position, left side or back, 153; restless, 272, 309, 322–323; troubled, 152–153; with light on, 11, 65, 190, 231, 272; windows closed and socks on, 80; with parents, 65; at friends, and enuresis, 240
Sleepwalking, 17, 190; *Nat. mur.* and *Phos.* compared, 153

Sleepy after lunch and before supper, 272
Slimy creatures, fear of, 110; foods, aversion to, 120, 159
Sloppy-looking, 267
Slow learner, perfectionist, 106; sense, diminished or loss, 235; sense, acute, 194
Smiles, involuntarily, 149
Smirks, 62
Snacks all day, 159, 199–200, 283
Snakes, fear of, 65, 151, 229–230
Sneezing, 234; in paroxysms, 194, 277; paroxysmal attacks < in spring or fall, 156
Snuffles, 69–70, 81; chronic, 37
Sobs, loud, racking, 227
Social, norms, inability to be subservient to, 265, 267; standing, painful awareness of, 60; status, maintaining appearance, 55–56
Socially active, 270
Soda pop, craved, 73
Soft boiled eggs, 27
Soft drinks, thirst for, 157
Soils pants in exciting play, 202
Soles, pain, itch and perspire, 124; swell, 123
Somaticized, fears, 56–58; symptoms, 221
Somnambulism, 190; see also Sleepwalking
Songs, sings sad, 139, 147
Sore throats, right to left, > warm drinks, 71; repeated, 26; < talking and coughing, 196
"Soul," lacking, 57
Sour, desired, 159; fruit craved, 119
Sour foods, aversion to, 282, craved, 198; <, 238
"Spacing out", 103, 270
Sparkle and sadness in eyes, 156
Speak, forget what about to, 94
Spelling mistakes, 104
Spices, craved, 282, 331
Spider hemangiomas, 117
Spiders, fear of, 4, 11, 65, 151, 187,
Spina bifida, 32, 37
Spinning games, cause nausea, 160

Splenic flexure, pain, 160
Split nails, 336
Sports, 144; slow at, 5
Spots, black/white floating, 192
Spotting, 161
Spying, 101
Squash, aversion to, 282
Stairs, climbing, <, 27
Stammering, 93
Staph infections, 277, 289; *Med.* like *Sul.*, 115
Stare, distrustful, 50; strong, serious, 9, 21
Startled, by auditory intrusion, 111
Starves self, 55
Starving children, resembles, 19
Status, fears loss of, 63
Sternocleidomastoid muscles weak, 72
Sternum, itches and feels tight, 197
Stiff neck, *Nat. mur.* and *Ign.* compared, 163
Stimulation, seeks, 309
Stitches, in chest, during growth spurts, 329
Stomach aches, constant in pregnancy, 55; during illness, 74; from fear, 189; fictitious fabrication of, 201; since mononeucleosis, 72; vomiting, as drink warms, 199
Stomps, 8
Stool passage, leaning backwards, 121; to get rewards, 202
Stools, black, tarry, 200; explosive, *Tub.* and *Sul.* compared, 333; hard then soft, 77; hard, large, *Calc.* and *Puls.* compared, 240; large and hard, 30; little balls, 333; mucous yellow-green, 129; no two alike, 240; no urge to, 76; plays with, 268–269; white and bileless, 30
"Stork bites," red, on forehead, 25
Strabismus, from birth, 326
Strangers, fear of, 4, 64, 80, 304; cause anxiety, 50
Strawberries, skin <, 126
Streptococcal infection, 6, 289; repeated, 26
Striking, siblings and parents, 308

String bean body, 203
Strokes, in utero, 340
Structure and scheduling, important, 7; needs, 4
Stubbornness, 259
Study, difficult, 306; *Calc., Nat. mur., Puls.,* and *Sul.* compared, 269–270; headaches from, 305
Stuffed animals, carrying, 229
Stunted, physically, emotionally, or mentally, 128
Stupid, calls parent, 62
Stuttering, 105
Styes, 68, 326; recurring, 233
Subacute disorders, 292
Subconjunctival hemorrhages, 205; *Phos.* and *Arn.* compared, 193
Submissive, 217, 227
Sucking reflexes, poor, 82
Sugar, craved, 67; intense reaction to, 308
Suicide, and inconsolability, 222; dwelling on, 108
Sulkiness, 149
Sung to, desires to be, 177
Sunglasses, 156
Sunshine, craved, 205
Supernatural phenomena, interest in, 14
Supernumerary teeth, 328
Surgical repair, side effects of, 82
Sweat, profuse, 325
Sweet, 220, 227; aversion/desire, 198; craved, 27, 73, 119, 159, 198, 238, 282, 331; craved, in headache, 192; craves, screaming, "Give me! Give me!", 64
"Swimmer's ear," 234
Sycotic miasm and *Nat. mur.,* 142; and masturbation, 286
Sympathetic nature, 182–183, 188
Sympathy, in extreme becomes illness, 189
Symptomatolgy confused, 292

Talking, and lean for age, 200; delayed, 3; in sleep, 66, 152, 231
Tall, thin girls, and menses, 202
Tantrums, 8, 96, 98

Tart fruit, craved, 119
Task oriented, *Nat. mur.* and *Calc.* compared, 150
Tattle-tales, 101
Tears, acrid, 235; of rage, 311; suppressed and asthma, 158
Teasing, of siblings, 319
Teeth, feel as if jammed together, 328; long and thin, 195; many sets of, 328; serrated, 328; serrated, soft, discolored, *Med., Tub.,* and *Lyc.* compared, 116; soft, lacking enamel, 26; tardy eruption, 328; yellowing, 71
Teeth grinding, 17, 309, 341; in sleep, 322; in dentition, 328
Teething, and temper, 7; with colds, colic and diarrhea, 26
Temper tantrums, 311, 313
Temper, from tenderhearted boys, 227
Tendonitis, easily induced, 162
Tense, against errors, 144; with anxiety, *Nat. mur.* and *Phos.* compared, 186
Terror, of severe disease, 188
Testicles, undescended, 78, 82
Thrive, failure to, 25; intense, 157
Thirstlessness, with dry mouth or fever, 238
Thirstiness, 198
Thoracic vertebrae, scoliosis of, 32
Thoughtlessness, 101
Threatening, 98
Three p.m. to six p.m. time aggravation, 165
Throat, raw, dry, and burning, 196; sensation of closing at larynx, 237; tickles, 198
Throwing, at parent's face, 98; self on ground, 311; things, 95; things at people liked, 99
Thrush, 25
Thumb sucking, as regression, 221
Thunder, fear of, 205
Thunderstorms, fear of, 12, 151, 322
Thuja and *Med.* as complementaries, 100, 103, 111
Thyroid 25–27, 35, 341; and calcium

metabolism, 3

Tidiness, 217

Tigers, fear of, 321

Time, passes too slowly, 102–103

Timidity, 216, 227; *Lyc.*, *Puls.*, and *Nat. mur.* compared, 58; see also Shyness

Tissue, shrinking, 163

Tittering, tense and nervous, 149

Toads, fear of, 110

Tobacco smoke and headaches, 192

Toenails, ingrown, 163

Toes, curled under foot, 216

Toilet training, 122; early, 141; by self, 10; as stress causing regression, 221

Tomatoes, aggravating dry skin, 80

Tongue, geographically mapped, with red and white areas, 157; long and thin, 195; red tip, 279

Tongue-tied, 102

Tonsillitis, chronic, 279–280; from suppression, 24; when swallowing, sharp pains, 328; with hard, smelly, white pus, 71

Tonsils, enormous, red, *Calc.* and *Bell.* compared, 26; swollen, 117

Tooth, eruption, painful, 25

Torticollis, 72

Torture, of animals, 95

Touch, aversion to, 15

Touches everything, 10

Trachea, dry, tickle in, 237

Trance-like state, immobilized in, 184

Transgressions, perceived, 98

Translucent, children, 204; greenish skin, 72

Traumatic event, causes fear, 189

Travelling, love of, 309–310

Trifles, worries over, 321

Truss, of yarn and knot, 29

Truth-stretching, 258

Tubercular miasm and *Calc*, 10

Tubercular type of *Sul.*, 262, 271, 273–274

Tuberculosis, family history of, 339

Tucked in, desire to be, 177, 190

Turkey, craved, 282

Twilight, <, 205

Twitches as falls asleep, 272

Tympanic membrane scarred, 23

Tyrant, 61

Ulcers, and emotional stress, 239; from fear, 189

Umbilical hernia, 304

Unconditional love to *Lyc.* children, 58

Uncooperative, 325

Unknowable things, interest in, 15

Upside-down drawing, 104

Uric acid diathesis, 77

Urinary, red sand, 77

Urination, frequency in evening, 77; frequent, night, and burning, 241; in public place difficult, 161

Urine, acidic, 129; burning, 122; dribbling, 77; strong odor, 122

Urticaria, 126, 157, 290; from nearby disliked animal, 321

Vaccinations, after, 291; aversion to touch, after, 15

Vagina, picks at, 93

Vaginal, infection and discharge, even in infants, 122; infections in very young, 129; odor, 241

Vaginitis, 262, 286; chronic, 241; nondescript, in young girls, 161; recurring, 31; with offensive leukorrhea, 122

Varicose veins, in pregnancy, 55

Vasomotor instability, 21

Vegetables, aversion, 282, 332

Vegetarian-fruitarian, conversion, 120

Vertigo, < sun, reading, walking and looking up, 154

Violence, after acute disorders, 314; *Med and Tub.* compared, 98; observed, love of, 99

Violent, 311

Visual distortions, 192–193; in fever, 114

Visual disturbances, precede headache, 274, 324, 326

Visual experiential concepts, 105

Visual field loss, 193

Vitiligo, 126

Voice loss, frequent, 196; soft, 216

Vomiting, 199, in headache, 192; > asthma attack, 118; chronic, painless, 28; from anticipation, 182; from fear, 189; after nursing, with yellow mucus, 120

Vomits milk, yet yogurt digested, 293

Wakes, hungry, 29, 205; in fright, and goes to parents bed, 51; irritable, 62; at night to eat, 199; not knowing where, *Stram., Lyc., Calc., and Puls.* compared, 66; refreshed, 17, 191, 231; to drink, 198; unrefreshed, 323

Walking, and talking, slow development, 162; delayed, 3, 9; late learners, 62; in sleep, 190

Wants, not knows what, 313–314

War, dreams of, 153

Warm food and drink, craved, 73; aversion to, 238

Warm-blooded, 165

Warm-hearted, 175

Warts, 125, 164; on hands, face, soles, 204; on penis, 122; on palms and fingers, in crops, 34

Wasting and wrinkling of flesh, 70

Water, asks for at night, *Phos.* and *Puls.* compared, 180; cool or cold craved, 28, 332; fear of, *Stram. and Med.* compared, 110; ice cold, thirst for, 157

Weaned, with fussing and crying, 245

Weather changes, and colds, 277

Weeping, 148–149; from anger, 311–312; from pain, 225; in older boys, 224; in sleep, 231; *Nat. mur., Phos., and Puls. compared,* 185; involuntary, 224; >, 106; > illness, 245

Weepy, 198; and morose before menses, 242

Weight loss, and acute diseases, 204; with appetite, *Lyc., Nat. mur., Tub. and Calc.* compared, 80

Weight on chest, obstructs breathing, 197

Wens, 126

Wheat cereal and colic, 160

Wheezing, when lying down, 198

When, what and where forgotten, 270

Whimper, 14, 223

Whine, 222, 312

Whispering, 106, 140, 185

Whooping cough, 329

Wide-eyed, with glimmer, 192

Willfully slow information assimilation, 3

Witches, perceives, 187

Wolves, fear of, 321

Wool, < skin, 244

Word order in speech confused, 181

Words, forgets, 94, 270; swallowed, 93; uses wrong, 63

Worms, feeling as if in ears, 114

Worrying, 186

Wrinkled

Wrinkling, of body and weight loss, 25; of forehead, 50

Writing, hurriedly, and not wanting to read it, 63; mistakes in, 63, 306

Yeast, infection, at genitals, perineum, and anus, 121

Yellow tinge of skin, 70, 79

Yielding, 217

Yogurt, desired, 159, 331; frozen yogurt, desired, 198

"Youth is wasted on the young.", 139

About the Author

Paul Herscu, N.D., a native of Rumania, is a graduate of the National College of Naturopathic Medicine in Portland, Oregon. He resides in Amherst, Massachusetts, with his wife and partner Amy Rothenberg, N.D., daughter Sophia, and son Misha, where he practices, teaches, and writes about homeopathy.

Dr. Herscu teaches a five-year course in homeopathy at the Swedish Academy of Classical Homeopathy in Goteborg, Sweden. In addition, Dr. Herscu lectures in England, Canada, and the United States. He was instrumental in the development of the Homeopathic Academy of Naturopathic Physicians (HANP), a pacesetting organization of classical homeopaths, where he currently sits on the board. He is the founder and director of the New England School of Homeopathy.

Dr. Herscu's articles have appeared in many homeopathic journals. He regularly contributes columns to *Homeopathy Today*, the newsletter of the National Center of Homeopathy, and *Simillimum*, the journal of the HANP.

He may be contacted at:
The New England School of Homeopathy
356 Middle Street
Amherst, MA 01002